AF864030

theclinics.com

SURGICAL ONCOLOGY CLINICS OF NORTH AMERICA

Metastasectomy and Cytoreductive Surgery

GUEST EDITOR
Pascal Fuchshuber, MD, PhD

CONSULTING EDITOR
Nicholas J. Petrelli, MD

July 2007 • Volume 16 • Number 3

SAUNDERS
An Imprint of Elsevier, Inc.
PHILADELPHIA LONDON TORONTO MONTREAL SYDNEY TOKYO

W.B. SAUNDERS COMPANY
A Division of Elsevier Inc.

1600 John F. Kennedy Boulevard, Suite 1800 • Philadelphia, PA 19103-2899

http://www.theclinics.com

SURGICAL ONCOLOGY CLINICS OF NORTH AMERICA
July 2007
Editor: Catherine Bewick

Volume 16, Number 3
ISSN 1055-3207
ISBN-13: 978-1-4160-5128-2
ISBN-10: 1-4160-5128-7

Copyright © 2007 by Elsevier Inc. All rights reserved. No part of this publication may be reproduced or transmitted in any form or by any means, electronic or mechanical, including photocopy, recording, or any information storage and retrieval system, without written permission from the publisher.

Single photocopies of single articles may be made for personal use as allowed by national copyright laws. Permission of the publisher and payment of a fee is required for all other photocopying, including multiple or systematic copying, copying for advertising or promotional purposes, resale, and all forms of document delivery. Special rates are available for educational institutions that wish to make photocopies for non-profit educational classroom use. Permissions may be sought directly from Elsevier's Rights Department in Philadelphia, PA, USA; phone: (215) 239-3804, fax: (215) 239-3805, e-mail: healthpermissions@elsevier.com. Requests may also be completed on-line via the Elsevier home page (http://www.elsevier.com/locate/permissions). In the USA, users may clear permissions and make payments through the Copyright Clearance Center, Inc., 222 Rosewood Drive, Danvers, MA 01923, USA; phone: (978) 750-8400, fax: (978) 750-4744, and in the UK through the Copyright Licensing Agency Rapid Clearance Service (CLARCS), 90 Tottenham Court Road, London WIP 0LP, UK; phone: (+44) 171 436 5631; fax: (+44) 171 436 3986. Other countries may have a local reprographic rights agency for payments.

The ideas and opinions expressed in the *Surgical Oncology Clinics of North America* do not necessarily reflect those of the Publisher. The Publisher does not assume any responsibility for any injury and/or damage to persons or property arising out of or related to any use of the material contained in this periodical. The reader is advised to check the appropriate medical literature and the product information currently provided by the manufacturer of each drug to be administered to verify the dosage, the method and duration of administration, or contra-indications. It is the responsibility of the treating physician or other health care professional, relying on independent experience and knowledge of the patient, to determine drug dosages and the best treatment for the patient. Mention of any product in this issue should not be construed as endorsement by the contributors, editors, or the Publisher of the product or manufacturers' claims.

Surgical Oncology Clinics of North America (ISSN 1055-3207) is published quarterly by Elsevier Inc., 360 Park Avenue South, New York, NY 10010-1710. Months of publication are January, April, July, and October. Business and editorial offices: 1600 John F. Kennedy Boulevard, Suite 1800, Philadelphia, PA 19103-2899. Customer service office: 6277 Sea Harbor Drive, Orlando, FL 32887–4800. Periodicals postage paid at New York, NY, and additional mailing offices. Subscription prices are $187.00 per year (US individuals), $275.00 (US institutions) $94.00 (US student/resident), $215.00 (Canadian individuals), $335.00 (Canadian institutions), $127.00 (Canadian student/resident), $253.00 (foreign individuals), $335.00 (foreign institutions), and $127.00 (foreign student/resident). Foreign air speed delivery is included in all *Clinics* subscription prices. All prices are subject to change without notice. POST-MASTER: Send address changes to *Surgical Oncology Clinics of North America*, Elsevier Periodicals Customer Service, 6277 Sea Harbor Drive, Orlando, FL 32887–4800. **Customer Service: 1-800-654-2452 (US). From outside the United States, call 1-407-345-4000. E-mail: hhspcs@wbsaunders.com.**

Reprints. For copies of 100 or more, of articles in this publication, please contact the Commercial Reprints Department, Elsevier Inc., 360 Park Avenue South, New York, New York 10010-1710. Tel. (212) 633-3813 Fax: (212) 462-1935 email: reprints@elsevier.com.

Surgical Oncology Clinics of North America is covered in *Index Medicus and EMBASE/Excerpta Medica, Current Contents/Clinical Medicine, and ISI/BIOMED.*

Printed in the United States of America.

CONSULTING EDITOR

NICHOLAS J. PETRELLI, MD, Bank of America Endowed Medical Director, Helen F. Graham Cancer Center at Christiana Care Health System, Newark, Delaware; and Professor of Surgery, Thomas Jefferson University, Philadelphia, Pennsylvania

GUEST EDITOR

PASCAL FUCHSHUBER, MD, PhD, Associate Clinical Professor of Surgery, University of California San Francisco, San Francisco; and Chief of Surgical Oncology, Department of Surgery, The Permanente Medical Group, Kaiser Medical Center, Walnut Creek, California

CONTRIBUTORS

EDDIE K. ABDALLA, MD, Assistant Professor, Hepatobiliary Surgery and Surgical Oncology, The University of Texas M.D. Anderson Cancer Center, Department of Surgical Oncology, Houston, Texas

RENÉ ADAM, MD, PhD, AP-HP Hopital Paul Brousse, Centre Hépato-Biliare; Université Paris-Sud; and Inserm, Villejuif, France

THOMAS ALOIA, MD, AP-HP Hopital Paul Brousse, Centre Hépato-Biliare, Villejuif, France

HORACIO J. ASBUN, MD, Director of Advanced Minimal Access Surgery, John Muir Health, Walnut Creek; and Director of Hepatobiliary and Pancreas Cancer Program, John Muir Cancer Center, Walnut Creek, California

EMILY K. BERGSLAND, MD, Associate Professor of Medicine, Department of Medicine, Division of Hematology/Oncology, University of California, UCSF Comprehensive Cancer Center, San Francisco, California

ANTON J. BILCHIK, MD, PhD, FACS, Assistant Director of Surgical Oncology, Department of Surgical Oncology, John Wayne Cancer Institute at Saint John's Health Center, Santa Monica, California

GEORGIA BITSAKOU, MD, AP-HP Hopital Paul Brousse, Centre Hépato-Biliare, Villejuif, France

EUGENE A. CHOI, MD, Clinical Fellow, The University of Texas M.D. Anderson Cancer Center, Department of Surgical Oncology, Houston, Texas

TODD L. DEMMY, MD, Clinical Chair, Department of Thoracic Surgery, Roswell Park Cancer Institute; and Associate Professor, Department of Surgery, State University of New York—Buffalo, Buffalo, New York

KELLI BULLARD DUNN, MD, Associate Professor, Department of Surgical Oncology, Roswell Park Cancer Institute; and Department of Surgery, State University of New York—Buffalo, Buffalo, New York

JESUS ESQUIVEL, MD, FACS, Director, Peritoneal Surface Malignancy Program, Surgical Oncology, St. Agnes Hospital, Baltimore, Maryland

PASCAL FUCHSHUBER, MD, PhD, Associate Clinical Professor of Surgery, University of California San Francisco, San Francisco; and Chief of Surgical Oncology, Department of Surgery, The Permanente Medical Group, Kaiser Medical Center, Walnut Creek, California

ROBBERT J. DE HAAS, MD, AP-HP Hopital Paul Brousse, Centre Hépato-Biliare, Villejuif, France; Department of Surgery, University Medical Center Utrecht, Utrecht, the Netherlands

DANIEL M. JAECK, MD, PhD, FRCS, Professor, Centre de Chirurgie Viscérale et de Transplantation, Hopital de Hautepierre, Hopitaux Universitaires Strasbourg, Université Louis Pasteur, Strasbourg, France

DONALD L. KLIPPENSTEIN, MD, Associate Professor, Clinical Radiology, State University of New York at Buffalo, School of Medicine and Biomedical Sciences; and Vice Chairman of Diagnostic Radiology and Director of CT, Roswell Park Cancer Institute, Buffalo, New York

DOMINICK M. LAMONICA, MD, Assistant Professor, Radiology, State University of New York at Buffalo, School of Medicine and Biomedical Sciences; and Director of Nuclear Medicine, Roswell Park Cancer Institute, Buffalo, New York

CHRIS C. LEE, MD, Fellow in Surgical Oncology, Department of Surgical Oncology, John Wayne Cancer Institute at Saint John's Health Center, Santa Monica, California

LAWRENCE LEICHMAN, MD, FACP, Director of GI Cancer, Aptium Oncology, Comprehensive Cancer at Desert Regional Medical Center, Palm Springs, California

RENATO LUPINACCI, MD, Service de Chirurgie Digestive, Hopital Ambroise-Paré, Boulogne Billancourt, France

JAMES M. McLOUGHLIN, MD, Assistant Professor of Surgery, Division of Surgical Oncology, Department of Surgery, Medical College of Georgia, Augusta, Georgia

RAFAEL MILLER, MD, AP-HP Hopital Paul Brousse, Centre Hépato-Biliare, Villejuif, France; Department of Surgery, Kaplan Medical Center Rehovot and Hebrew University, Jerusalem, Israel

ERIC K. NAKAKURA, MD, PhD, Assistant Professor of Surgery, Department of Surgery, Division of Surgical Oncology, University of California, UCSF Comprehensive Cancer Center, San Francisco, California

BERNARD NORDLINGER, MD, AP-HP, Hopital Ambroise-Paré, Service de chirurgie digestive, Boulogne and Université Versailles, Saint-Quentin, France

ELIE OUSSOULTZOGLOU, MD, Centre de Chirurgie Viscérale et de Transplantation, Hopital de Hautepierre, Hopitaux Universitaires Strasbourg, Université Louis Pasteur, Strasbourg, France

CHRISTOPHE PENNA, MD, AP-HP, Hopital Ambroise-Paré, Service de chirurgie digestive, Boulogne and Université Versailles, Saint-Quentin, France

NICHOLAS J. PETRELLI, MD, Bank of America Endowed Medical Director, Helen F. Graham Cancer Center at Christiana Care Health System, Newark, Delaware; and Professor of Surgery, Thomas Jefferson University, Philadelphia, Pennsylvania

MARCOS PITOMBO, MD, AP-HP Hopital Paul Brousse, Centre Hépato-Biliare, Villejuif, France

C. BETHAN POWELL, MD, Clinical Professor of Obstetrics and Gynecology, Division of Gynecologic Oncology, University of California, San Francisco, California

EDOARDO ROSSO, MD, Centre de Chirurgie Viscérale et de Transplantation, Hopital de Hautepierre, Hopitaux Universitaires Strasbourg, Université Louis Pasteur, Strasbourg, France

VERNON K. SONDAK, MD, Chief, Division of Cutaneous Oncology, H. Lee Moffitt Cancer Center and Research Institute; and Professor of Surgery, Departments of Interdisciplinary Oncology and Surgery, University of South Florida College of Medicine, Tampa, Florida

MICHAELA STRAZNICKA, MD, Director of Thoracic Oncology Program, John Muir Cancer Center, Walnut Creek, California

VIVIAN E. STRONG, MD, Assistant Attending Surgeon, Memorial Sloan-Kettering Cancer Center; and Assistant Professor of Surgery, Weill Medical College of Cornell University, New York, New York

ELIZABETH SUH-BURGMANN, MD, Gynecologic Oncology, The Permanente Medical Group, Walnut Creek, California

ALAN P. VENOOK, MD, Professor of Medicine, Department of Medicine, Division of Hematology/Oncology, University of California, UCSF Comprehensive Cancer Center, San Francisco, California

DENNIS A. WICHERTS, MD, AP-HP Hopital Paul Brousse, Centre Hépato-Biliare, Villejuif, France; Department of Surgery, University Medical Center Utrecht, Utrecht, the Netherlands

BYRON E. WRIGHT, MD, FACS, Fellow in Surgical Oncology, Department of Surgical Oncology, John Wayne Cancer Institute at Saint John's Health Center, Santa Monica, California

JONATHAN S. ZAGER, MD, Division of Cutaneous Oncology, H. Lee Moffitt Cancer Center and Research Institute; and Assistant Professor of Surgery, Department of Interdisciplinary Oncology, University of South Florida College of Medicine, Tampa, Florida

CONTENTS

FORTHCOMING ISSUES

October 2007

Tumor Immunology
Robert P. Sticca, MD, *Guest Editor*

January 2008

Translational Research in Surgical Oncology
Ben Li, MD, *Guest Editor*

April 2008

Thyroid Cancer
Robert Witt, MD, *Guest Editor*

RECENT ISSUES

April 2007

Pre and Postoperative Cancer Imaging: Practical and Innovative Approaches
Scott H. Kurtzman, MD, *Guest Editor*

January 2007

Lymphadenectomy in Surgical Oncology: Staging and Therapeutic Role
Vijay P. Khatri, MBChB, FACS, *Guest Editor*

October 2006

Adenocarcinoma of the Gastroesophageal Junction
Martin S. Karpeh, Jr, MD, *Guest Editor*

THE CLINICS ARE NOW ONLINE!

Access your subscription at:
http://www.theclinics.com

ELSEVIER
SAUNDERS

Surg Oncol Clin N Am
16 (2007) xiii–xiv

SURGICAL
ONCOLOGY CLINICS
OF NORTH AMERICA

Foreword

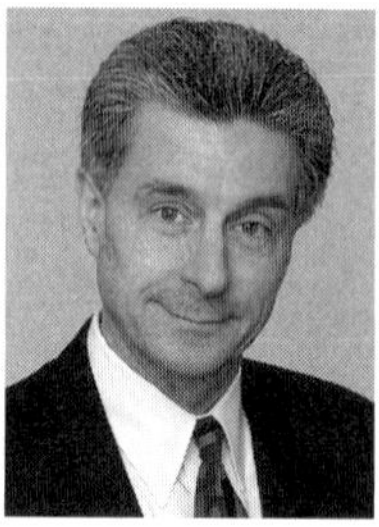

Nicholas J. Petrelli, MD
Consulting Editor

This edition of *Surgical Oncology Clinics of North America* contains two parts: the first deals with metastasectomy and the second with cytoreductive surgery. The guest editor for this edition is Pascal Fuchshuber, MD, PhD, Associate Clinical Professor of Surgery at the University of California at San Francisco, and Chief of Surgical Oncology at The Permanente Medical Group, Walnut Creek, California. Dr. Fuchshuber completed his surgical oncology fellowship at the Roswell Park Cancer Institute in Buffalo, New York.

Both parts in this edition of *Surgical Oncology Clinics of North America* have contributions from individuals who have had extensive experience in the areas of metastasectomy and cytoreductive surgery. This edition is also very timely since with the recent development of new chemotherapeutic and targeted agents in colorectal cancer, about 15% of patients who present with unresectable hepatic metastases are converted to resectable metastases. Recent publications have also demonstrated an improvement in survival for patients who undergo hepatic resection for colorectal metastases in the presence of extrahepatic disease. However, I would emphasize to our readers that the latter should be performed only in the context of a clinical trial. There is also an excellent discussion in this edition of *Surgical Oncology Clinics of North America* concerning the outcome of hepatic resection for non-neuroendocrine liver metastases by Drs. Choi and Abdalla from the M.D. Anderson Cancer Center in Houston, Texas. Also in part one is a discussion by Drs. Demmy and Dunn from the Roswell Park Cancer Institute

1055-3207/07/$ - see front matter © 2007 Elsevier Inc. All rights reserved.
doi:10.1016/j.soc.2007.04.018

on the indications and outcomes for both surgical and nonsurgical treatment of lung metastases.

In part two of *Surgical Oncology Clinics of North America* is a discussion of cytoreductive surgery. This section is especially timely in view of the session held at the Society of Surgical Oncology meeting in Washington, DC, in 2007 dealing with the current status of the surgical therapy for peritoneal carcinomatosis, which was moderated by Drs. Edward A. Levine and Jesus Esquivel. Dr. Esquivel has an excellent discussion in this edition of *Surgical Oncology Clinics of North America* dealing with the development of standards of care for the community for cytoreductive surgery of peritoneal malignancies. He has taken a leadership role in this area. Cytoreductive surgery is also discussed in the context of neuroendocrine cancers, gynecologic malignancies, and melanoma.

Dr. Fuchshuber emphasizes in his preface that reports from centers throughout the world have demonstrated that long-term survival is possible in individuals who undergo extensive and repeated metastasectomy and cytoreductive surgery as part of a multimodality treatment approach. However, he also emphasizes that the price patients may pay is potentially high in that the long-term effects of chemotherapy and repeated surgery must be weighed against the benefits of this multimodality treatment approach.

A committed multidisciplinary team with experience and resources can successfully build these multimodality treatment programs, whether in academic centers or the community cancer center setting. However, it demands a multidisciplinary team that stays on the cutting edge of cancer treatment.

I congratulate Dr. Fuchshuber for a timely and outstanding collection of educational chapters in this edition of *Surgical Oncology Clinics of North America.*

Nicholas J. Petrelli, MD
Helen F. Graham Cancer Center
Christiana Care Health Services
4701 Ogletown-Stanton Road
Suite 1213, Newark, DE 19713, USA

Thomas Jefferson University
College Building
1025 Walnut Street
Philadelphia, PA 19107, USA

E-mail address: npetrelli@christianacare.org

ELSEVIER
SAUNDERS

Surg Oncol Clin N Am
16 (2007) xv–xvi

SURGICAL
ONCOLOGY CLINICS
OF NORTH AMERICA

Preface

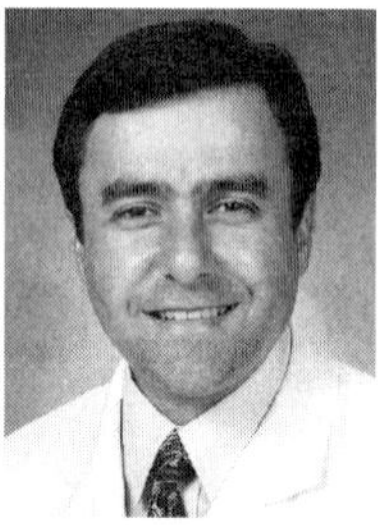

Pascal Fuchshuber, MD, PhD
Guest Editor

We can identify two recent developments that have propelled cytoreductive surgery and metastasectomy from relative obscurity to the forefront of a rapidly evolving field of surgical oncology: advances in systemic and regional cytotoxic and biologic therapy and the establishment of safe and effective surgical techniques for metastasectomy and cytoreduction. Nowhere is this better illustrated than in the treatment of colorectal cancer metastases and peritoneal malignancies. It is therefore not surprising that a large part of this issue of *Surgical Oncology Clinics of North America* is dedicated to these disease entities.

It is particularly for colorectal cancer metastases that a paradigm shift has occurred for the role of surgical resection. The boundary that existed between R0 and R1 resection for the indication of surgical therapy is being challenged by effective systemic chemotherapy and targeted biologic therapy. With long-term survival now seen after metastasectomy even in the presence of extrahepatic disease and metastatic disease in multiple organs, traditional indications for surgery have given way to new criteria for resectability. Surgical limitations based on disease burden have been replaced by a strategy in which metastasectomy is limited only by the function of the remnant organ. The goal of maximum cytoreduction has vastly increased the number of patients eligible for metastasectomy. Recent data from centers throughout the world show that extensive and repeat metastasectomy and cytoreductive surgery as part of a multimodality treatment plan can lead to long-term survival in a sizable percentage of patients. The price,

1055-3207/07/$ - see front matter © 2007 Elsevier Inc. All rights reserved.
doi:10.1016/j.soc.2007.04.020

however, is high and one must be cognizant of the toll that long-term chemotherapy and repeat surgery demand of these patients. As surgeons, we need to remind ourselves that we owe the expanded indications for surgery in the metastatic setting to the scientific accomplishments in the development of effective systemic and regional therapy. We should also familiarize ourselves with the advances in surgical techniques that allow us to expand the limits of organ resection for metastatic disease and cytoreductive surgery. Repeat hepatectomy and peritonectomy is not for the faint of heart. It demands special attention to modern surgical principles. Simply knowing one technique is not sufficient.

Cure remains elusive for most patients afflicted by metastatic cancer, but we are a step closer to making solid cancer disease a chronic condition. There is a roadmap to achieve this goal where there used to be none a decade or two ago. It is our responsibility to seize this opportunity to give our patients appropriate choices in the treatment of their ailment. This issue is dedicated to modern multimodality treatment of advanced cancer and attempts to demonstrate that, even though biology certainly remains king, our chance to at least delay defeat and maybe outright win has significantly increased.

I wish to thank all authors for their willingness and effort to contribute to this edition. My hope is that the reader will be encouraged to apply and further the knowledge that has improved the fate of those afflicted by metastatic cancer.

Pascal Fuchshuber, MD, PhD
Kaiser Medical Center
1425 South Main
Walnut Creek, CA 94596, USA

E-mail address: pascal.fuchshuber@kp.org

ELSEVIER
SAUNDERS

Surg Oncol Clin N Am
16 (2007) 471–492

SURGICAL
ONCOLOGY CLINICS
OF NORTH AMERICA

Preoperative Imaging for Metastasectomy

Donald L. Klippenstein, MD[a,b,*],
Dominick M. Lamonica, MD[a,b]

[a] *State University of New York at Buffalo, School of Medicine and Biomedical Sciences, Buffalo, NY 14214, USA*
[b] *Roswell Park Cancer Institute, Elm & Carlton Streets, Buffalo, NY 14263, USA*

For most solid neoplasms, medical imaging is a vital component of tumor staging and surveillance. Imaging strategies vary according to the type and grade of primary neoplasm, tumor stage at diagnosis, tumor markers, previous therapies, and patient symptoms. Preoperative imaging for metastasectomy differs from standard surveillance and follow-up imaging of metastatic disease. An imaging modality or technique that is adequate for monitoring tumor response to chemotherapy may not be accurate enough to guide planning for metastasectomy. Preoperative imaging strategies for metastasectomy tend to concentrate on maximizing sensitivity for detection of metastases throughout the body and within the individual organ(s) or body part where the surgery is planned. Maximum sensitivity during preoperative imaging is especially important in organs such as lung and liver where detection of additional metastases determines the feasibility of metastasectomy and influences the type and extent of surgery. In this article, we address imaging of individual organs (lung, liver, adrenals) and outline imaging strategies for specific types of neoplasms.

Pulmonary imaging

Since 1977, when axial CT was first compared with conventional whole-lung tomography, successive "generations" of CT technology have provided the most sensitive imaging method for detecting pulmonary nodules [1]. The

* Corresponding author. Roswell Park Cancer Institute, Elm & Carlton Streets, Buffalo, NY 14263.
E-mail address: donald.klippenstein@roswellpark.org (D.L. Klippenstein).

1055-3207/07/$ - see front matter © 2007 Elsevier Inc. All rights reserved.
doi:10.1016/j.soc.2007.04.004 **surgonc.theclinics.com**

high contrast between air in the lungs and soft tissue structures is ideal for the detection of focal nodules, and even low-dose CT accurately identifies solid nodules [2,3]. Metastases to the lungs usually appear as focal solid, soft tissue density, parenchymal, pleural, or endobronchial nodules. More diffuse metastatic involvement may appear as thickening of the pleura or interstitium and lymphatics. Homogeneous or central dense calcification or lamellated calcifications within a pulmonary nodule imply prior granulomatous disease, whereas "popcorn calcifications" with or without fat are highly suggestive of a hamartoma. These characteristics are best evaluated on thin images of less than 3 mm. Metastatic osteogenic sarcoma to the lung may mimic the classic attributes of benign calcified pulmonary nodules.

The development of helical CT eliminated false-negative results due to inconsistent patient breathing during nonhelical CT (misregistration artifact) and increased pulmonary nodule detection rates significantly [4]. The thinner images and overlapping images reconstructed from the helical 3D data set increase image resolution and pulmonary nodule detection rates [5,6]. In a small series of patients undergoing pulmonary metastasectomy, preoperative single-detector CT was 100% sensitive for histologically proven intrapulmonary metastases 6 mm or larger. Detection of intrapulmonary nodules less than 6 mm in diameter was 69% accurate, and sensitivity for pleural nodules less than 6 mm in diameter was only 17% accurate [7]. More recent studies have included larger cohorts assessed by CT before pulmonary metastasectomy. Although CT was found to underestimate the number of viable pulmonary metastases in 22% to 26% of patients, the majority of the preoperative CT scans in these studies were with single-detector helical CT, and no scans were performed with images less than 5 mm in thickness [8,9].

Multidetector CT (MDCT) with 4 to 64 detectors is able to image the entire chest at 1 mm or less slice thickness in a single breath-hold. The higher number of detectors enables faster image acquisition, which reduces motion artifact. These thin images increase resolution in the Z-axis (perpendicular to the imaging plane) and virtually eliminate partial volume artifact for objects in the lung larger than 2 mm. This increase in resolution makes it unnecessary to reconstruct overlapping images for nodule detection and may help in distinguishing benign entities from potential malignancies. With the large number of images generated by MDCT, it becomes necessary to view the study at a computer or a picture archiving and communication system (PACS) workstation. Cine viewing of lung images at a work station has been shown to improve nodule detection over film-based image reading [10].

Additional recent CT developments that provide increased sensitivity for pulmonary nodule detection have not been examined in published studies of patients having pulmonary metastasectomy. Maximum intensity projection displays made from images acquired at 1 mm thickness have been shown to significantly increase detection of pulmonary nodules 5 mm or less in diameter [11,12]. Double-reading chest CT scans by a second radiologist also increases sensitivity for nodule detection [13,14]. Recently, several versions of computer-aided detection (CAD) software have been developed and tested for pulmonary nodule detection. The most accurate results with CAD in the lung require CT images to be acquired at 1 mm thickness or less [15,16]. Even with these very thin images, nodule detection with CAD alone has been for the most part no better than that by radiologists [17,18]. CAD software also suffers from relatively high false-positive rates [7,15,17]. CAD tends to be more sensitive than a radiologist at detecting small central nodules in the lungs. Therefore, CAD used as a second reader (after primary reading by radiologist) has been shown to be significantly more sensitive at detecting pulmonary nodules than radiologist or CAD reading alone and more sensitive than a radiologist as a second reader [13,14,19].

Therefore, if high sensitivity for pulmonary nodule detection is required, as in preoperative imaging for metastasectomy, MDCT should be used with images acquired at 1 mm thickness or less. The CT study should be viewed at a computer workstation using maximum intensity projection images with the thin references images available for review. CAD as a second reader will also likely increase the number of nodules detected.

Although recent developments in CT technology have increased the sensitivity for nodule detection, the specificity for small, noncalcified, pulmonary nodules on a single CT scan remains low. Nodule contrast enhancement after intravenous administration of iodinated contrast media may be measured to increase specificity. A multicenter trial showed that single-detector helical CT and 3 mm collimation distinguished solid malignant nodules 7 mm or greater in diameter from solid benign nodules with 98% sensitivity and 58% specificity when contrast enhancement increased pulmonary nodule density by more than 15 Hounsfield units (HU) [20]. Although MDCT with thinner images may make it possible to accurately evaluate contrast enhancement in nodules less than 7 mm in diameter, the specificity will likely remain relatively low due to the fact that granulomas and benign tumors may have enhancement greater than 15 HU. Because interval nodule growth over a course of weeks to months is highly predictive of malignancy, pulmonary nodules are often followed by CT to assess for growth. Depending on the rate of growth, the diagnosis of malignancy may remain uncertain or be delayed for a few months. CT tumor volume estimates for solid nodules based on three-dimensional models are more accurate in detecting subtle nodule growth than standard two-dimensional measurements. This allows for earlier diagnosis of malignancy based on nodule growth [21–23].

When pulmonary nodules are 10 mm or more in diameter, fluorodeoxyglucose positron emission tomography (FDG-PET) scanning is highly accurate in distinguishing malignant tumor from benign disease [24]. For single pulmonary nodules, positron emission tomography (PET)/CT has shown to provide better characterization than PET or CT alone [25]. If preoperative knowledge of lymph node involvement in the mediastinum is critical, PET/CT may be the most accurate noninvasive method of assessing these patients, depending on the type of their primary tumor [26,27].

Relatively little data are available comparing MRI with MDTC in pulmonary nodule detection. A recent study showed that MRI is similar to CT for the detection of pulmonary nodules 6 mm or greater in diameter. Because over 60% of the nodules in this study were less than 6 mm in diameter, MRI detected only 85% of nodules seen on MDCT [28].

Hepatic imaging

Imaging of the liver for metastatic disease is most frequently performed with contrast-enhanced CT using an iodine-containing intravenous contrast media. The development of helical CT has made it possible to image the liver with thin slices during "arterial" and "portal venous" phases of contrast enhancement. Arterial-phase imaging is performed during maximum opacification of the hepatic arteries. During the late arterial phase, hypervascular metastases have more contrast enhancement than the surrounding normal liver. Liver metastases from melanoma, renal cell carcinoma, neuroendocrine, and breast carcinoma and some sarcomas may be hypervascular. The portal venous or hepatic venous phase of liver contrast enhancement occurs when the liver achieves maximum density as opacified blood fills the portal veins and the contrast diffuses into the extracellular space of the liver parenchyma. The portal venous phase is optimal for imaging hypovascular metastases to the liver, such as those from colorectal carcinoma. Maximum tumor enhancement in hypervascular metastases and maximum liver enhancement during the portal venous phase require a rapid infusion of iodinated contrast (preferably 4–5 mL/s) and sufficient iodine load per patient body weight (520–600 mg/kg) [29]. MDCT with thin-slice imaging down to 2.5-mm thickness (with overlapping images) maximizes sensitivity for liver lesion/tumor detection [30,31].

There have been several preoperative imaging studies evaluating the detection of primary and secondary malignancies in the liver by single-detector CT. Although the patient populations and methods for determining the true number of liver lesions have varied, the sensitivity for detection of metastases has usually been between 60% and 80%. Almost invariably, these imaging studies from the 1990s found that contrast-enhanced MRI was more sensitive than contrast-enhanced CT for the detection of metastases [32–35]. With more recent studies including MDCT preoperatively for metastasectomy, sensitivities of greater than 75% (some >90%) for liver metastases are more typical [36–40]. Although one recent study found only 48% sensitivity for MDCT, it was not significantly different then the sensitivity of contrast-enhanced MRI (43%) [41]. Some of these studies also suggest that state-of-the-art MDCT may be at least as sensitive as gadolinium-enhanced

MRI (Gd-MRI) in patients undergoing liver resection. MRI is usually better at differentiating benign from malignant liver lesions than contrast-enhanced CT or CT arterial portography. Therefore, preoperative MRI may provide additional useful information that alters surgical planning.

There are three major categories of MRI contrast agents available. The most widely used gadolinium (Gd) agents are not tissue specific and distribute themselves in the extracellular space of the liver and other organs in a fashion similar to iodinated contrast media in CT. As in contrast-enhanced CT, Gd-MRI may be used to characterize lesions by their enhancement patterns. T1-weighted dynamic breath-hold Gd-MRI of the liver is usually performed during hepatic artery, portal venous, and delayed phases of contrast enhancement. Superparamagnetic iron oxide (SPIO) agents injected intravenously are taken up by the Kupffer cells in the liver, and the iron in these cells causes loss of signal on delayed T2-weighted images. Because metastases do not take up the SPIO agents, conspicuity of these tumors is increased. One of the SPIO agents, ferucarbotran, may be used to obtain dynamic T1-weighted images in the first few minutes after injection, in addition to the delayed T2-weighted images. Optimized gradient echo sequences allow for more accurate depiction of small metastases when performing SPIO-MRI [42,43]. Manganese-based (Mn-DPDP) and Gd-based (Gd-BOPTA and Gd-EOB-DPTA) hepatocyte-specific agents are selectively taken up by the normal liver but not by the metastases. Delayed T1-weighted images show increased signal in the liver parenchyma, whereas the metastases remain intermediate to low signal. Gd-BOPTA and Gd-EOB-DPTA agents may be used to obtain dynamic T1-weighted imaging for a few minutes after bolus injection, but it is the delayed imaging that is most sensitive for detection of metastatic disease [44]. Mn-DPDP is usually imaged at 15 minutes to 2 hours after injection, but 24-hour delayed imaging may improve identification of metastases, showing specific ring enhancement from delayed excretion of the contrast agent due to compressed liver parenchyma [45]. Gd-MRI, SPIO-MRI, and hepatocyte specific contrast MRI show greater sensitivity and specificity for lesion detection than MRI without contrast [42,46–48]. Although one study showed equivalent sensitivity between Gd-MRI and SPIO-MRI for detection of colorectal cancer metastases, other comparative studies indicate that SPIO-MRI may have an advantage over Gd-MRI [38,49,50]. SPIO-MRI and MRI with hepatocyte specific agents seem to have similar accuracy in imaging metastases [44,51–53]. Mn-DPDP has recently become commercially unavailable.

Contrast-enhanced MRI has largely replaced CT arterial portography (CTAP) in preoperative imaging for metastasectomy. CTAP is sensitive for the detection of liver lesions, but it suffers from flow-related artifacts (uneven mixing of opacified and unopacified blood) and relatively low specificity. CTAP is an invasive procedure requiring arterial catheterization of the superior mesenteric artery or the splenic artery. Multiple studies have shown a similar sensitivity and superior specificity of MRI over CTAP [47,54,55]. A recent small trial of mostly colorectal and breast cancer patients has shown superiority of Gd-MR arterial portography over CTAP in liver lesion sensitivity and specificity [56]. It is unknown whether Gd-MR arterial portography will prove superior to the liver specific MR contrast agents and whether any incremental improvement will justify the added expense and the additional invasive procedure for the patient.

For many years, intraoperative ultrasound (IOUS) in conjunction with palpation and visual inspection of the liver by the surgeon has been considered the gold standard for the evaluation of liver metastases. Although few studies have blinded the intraoperative sonographer from preoperative imaging studies, almost all series show that IOUS detects more liver metastases than any method of preoperative imaging [57,58]. A new gold standard for intraoperative liver imaging is emerging with the advent of contrast-enhanced IOUS. The combination of pulse-inversion harmonic imaging and bolus intravenous injection of a microbubble contrast agent results in better lesion conspicuity and increased sensitivity and specificity of IOUS [59].

The role of FDG-PET imaging specific to the liver has changed as CT and MRI equipment and techniques have improved. Most studies comparing PET and CT in preoperative imaging for metastasectomy were performed at a time when nonhelical CT or single-detector helical CT were standard. Many of these studies did not state the CT or MRI scanning techniques used, accepted outside CT or MRI scans where the equipment and techniques were not standardized, or used the results of the CT and MRI studies to interpret the PET scan. Many of these earlier studies concluded that PET was more accurate than conventional diagnostic modalities in imaging metastases in the liver. A meta-analysis of the medical literature during the years 1985 to 2000 evaluating noninvasive imaging methods for detection of hepatic metastases from gastrointestinal tract cancers concluded that FDG-PET was more sensitive than MR, CT, and ultrasound for the detection of liver metastases [60]. Preoperative imaging studies using early MDCT equipment and imaging techniques somewhat suboptimal to current state-of-the-art techniques showed equivalent accuracy for detection of liver metastases by FDG-PET and CT [61,62]. Recent studies comparing MRI with PET demonstrate the superior diagnostic accuracy of MRI for liver metastases from a variety of primary malignancies [63–66]. With improvements in CT and MRI, the major utility of PET imaging before liver resection is in the detection of extrahepatic tumor rather than liver metastases.

Adrenal imaging

Adrenal masses are relatively common in the general population, with a postmortem incidence of adrenal adenoma of up to 8.7% [67]. Even in patients who have a history of cancer, these unilateral or bilateral masses are frequently benign. Differentiation of benign from malignant lesions may determine the need for adrenalectomy. Adrenal adenomas contain varying amounts of lipid. "Lipid-rich" adenomas are classified as those with density 10 HU or less on unenhanced CT because essentially all malignant adrenal lesions have been found to have densities greater than 10 HU [68–70]. Approximately 30% of adrenal adenomas are lipid poor (density > 10 HU) and therefore cannot be distinguished from malignant lesions on noncontrast CT [70,71]. By imaging the adrenals before intravenous contrast, during the portal venous phase of contrast enhancement, and at 10 to 15 minutes after contrast injection, relative and absolute values of contrast washout from the adrenal mass can be calculated. Adrenal adenomas have a rapid washout of contrast relative to adrenal malignancies. By using cutoff values in adrenal masses of 52% or 60%, absolute contrast washout for 10- or 15-minute delayed CT images, respectively, sensitivities of 98% to 100% and specificities of 92% to 98% can be achieved [68,69].

MRI is able to characterize adrenal masses as adenomatous or nonadenomatous by using chemical shift imaging. Adenomas that contain lipid have signal drop out on out-of-phase images due to cancellation of signal from lipid and water containing tissue relative to in-phase images. This can usually be assessed qualitatively because signal drop out in adenomas is frequently dramatic. By using quantitative methods to measure the signal drop out, some series have achieved 100% accuracy in distinguishing adenomas from malignancies [72,73]. One study found that in a small subset of patients who had adenomas with CT density measurements of greater than 30 HU, only 1 of 8 masses could be accurately characterized on chemical shift MRI imaging [74].

FDG-PET imaging of adrenal masses is highly accurate in distinguishing malignant from benign lesions. After excluding diabetic patients, qualitative assessment of FDG uptake has resulted in sensitivities of 100% and specificities of 93% or greater [75–78]. This high accuracy has been attained by classifying malignant adrenal masses as those with FDG uptake greater than or equal to liver or by assessing for abnormal uptake within the adrenal mass greater than the blood pool and background.

Colorectal carcinoma

Preoperative imaging for possible liver resection (or combination liver and pulmonary resection) in metastatic colorectal carcinoma patients should include FDG-PET; MDCT of the chest, abdomen, and pelvis; and preferably liver MRI with SPIO contrast or tissue-specific contrast agents targeting the Kupffer cells or hepatocytes. If pulmonary metastasectomy only is being considered, liver MRI may be unnecessary. As shown in recent studies, PET provides more accurate staging of extrahepatic intra-abdominal tumor burden with higher sensitivity compared with CT scan (92% for PET versus 61% for CT for abdominal or pelvic metastases). In 20% to 30% of patients, these preoperative PET findings will alter the treatment plan [79]. The use of PET should result in better patient selection with fewer unnecessary laparotomies [80,81]. Although chest CT is more sensitive than PET for detection of pulmonary metastases, FDG-PET may differentiate benign from malignant nonspecific–appearing, noncalcified pulmonary nodules seen on CT. When CEA levels were abnormal and contrast CT was negative for tumor recurrence, PET was shown to carry a positive predictive value of 89% and a negative predictive value of 100% for tumor recurrence in one study [82]. FDG-PET seems to be less sensitive in detecting metastases from mucinous carcinoma. It is unclear whether this should alter the imaging scheme in patients who have known mucinous colorectal carcinoma [83].

Melanoma

Because melanoma metastases may involve many different organs, strategies for preoperative imaging before metastasectomy must include the entire patient [84]. A group of 18 patients who had stage IV melanoma underwent preoperative MDCT of the chest, abdomen, and pelvis with and without intravenous contrast and whole-body FDG-PET. Three of these patients had further assessment with Gd-MRI of the liver. There was no significant difference in sensitivity and specificity between CT/MR and PET. When CT/MR and PET were interpreted together, there was a significant increase in accuracy, with sensitivity of 88% and specificity 91% (lesion-by-lesion analysis) [85]. A larger study with a more heterogeneous patient population showed that PET was more accurate than CT in staging melanoma for chest, abdomen, and pelvis (90% versus 69%). No information was provided regarding the methods or equipment used for CT scanning. Despite these limitations, CT showed similar accuracy to FDG-PET when evaluating lungs, bones, kidneys, and adrenals [86]. A recent imaging study comparing whole-body MDCT with whole-body Gd-MRI in patients who had stage III-IV melanoma showed superior detection of brain, bone marrow, subcutaneous tissues, liver, muscle, and splenic metastases by MRI. MDCT detected more lung metastases than MRI, and the modalities were similar in assessing lymph nodes, kidneys, and adrenals [87]. A comparison of FDG-PET/CT with whole-body Gd-MRI showed overall accuracy of 87% and 79%, respectively. PET/CT was more sensitive in detection of skin/subcutaneous and lymph node metastases, and MRI was superior at detection of brain, liver, and bone metastases [88]. FDG-PET/CT is more accurate than FDG-PET for detecting melanoma metastases [89]. Although whole-body MRI has advantages over whole-body CT, many institutions do not have the equipment or expertise to perform state-of-the-art whole-body MRI. Even if FDG-PET/CT and whole-body Gd-MRI are performed for staging, chest MDCT may add useful clinical information. If state-of-the-art whole-body MRI is not available, accurate staging may be obtained with FDG-PET/CT; MDCT of the chest, abdomen, and pelvis; and MRI of the brain. Imaging of the liver with MDCT should be performed during hepatic artery and portal venous phases of contrast enhancement. Precontrast images can substitute for the hepatic artery phase [90].

Gastrointestinal endocrine tumors

Most neuroendocrine tumors are well differentiated and express the somatostatin receptor. Therefore, gastro-entero-pancreatic (GEP) tumors can be effectively imaged using somatostatin receptor scintigraphy (SRS) with the radiolabeled somatostatin-analog In-111 octreotide [91]. The presence of the somatostatin receptor seen on SRS may also predict the efficacy of octreotide for therapy. Somatostatin receptor expression can be variable between tumor subtypes and patients and within an individual, possibly as a result of dedifferentiation [92]. When dedifferentiation occurs, the tumor not only becomes detectable by FDG-PET but often behaves more aggressively [93]. Fig. 1 depicts the differences between SRS and FDG-PET in patients who have low- and high-grade GEP tumors. SRS in combination with CT, with or without image fusion, adds anatomic detail and increases accuracy of tumor detection [94,95]. Recent advances in MDCT have resulted in 94% sensitivity for detection of primary pancreatic insulinoma using thin section biphasic contrast enhanced imaging [96]. This is a neoplasm that SRS does not accurately detect. CT of the liver for detection of carcinoid metastases must include hepatic arterial and portal venous phases for maximum sensitivity [97]. A study to assess the detection of liver metastases from well differentiated GEP tumors showed that MR depicted more liver metastases than single-detector CT or SRS [98]. Therefore, SRS and MDCT should be the first imaging procedures performed for GEP tumors. If the tumor is not well differentiated or if it is poorly depicted on SRS, FDG-PET may be helpful. MRI is the most sensitive method for detection of liver metastases and should be performed before considering liver resection or ablation.

Other radioligands are under investigation in the United States and Europe for the diagnosis and therapy of GEP tumors. These are somatostatin analogs coupled with conventional single–photon, gamma-emitting or beta-emitting radioisotopes. Some of these have dual purpose for diagnosis and therapy. Examples of these compounds include indium-111 and yttrium-90 DOTA-Tyr^3-octreotide (DOTATOC) and lutetium-177 DOTA-Tyr^3-octreotate [99]. Yttrium-90 DOTATOC is a pure gamma-emitting radiopharmaceutical used only in therapy of receptor-expressing neuroendocrine tumor. Positron-emitting preparations, such as gallium-68 DOTATOC, indium-110m pentetreotide, and copper-64 TETA-octreotide, have the potential to more accurately depict the true extent of disease using PET [91]. Other positron-emitting radiopharmaceuticals under investigation for diagnostic imaging of GEP tumors and potentially more accurate than SRS are carbon-11-5-hydroxytryptophan and fluorine-18 fluorodopa [100,101].

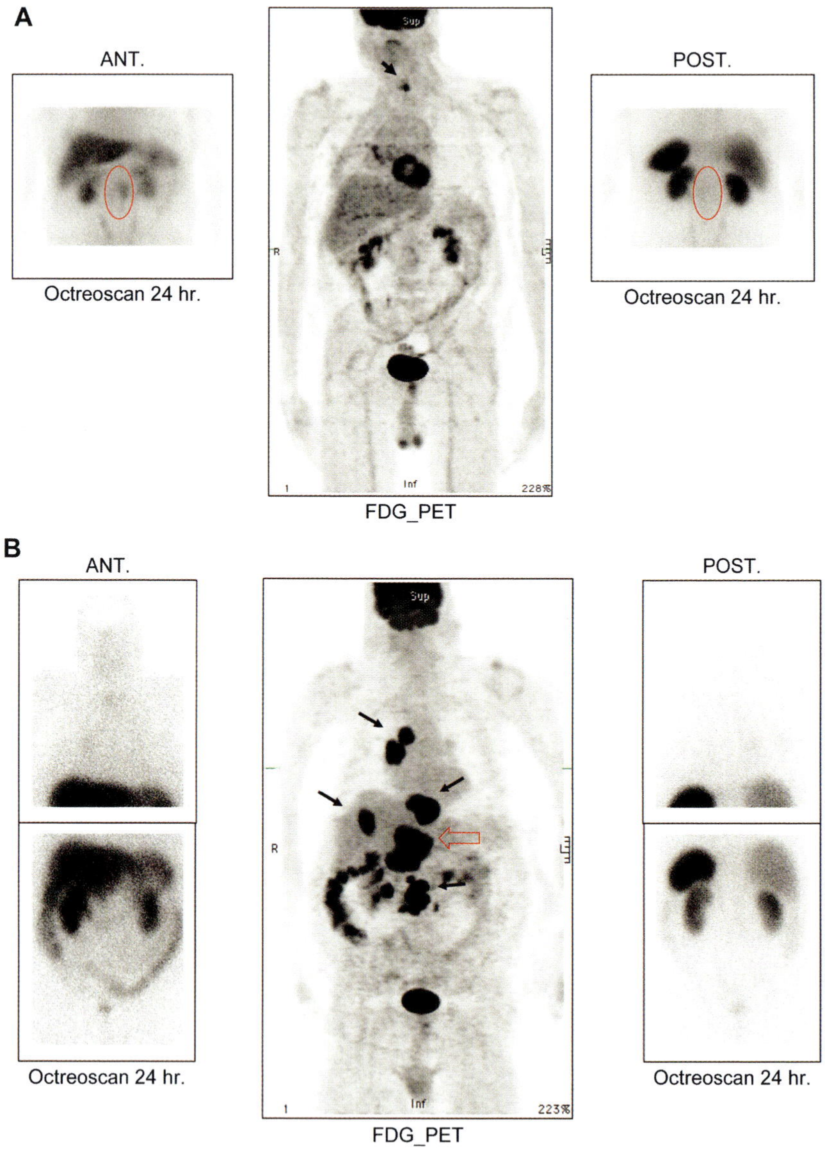

Fig. 1. (*A*) Low-grade neuroendocrine tumor. Right pneumonectomy for non-small cell lung carcinoma. Right vocal cord paralysis (*arrow*). Retroperitoneal and pancreatic lymph nodes positive for metastases from low-grade neuroendocrine tumor of pancreatic origin. Receptor-bearing neoplasm within the central abdomen (*circle*) is not evident on restaging PET scan for management of lung tumor. (*B*) High-grade neuroendocrine tumor. FDG-PET reveals a large mass in region of the porta hepatis, pancreas, and celiac axis (*red arrow*) and metastases within the retroperitoneum, liver, mediastinum, and right lung hilum (*black arrows*). None of this is evident on subsequent OctreoScan done before systemic therapy.

Sarcoma

Soft tissue and primary bone sarcomas are a heterogeneous group of malignancies. Chest CT is the most sensitive method for detecting pulmonary metastases. A recent study confirms that CT is more sensitive than PET for detecting pulmonary metastases up to 2.2 cm from musculoskeletal sarcomas [102]. FDG-PET is potentially more sensitive for soft tissue sarcoma recurrence in other parts of the body [103]. Within the pediatric and young adult population, FDG-PET can accurately detect metastases from Ewing's sarcoma but is less accurate in assessing metastatic osteogenic sarcoma [104,105]. This is likely due to the osteoblastic or sclerotic nature of osteogenic sarcoma metastases. Evaluation of osteoblastic bone metastases such as osteogenic sarcoma may therefore require bone scintigraphy or whole-body MRI. Fig. 2 is an example of a young male patient who has rhabdomyosarcoma and numerous metastases to the bone marrow seen on FDG-PET/CT but not depicted on bone scan and not obvious on the accompanying noncontrast CT.

A

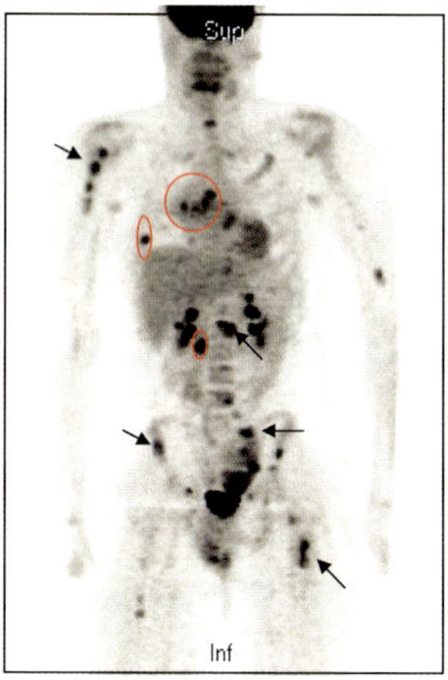

FDG_PET/CT

Fig. 2. (*A*) Rhabdomyosarcoma. In addition to soft tissue metastases (*circled in red*), FDG-PET reveals multiple skeletal lesions (*arrows*) not evident on bone scan. (*B*) Rhabdomyosarcoma. The most prominent skeletal lesion in the sacrum and left sacroiliac joint was imaged on CT. The remaining bone disease was described only on FDG-PET. Anterior oblique views on bone scan (not shown) did not show the humeral lesions revealed on PET. (*C*) Rhabdomyosarcoma. Prominent bone lesions at L2 and in the right distal femur. This is obvious on FDG-PET but not on CT scan.

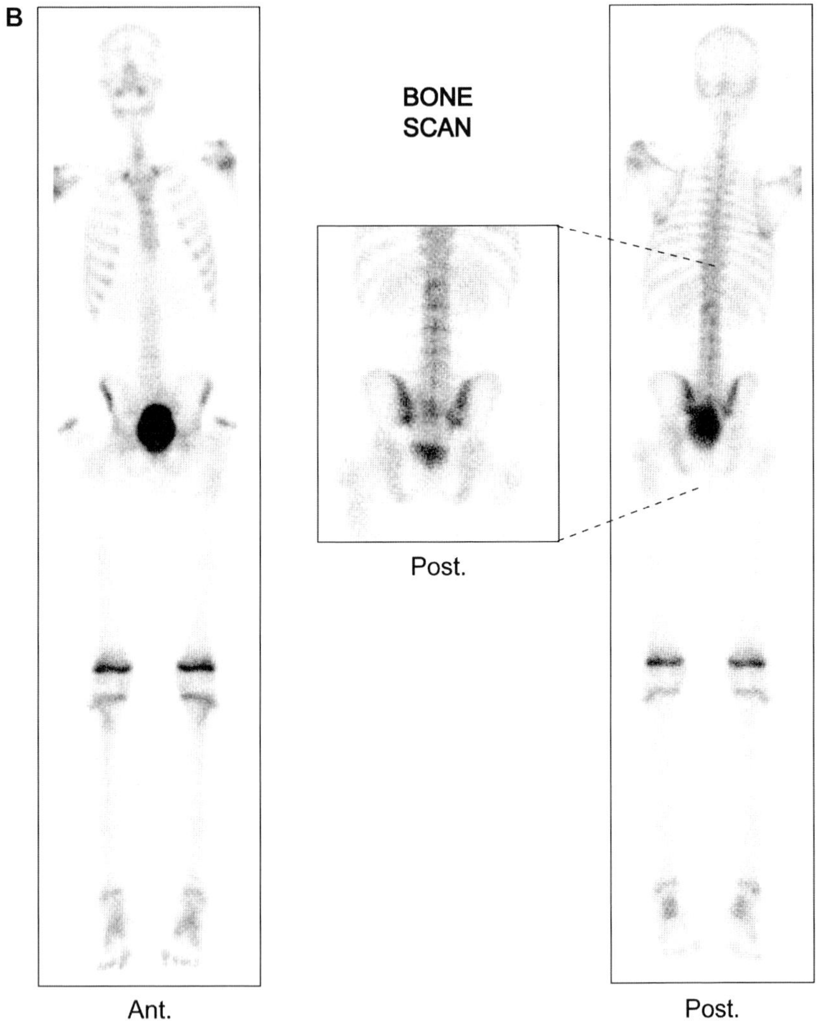

Fig. 2 (*continued*)

Peritoneal carcinomatosis

Early attempts at assessing the extent of peritoneal carcinomatosis by CT revealed severe limitations in detecting small-volume disease. A 1993 study using nonhelical CT in patients who had metastatic appendiceal and colorectal carcinoma showed sensitivity of 90%, 72%, and 28% for peritoneal tumor masses greater than 5 cm, 0.5 to 5 cm, and less than 0.5 cm, respectively [106]. In another early study with patients who had colorectal carcinoma, the overall sensitivity for tumor involvement per region of the

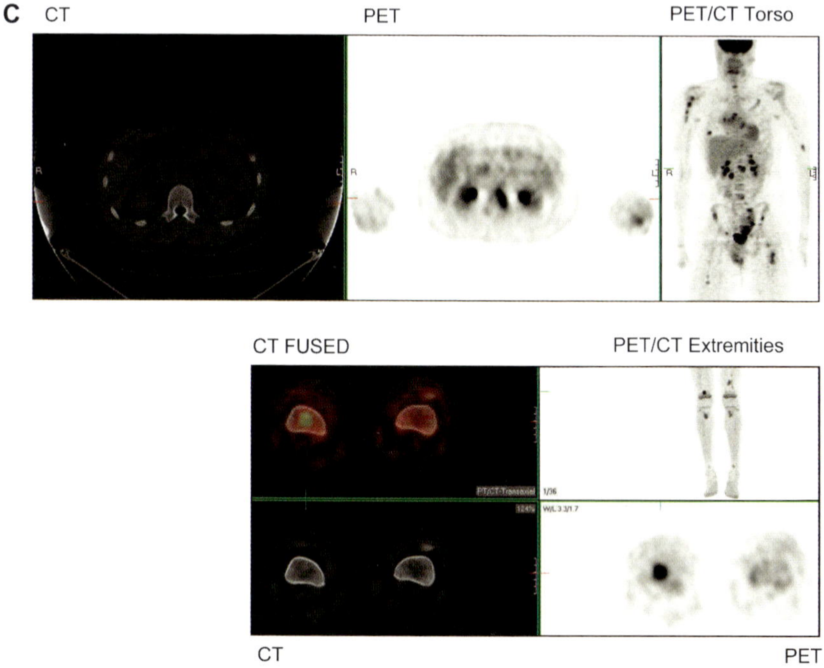

Fig. 2 (*continued*)

abdomen and pelvis was 25% to 37% [107]. A larger study of patients who had gastric cancer enrolled over 12 years showed a per-patient sensitivity of only 28% for CT [108]. In the era of nonhelical CT, there was limited success at improving detection of peritoneal tumor by the addition of water-soluble contrast or air into the peritoneal cavity before CT [109–111]. More encouraging results were obtained using single-detector helical CT to evaluate peritoneal metastases in ovarian cancer, with per patient sensitivity of 85% to 93% and specificity of 78% to 96% [112]. A recent small series of primary and previously treated patients who had ovarian cancer undergoing preoperative MDCT showed a 92% sensitivity for peritoneal tumor per patient [113]. Even with thin section axial images and multiplanar reconstruction in this study, detection of peritoneal metastases in some regions (pelvis, porta hepatis, subphrenic) was relatively low. Despite the previous technical limitations of CT, there is prognostic value in preoperative CT scans for predicting suboptimal cytoreduction in ovarian and colorectal carcinoma and peritoneal mesothelioma [114–117].

MRI seems to be at least as accurate as CT for the detection of peritoneal metastases. A multi-institutional study over 10 years ago found CT and MRI to have similar sensitivity for peritoneal disease in ovarian cancer [118]. A single-institution study showed CT and MRI to be equally accurate in the detection of inoperable tumor and the prediction of suboptimal cytoreduction in newly diagnosed ovarian cancer [114]. When Gd-MRI was compared with CT in patients who had mostly gastrointestinal and ovarian malignancies, MRI was found to have significantly better depiction of tumor involvement of the peritoneum, bowel, and mesentery [119]. In a small series of patients, MRI was accurate in demonstrating extensive mesenteric tumor or bladder implants (when the bladder was distended); the investigators considered these findings to be contraindications to cytoreductive surgery [120]. Gd-MRI with the addition of dilute barium oral contrast was superior to CT in sensitivity by tumor site (84% versus 54%) and in the detection of tumors less than 1 cm (75%–80% versus 22%–33%) [121]. In previously treated patients who had ovarian cancer with a negative CT and rising Ca-125, MRI detected tumor in 16 of the 19 patients subsequently proven to have recurrent disease [122]. As more data become available, lymphotropic nanoparticle–enhanced MRI may soon play a role in lymph node staging before cytoreductive surgery for a variety of neoplasms [123–125].

FDG-PET has the potential to significantly contribute to tumor staging in peritoneal carcinomatosis. In two studies that showed better sensitivity for CT than PET for peritoneal metastases, PET had higher specificity [126,127]. PET is more sensitive than CT or Gd-MRI in the detection of lymph node metastases during preoperative evaluation for cytoreductive surgery [127,128]. The accuracy of FDG-PET plus CT for the detection of peritoneal tumor is greater than the accuracy of PET or CT alone [129–131]. Integrated PET/CT was shown to be significantly more sensitive than CT in the detection of peritoneal metastases in a large group of patients who had gastric cancer [132] and had lesion-based sensitivity and specificity of 78% and 75% in patients who had persistent ovarian cancer [133]. FDG-PET and PET/CT have been highly accurate in evaluating patients who had ovarian cancer with negative or equivocal CT scans and rising Ca-125 levels. In this clinical setting, the patient-based accuracy of PET/CT for the detection of recurrent disease greater than or equal to 1 cm was 82% in a single study [134]. Under similar clinical circumstances, pooled data from three separate studies gave PET a sensitivity and specificity of 96% and 80% [135]. During the early follow-up period after therapy or in patients who have small volume residual disease, PET has limited utility in ovarian cancer [136,137]. In ovarian or peritoneal carcinoma patients with complete clinical remission (including negative CT), FDG-PET detected disease in only 1 of 10 patients found to have peritoneal disease at surgery [138]. PET/CT was only 13% sensitive for the detection of residual peritoneal metastases less than or equal to 1 cm in a small group of patients who had ovarian cancer after initial cytoreductive surgery [128].

Contrast-enhanced MDCT or MRI of the abdomen and pelvis should be performed in addition to FDG-PET or PET/CT for staging of peritoneal carcinomatosis before cytoreductive surgery. A low-density oral contrast agent before MDCT is less likely to obscure calcified metastases in close proximity to the bowel than high-density barium oral contrast. For MDCT, the addition of arterial phase imaging and multiplanar reconstructions may be helpful in evaluation. MDCT of the chest should accurately exclude lung and pleural metastases. Gd-MRI with oral contrast (low signal on T1 images) and breath-hold T1-weighted, fat-suppressed gradient echo sequences optimize the detection of peritoneal tumor. Administration of glucagon may help eliminate artifact due to bowel peristalsis. A well distended urinary bladder and T2-weighted imaging aids in the evaluation of bladder wall involvement.

Summary

Strategies for preoperative imaging before metastasectomy will continue to evolve. During the next few years, it is likely that MDCT with 64 or more detectors, 3 Tesla MRI, lymphotropic nanoparticle–enhanced MRI, and new commercially available contrast agents and radiopharmaceuticals will continue to increase the sensitivity and specificity for solid-tumor imaging.

References

[1] Muhm JR, Brown LR, Crowe JK. Detection of pulmonary nodules by computed tomography. AJR Am J Roentgenol 1977;128(2):267–70.
[2] Wormanns D, Ludwig K, Beyer F, et al. Detection of pulmonary nodules at multirow-detector CT: effectiveness of double reading to improve sensitivity at standard-dose and low-dose chest CT. Eur Radiol 2005;15(1):14–22.
[3] Weng MJ, Wu MT, Pan HB, et al. The feasibility of low-dose CT for pulmonary metastasis in patients with primary gynecologic malignancy. Clin Imaging 2004;28(6):408–14.
[4] Remy-Jardin M, Remy J, Giraud F, et al. Pulmonary nodules: detection with thick-section spiral CT versus conventional CT. Radiology 1993;187(2):513–20.
[5] Paranjpe DV, Bergin CJ. Spiral CT of the lungs: optimal technique and resolution compared with conventional CT. AJR Am J Roentgenol 1994;162(3):561–7.
[6] Buckley JA, Scott WW Jr, Siegelman SS, et al. Pulmonary nodules: effect of increased data sampling on detection with spiral CT and confidence in diagnosis. Radiology 1995;196(2):395–400.
[7] Diederich S, Semik M, Lentschig MG, et al. Helical CT of pulmonary nodules in patients with extrathoracic malignancy. AJR Am J Roentgenol 1999;172:353–60.
[8] Parsons AM, Detterbeck FC, Parker LA. Accuracy of helical CT in the detection of pulmonary metastases: is intraoperative palpation still necessary? Ann Thorac Surg 2004;78(6):1910–6 [discussion: 1916–8].
[9] Kayton ML, Huvos AG, Casher J, et al. Computed tomographic scan of the chest underestimates the number of metastatic lesions in osteosarcoma. J Pediatr Surg 2006;41:200–6.
[10] Tillich M, Kammerhuber F, Reittner P, et al. Detection of pulmonary nodules with helical CT: comparison of cine and film-based viewing. AJR Am J Roentgenol 1997;169:1611–4.
[11] Gruden JF, Ouanounou S, Tigges S, et al. Incremental benefit of maximum-intensity-projection images on observer detection of small pulmonary nodules revealed by multidetector CT. AJR Am J Roentgenol 2002;179:149–57.

[12] Valencia R, Denecke T, Lehmkuhl L, et al. Value of axial and coronal maximum intensity projection (MIP) images in the detection of pulmonary nodules by multislice spiral CT: comparison with axial 1-mm and 5-mm slices. Eur Radiol 2006;16:325–32.
[13] Rubin GD, Lyo JK, Paik DS, et al. Pulmonary nodules on multi-detector row CT scans: performance comparison of radiologists and computer-aided detection. Radiology 2005; 234:274–83.
[14] Wormanns D, Beyer F, Diederich S, et al. Diagnostic performance of a commercially available computer-aided diagnosis system for automatic detection of pulmonary nodules: comparison with single and double reading. Rofo 2004;176(7):953–8.
[15] Kim JS, Kim JH, Cho G, et al. Automated detection of pulmonary nodules on CT images: effect of section thickness and reconstruction interval—initial results. Radiology 2005;236: 295–9.
[16] Gurung J, Maataoui A, Khan M, et al. Automated detection of lung nodules in multidetector CT: influence of different reconstruction protocols on performance of a software prototype. Rofo 2006;178(1):71–7.
[17] Lee JW, Goo JM, Lee HJ, et al. The potential contribution of a computer-aided detection system for lung nodule detection in multidetector row computed tomography. Invest Radiol 2004;39:649–55.
[18] Yuan R, Vos PM, Cooperberg PL. Computer-aided detection in screening CT for pulmonary nodules. AJR Am J Roentgenol 2006;18:1280–7.
[19] Bae KT, Kim JS, Na YH, et al. Pulmonary nodules: automated detection on CT images with morphologic matching algorithm—preliminary results. Radiology 2005;236: 286–94.
[20] Swensen SJ, Viggiano RW, Midthun DE, et al. Lung nodule enhancement at CT: multicenter study. Radiology 2000;214:73–80.
[21] Goodman LR, Gulsun M, Washington L, et al. Inherent variability of CT lung nodule measurements in vivo using semiautomated volumetric measurements. AJR Am J Roentgenol 2006;186:989–94.
[22] Revel MP, Bissery A, Bienvenu M, et al. Are two-dimensional CT measurements of small noncalcified pulmonary nodules reliable? Radiology 2004;231:453–8.
[23] Kostis WJ, Yankelevitz DF, Reeves AP, et al. Small pulmonary nodules: reproducibility of three-dimensional volumetric measurement and estimation of time to follow-up CT. Radiology 2004;231:446–52.
[24] Gould MK, Maclean CC, Kuschner WG, et al. Accuracy of positron emission tomography for diagnosis of pulmonary nodules and mass lesions: a meta-analysis. JAMA 2001;285(7): 914–24.
[25] Nie Y, Li Q, Li F, et al. Integrating PET and CT information to improve diagnostic accuracy for lung nodules: a semiautomatic computer-aided method. J Nucl Med 2006;47: 1075–80.
[26] Pfannschmidt J, Klode J, Muley T, et al. Nodal involvement at the time of pulmonary metastasectomy: experiences in 245 patients. Ann Thorac Surg 2006;81:448–54.
[27] Ercan S, Nichols FC, Trastek VF, et al. Prognostic significance of lymph node metastasis found during pulmonary metastasectomy for extrapulmonary carcinoma. Ann Thorac Surg 2004;77:1786–91.
[28] Schroeder T, Ruehm SG, Debatin JF, et al. Detection of pulmonary nodules using a 2D HASTE MR sequence: comparison with MDCT. AJR Am J Roentgenol 2005;185:979–84.
[29] Johnson PT, Fishman EK. IV contrast for MDTC: current thoughts and practice. AJR Am J Roentgenol 2006;186:406–15.
[30] Weg N, Scheer MR, Gabor MP. Liver lesions: improved detection with dual-detector-array CT and routine 2.5-mm thin collimation. Radiology 1998;209:417–26.
[31] Haider MA, Amitai MM, Rappaport DC, et al. Multi-detector row helical CT in preoperative assessment of small ($\leq$1.5 cm) liver metastases: Is thinner collimation better? Radiology 2002;225:137–42.

[32] Bhattacharjya S, Bhattacharjya T, Baber S, et al. Prospective study of contrast-enhanced computed tomography, computed tomography during arterioportography, and magnetic resonance imaging for staging colorectal liver metastases for liver resection. Br J Surg 2004;91:1361–9.
[33] Ward J, Naik KS, Guthrie JA, et al. Hepatic lesion detection: comparison of MR imaging after the administration of superparamagnetic iron oxide with dual-phase CT by using alternative-free response receiver operating characteristic analysis. Radiology 1999;210: 459–66.
[34] Reimer P, Jahnke N, Fiebich M, et al. Hepatic lesion detection and characterization: value of nonenhanced MR imaging, superparamagnetic iron oxide-enhanced MR imaging, and spiral CT: ROC analysis. Radiology 2000;217:152–8.
[35] Oudkerk M, Torres CG, Song B, et al. Characterization of liver lesion with mangafodipir trisodium-enhanced MR imaging: multicenter study comparing MR and dual-phase spiral CT. Radiology 2002;223:517–24.
[36] Kim KW, Kim AY, Kim TK, et al. Small ($\leq$2 cm) hepatic lesions in colorectal cancer patients: detection and characterization on mangafodipir trisodium-enhanced MRI. AJR Am J Roentgenol 2004;182:1233–40.
[37] Soyer P, Poccard M, Boudiaf M, et al. Detection of hypovascular hepatic metastases at triple-phase helical CT: sensitivity of phases and comparison with surgical and histopathologic findings. Radiology 2004;231:413–20.
[38] Ward J, Robinson PJ, Guthrie JA, et al. Liver metastases in candidates for hepatic resection: comparison of helical CT and gadolinium- and SPIO- enhanced MR imaging. Radiology 2005;237:170–80.
[39] Holalkere NS, Sahani DV, Blake MA, et al. Characterization of small liver lesions: added role of MR after MDCT. J Comput Assist Tomogr 2006;30(4):591–6.
[40] Numminen K, Isoniemi H, Halavaara J, et al. Preoperative assessment of focal liver lesions: multidetector computed tomography challenges magnetic resonance imaging. Acta Radiol 2005;46(1):9–15.
[41] Onishi H, Murakami T, Kim T, et al. Hepatic metastases: detection with multi-detector row CT, SPIO-enhanced MR imaging, and both techniques combined. Radiology 2006;239(1): 131–8.
[42] Ward J, Guthrie JA, Wilson D, et al. Colorectal hepatic metastases: detection with SPIO-enhanced breath-hold MR imaging: comparison of optimized sequences. Radiology 2003; 228:709–18.
[43] Ward J. New MR techniques for the detection of liver metastases. Cancer Imaging 2006;6: 33–42.
[44] Kim YK, Lee JM, Kim CS, et al. Detection of liver metastases: gadobenate dimeglumine-enhanced three-dimensional dynamic phases and one-hour delayed phase MR imaging versus superparamagnetic iron oxide-enhanced MR imaging. Eur Radiol 2005; 15(2):220–8.
[45] Chung JJ, Kim MJ, Kim KW. Mangafodipir trisodium-enhanced MRI for the detection and characterization of focal hepatic lesions: is delayed imaging useful? J Magn Reson Imaging 2006;23(5):706–11.
[46] Bartolozzi C, Donati F, Cioni D, et al. Detection of colorectal liver metastases: a prospective multicenter trial comparing unenhanced MRI, MnDPDP-enhanced MRI, and spiral CT. Eur Radiol 2004;14:14–20.
[47] Vogl TJ, Schwarz W, Blume S. Preoperative evaluation of malignant liver tumors: comparison of unenhanced and SPIO (Resovist)-enhanced MR imaging with biphasic CTAP and intraoperative US. Eur Radiol 2003;13:262–72.
[48] Vidiri A, Carpanese L, D'Annibale M, et al. Evaluation of hepatic metastases from colorectal carcinoma with MR-superparamagnetic iron oxide. J Exp Clin Cancer Res 2004; 23(1):53–60.

[49] Del Frate C, Bazzocchi M, Mortele KJ. Detection of liver metastases: comparison of gadobenate dimeglumine-enhanced and ferumoxides-enhanced MR imaging examinations. Radiology 2002;225:766–72.
[50] Vogl TJ, Hammerstingl R, Schwarz W, et al. Magnetic resonance imaging of focal liver lesions: comparison of the superparamagnetic iron oxide resovist versus gadolinium-DTPA in the same patient. Invest Radiol 1996;31(11):696–708.
[51] Kim MJ, Kim JH, Lim JS, et al. Detection and characterization of focal hepatic lesions: mangafodipir vs. superparamagnetic iron oxide-enhanced magnetic resonance imaging. J Magn Reson Imaging 2004;20(4):612–21.
[52] Choi JY, Kim MJ, Kim JH. Detection of hepatic metastasis: manganese- and ferucarbotran-enhanced MR imaging. Eur J Radiol 2006;60(1):84–90.
[53] Kim HJ, Kim KW, Byun JH, et al. Comparison of mangafodipir trisodium- and ferucarbotran-enhanced MRI for detection and characterization of hepatic metastases in colorectal cancer patients. AJR Am J Roentgenol 2006;186:1059–66.
[54] van Etten B, van der Sijp JRM, Kruyt RH, et al. Ferumoxide-enhanced magnetic resonance imaging techniques in pre-operative assessment for colorectal liver metastases. Eur J Surg Oncol 2002;28:645–51.
[55] Semelka RC, Cance WG, Marcos HB, et al. Liver metastases: comparison of current MR techniques and spiral CT during arterial portography for detection in 20 surgically staged cases. Radiology 1999;312(1):86–91.
[56] Hosch WP, Schmidt SM, Plaza S. Comparison of CT during arterial portography and MR during arterial portography in the detection of liver metastases. AJR Am J Roentgenol 2006;186:1502–11.
[57] Jarnagin WR, Bach AM, Winston CB, et al. What is the yield of intraoperative ultrasonography during partial hepatectomy for malignant disease? J Am Coll Surg 2001;192:577–83.
[58] Zacherl J, Scheuba C, Imhof M, et al. Current value of intraoperative sonography during surgery for hepatic neoplams. World J Surg 2002;26:550–4.
[59] Leen E, Ceccotti P, Moug SJ, et al. Potential value of contrast-enhanced intraoperative ultrasonography during partial hepatectomy for metastases. Ann Surg 2006;243:236–40.
[60] Kinkel K, Lu Y, Both M, et al. Detection of hepatic metastases from cancers of the gastrointestinal tract by using noninvasive imaging methods (US, CT, MR imaging, PET): a meta-analysis. Radiology 2002;224:748–56.
[61] Truant S, Huglo D, Hebbar M, et al. Prospective evaluation of the impact of [^{18}F]fluoro-2-deoxy-D-glucose positron emission tomography of resectable colorectal liver metastases. Br J Surg 2005;92:362–9.
[62] Wiering B, Ruers TJM, Krabbe PFM, et al. Comparison of multiphase CT, FDG-PET and intra-operative ultrasound in patients with colorectal liver metastases selected for surgery. Ann Surg Oncol 2007;14(2):818–26.
[63] Ghanem N, Altehoefer C, Hogerle S, et al. Detectability of liver metastases in malignant melanoma: prospective comparison of magnetic resonance imaging and positron emission tomography. Eur J Radiol 2005;54(2):264–70.
[64] Sahani DV, Kalva SP, Fischman AJ, et al. Detection of liver metastases from adenocarcinoma of the colon and pancreas: comparison of mangafodipir trisodium-enhanced liver MRI and whole-body FDG PET. AJR Am J Roentgenol 2005;185:239–46.
[65] Seemann MD, Meisetschlaeger G, Gaa G, et al. Assessment of the extent of metastases of gastrointestinal carcinoid tumors using whole-body PET, CT, MRI, PET/CT and PET/MRI. Eur J Med Res 2006;11(2):58–65.
[66] Schmidt GP, Baur-Melnyk A, Herzog P, et al. High-resolution whole- body magnetic resonance image tumor staging with the use of parallel imaging versus dual-modality positron emission tomography-computed tomography. Invest Radiol 2005;40:743–53.
[67] Hedeland H, Ostberg G, Hokfelt B. On the prevalence of adrenocortical adenomas in an autopsy material in relation to hypertension and diabetes. Acta Med Scand 1968;184(3): 211–4.

[68] Blake MA, Kalra MK, Sweeney A, et al. Distinguishing benign from malignant adrenal masses: multi-detector row CT Protocol with 10-minute delay. Radiology 2006;238(2): 578–86.
[69] Caoili EM, Korobkin M, Francis IR, et al. Adrenal masses: characterization with combined unenhanced and delayed enhanced CT. Radiology 2002;222:629–33.
[70] Korobkin M, Brodeur FJ, Yutzy GG, et al. Differentiation of adrenal adenomas from nonadenomas using CT attenuation values. AJR Am J Roentgenol 1996;166(3):531–6.
[71] Boland GW, Lee MJ, Gazelle GS, et al. Characterization of adrenal masses using unenhanced CT: an analysis of the CT literature. AJR Am J Roentgenol 1998;171(1):201–4.
[72] Savci G, Yazici Z, Sahin N, et al. Value of chemical shift subtraction MRI in characterization of adrenal masses. AJR Am J Roentgenol 2006;186:130–5.
[73] Tsushima Y, Ishizaka H, Matsumoto M. Adrenal masses: differentiation with chemical shift, fast low-angle shot MR imaging. Radiology 1993;186:705–9.
[74] Haider MA, Ghai S, Jhaveri K, et al. Chemical shift MR imaging of hyperattenuating (>10 HU) adrenal masses: does it still have a role? Radiology 2004;231:711–6.
[75] Yun M, Kim W, Alnafisi N, et al. ^{18}F-FDG PET in characterizing adrenal lesions detected on CT or MRI. J Nucl Med 2001;42:1795–9.
[76] Maurea S, Mainolfi C, Bazzicalupo L, et al. Imaging of adrenal tumors using FDG PET: comparison of benign and malignant lesions. AJR Am J Roentgenol 1999;173:25–9.
[77] Boland GW, Goldberg MA, Lee MJ, et al. Indeterminate adrenal mass in patients with cancer: evaluation at PET with 2-[F-18]-fluoro-2-deoxy-D-glucose. Radiology 1995;194:131–4.
[78] Blake MA, Slattery JM, Kalra MK, et al. Adrenal lesions: characterization with fused PET/CT image in patients with proved or suspected malignancy: initial experience. Radiology 2006;238(3):970–7.
[79] Wiering B, Krabbe PFM, Jager GJ, et al. The impact of Fluor-18-deoxyglucose-positron emission tomography in the management of colorectal liver metastases. Cancer 2005;104: 2658–70.
[80] Wiering B, Krabbe PFM, Dekker HM, et al. The role of FDG-PET in the selection of patients with colorectal liver metastases. Ann Surg Oncol 2007;2(14):771–9.
[81] Fernandez FG, Drebin JA, Linehan DC, et al. Five-year survival after resection of hepatic metastases from colorectal cancer in patients screened by positron emission tomography with F-18 Fluorodeoxyglucose (FDG-PET). Ann Surg 2004;240:438–50.
[82] Flanagan FL, Dehdashti F, Ogunbiyi OA, et al. Utility of FDG-PET for Investigating unexplained plasma CEA elevation in patients with colorectal cancer. Ann Surg 1998;227(3): 319–23.
[83] Whiteford MH, Whiteford HM, Yee LF, et al. Usefulness of FDG-PET scan in the assessment of suspected metastatic or recurrent adenocarcinoma of the colon and rectum. Dis Colon Rectum 2000;43(6):759–67 [discussion: 767–70].
[84] Essner R, Belhocine T, Scott AM, et al. Novel imaging techniques in melanoma. Surg Oncol Clin N Am 2006;15:253–83.
[85] Finkelstein SE, Carrasquillo JA, Hoffman JM, et al. A prospective analysis of positron emission tomography and conventional imaging for detection of stage IV metastatic melanoma in patients undergoing metastasectomy. Ann Surg Oncol 2004;11(8):731–8.
[86] Swetter SM, Carroll LA, Johnson DL, et al. Positron emission tomography is superior to computed tomography for metastatic detection in melanoma patients. Ann Surg Oncol 2002;9(7):646–3.
[87] Muller-Horvat C, Radny P, Eigentler TK, et al. Prospective comparison of the impact on treatment decisions of whole-body magnetic resonance imaging and computed tomography in patients with metastatic malignant melanoma. Eur J Cancer 2006;42(3):342–50.
[88] Pfannenberg C, Aschoff P, Schanz S, et al. Prospective comparison of ^{18}F-fluorodeoxyglucose positron emission tomography/computed tomography and whole-body magnetic resonance imaging in staging of advanced malignant melanoma. Eur J Cancer 2007;43:557–64.

[89] Reinhardt MJ, Joe AY, Jaeger U, et al. Diagnostic performance of whole body dual modality ^{18}F-FDG PET/C imaging for N- and M- staging of malignant melanoma: experience with 250 consecutive patients. J Clin Oncol 2006;24:1178–87.
[90] Blake SP, Weisinger K, Atkins MB, et al. Liver metastases from melanoma: detection with multiphasic contrast-enhanced CT. Radiology 1999;213(1):92–6.
[91] Kaltsas G, Rockall A, Papadogias D, et al. Recent advances in radiological and radionuclide imaging and therapy of neuroendocrine tumours. Eur J Endocrinol 2004;151:15–27.
[92] Jadvar H, Segall GM. False-negative fluorine-18-FDG PET in metastatic carcinoid. J Nucl Med 1997;38(9):1382–3.
[93] Belhocine T, Foidart J, Rigo P, et al. Fluorodeoxyglucose positron emission tomography and somatostatin receptor scintigraphy for diagnosing and staging carcinoid tumours: correlations with the pathological indexes p53 and Ki-67. Nucl Med Commun 2002;23(8): 727–34.
[94] Koopmans KP, de Vries EGE, Kema IP, et al. Staging of carcinoid tumours with ^{18}F-DOPA PET: a prospective, diagnostic accuracy study. Lancet Oncol 2005;7:728–34.
[95] Pfannenberg AC, Eschmann SM, Horger M, et al. Benefit of anatomical-functional image fusion in the diagnostic work-up of neuroendocrine neoplasms. Eur J Nucl Med Mol Imaging 2003;30:835–43.
[96] Gouya H, Vignaux O, Augui J, et al. CT, endoscopic sonography, and a combined protocol for preoperative evaluation of pancreatic insulinomas. AJR Am J Roentgenol 2003;181: 987–92.
[97] Paulson EK, McDermott VG, Keogan MT, et al. Carcinoid metastases to the liver: role of triple-phase helical CT. Radiology 1998;206:143–50.
[98] Dromain C, de Baere T, Lumbroso J, et al. Detection of liver metastases from endocrine tumors: a prospective comparison of somatostatin receptor scintigraphy, computed tomography, and magnetic resonance imaging. J Clin Oncol 2005;23:70–8.
[99] Virgolini I, Traub-Weidinger T, Decristoforo C. Nuclear medicine in the detection and management of pancreatic islet-cell tumours. Best Pract Res Clin Endocrinol Metab 2005;19(2):213–27.
[100] Orlefors H, Sundin A, Garske U, et al. Whole-body ^{11}C-5-hydroxytryptophan positron emission tomography as a universal imaging technique for neuroendocrine tumors: comparison with somatostatin receptor scintigraphy and computed tomography. J Clin Endocrinol Metab 2005;90(6):3392–400.
[101] Becherer A, Szabo M, Karanikas G, et al. Imaging of advanced neuroendocrine tumors with 18F-FDOPA PET. J Nucl Med 2004;45(7):1161–7.
[102] Iagaru A, Chawla S, Menendez L, et al. F-FDG PET and PET/CT for detection of pulmonary metastases from musculoskeletal sarcomas. Nucl Med Commun 2006;27: 795–802.
[103] Johnson GR, Zhuang H, Khan J, et al. Roles of positron emission tomography with fluorine-18-deoxyglucose in the detection of local recurrent and distant metastatic sarcoma. Clin Nucl Med 2003;28:815–20.
[104] Daldrup-Link H, Franzius C, Link TM, et al. Whole-body MR imaging for detection of bone metastases in children and young adults: comparison with skeletal scintigraphy and FDG PET. AJR Am J Roentgenol 2001;177:229–36.
[105] Kneisl JS, Patt JC, Johnson JC. Is PET useful in detecting occult nonpulmonary metastases in pediatric bone sarcomas? Clin Orthop Relat Res 2006;450:101–4.
[106] Jacquet P, Jelinek JS, Steves MA, et al. Evaluation of computed tomography in patients with peritoneal carcinomatosis. Cancer 1993;72(5):1631–6.
[107] De Bree E, Koops W, Kroger R, et al. Peritoneal carcinomatosis from colorectal or appendiceal origin: correlation of preoperative CT with intraopertaive findings and evaluation of interobserver agreement. J Surg Oncol 2004;86:64–73.
[108] Gretschel S, Siegel R, Estevez-Schwarz L, et al. Surgical strategies for gastric cancer with synchronous peritoneal carcinomatosis. Br J Surg 2006;93:1530–5.

[109] Frasci G, Contino A, Iaffaioli RV, et al. Computerized tomography of the abdomen and pelvis with peritoneal administration of soluble contrast (IPC-CT) in detection of residual disease for patients with ovarian cancer. Gynecol Oncol 1994;52(2):154–60.
[110] Caseiro-Alves F, Goncalo M, Abraul E, et al. Induced pneumoperitoneum in CT evaluation of peritoneal carcinomatosis. Abdom Imaging 1995;20(1):52–5 [discussion: 56–7].
[111] Gryspeerdt S, Clabout L, Van Hoe L, et al. Intraperitoneal contrast material combined with CT for detection of peritoneal metastases of ovarian cancer. Eur J Gynaecol Oncol 1998;19(5):434–7.
[112] Coakley FV, Choi PH, Gougoutas CA, et al. Peritoneal metastases: detection with spiral CT in patients with ovarian cancer. Radiology 2002;223:495–9.
[113] Pannu HK, Horton KM, Fishman EK. Thin section dual-phase multidetector-row computed tomography detection of peritoneal metastases in gynecologic cancers. J Comput Assist Tomogr 2003;27(3):333–40.
[114] Qayyum A, Coakley FV, Westphalen AC, et al. Role of CT and MR imaging in predicting optimal cytoreduction of newly diagnosed primary epithelial ovarian cancer. Gynecol Oncol 2005;96:301–6.
[115] Dowdy SC, Mullany SA, Brandt KR, et al. The utility of computed tomography scans in predicting suboptimal cytoreductive surgery in women with advanced ovarian carcinoma. Cancer 2004;101:346–52.
[116] de Bree E, Koops W, Kroger R, et al. Preoperative computed tomography and selection of patients with colorectal peritoneal carcinomatosis for cytoreductive surgery and hyperthermic intraperitoneal chemotherapy. Eur J Surg Oncol 2006;32:65–71.
[117] Yan TD, Haveric N, Carmignani CP. Abdominal computed tomography scans in the selection of patients with malignant peritoneal mesothelioma for comprehensive treatment with cytoreductive surgery and perioperative intraperitoneal chemotherapy. Cancer 2005;103: 839–49.
[118] Tempany CMC, Zou KH, Silverman SG. Staging of advanced ovarian cancer: comparison of imaging modalities: report from the Radiological Diagnostic Oncology Group. Radiology 2000;215:761–7.
[119] Low RN, Semelka RC, Worawattanakul S, et al. Extrahepatic abdominal imaging in patients with malignancy: comparison of MR imaging and helical CT, with subsequent surgical correlation. Radiology 1999;210:625–32.
[120] Cotton F, Pellet O, Gilly FN, et al. MRI evaluation of bulky tumor masses in the mesentery and bladder involvement in peritoneal carcinomatosis. Eur J Surg Oncol 2006;32: 1212–6.
[121] Low RN, Barone RM, Lacey C, et al. Peritoneal tumor: MR imaging with dilute oral barium and intravenous gadolinium-containing contrast agents compared with unenhanced MR imaging and CT. Radiology 1997;204:513–20.
[122] Balestreri L, Bison L, Sorio R, et al. Abdominal recurrence of ovarian cancer: value of abdominal MR in patients with positive CA 125 and negative CT. Radiol Med (Torino) 2002; 104(5–6):426–36.
[123] Koh DM, Brown G, Temple L, et al. Rectal cancer: mesorectal lymph nodes at MR imaging with USPIO versus histopathologic findings: initial observations. Radiology 2004;231(1): 91–9.
[124] Anzai Y, Piccoli CW, Outwater EK, et al. Evaluation of neck and body metastases to nodes with ferumoxtran 10-enhanced MR imaging: phase III safety and efficacy study. Radiology 2003;228(3):777–88.
[125] Saksena MA, Saokar A, Harisinghani MG. Lymphotropic nanoparticle enhanced MR imaging (LNMRI) technique for lymph node imaging. Eur J Radiol 2006;58:367–74.
[126] Lim JS, Kim MJ, Yun MJ, et al. Comparison of CT and 18F-FDG PET for detecting peritoneal metastasis on the preoperative evaluation for gastric carcinoma. Korean J Radiol 2006;7(4):249–56.

[127] Drieskens O, Stroobants S, Gysen M, et al. Positron emission tomography with FDG in the detection of peritoneal and retroperitoneal metastases of ovarian cancer. Gynecol Obstet Invest 2003;55(3):130–4.
[128] Pannu HK, Cohade C, Bristow RE, et al. PET-CT detection of abdominal recurrence of ovarian cancer: radiologic-surgical correlation. Abdom Imaging 2004;39:398–403.
[129] Turlakow A, Yeung H, Walmon HW, et al. Peritoneal carcinomatosis role of (18) F-FDG PET. J Nucl Med 2003;44(9):1407–12.
[130] Suzuki A, Kawano T, Takahashi N, et al. Value of 18F-FDG PET in the detection of peritoneal carcinomatosis. Eur J Nucl Med Mol Imaging 2004;31(10):1413–20.
[131] Picchio M, Sironi S, Messa C, et al. Advanced ovarian carcinoma: usefulness of [(18)F] FDG-PET in combination with CT for lesion detection after primary treatment. Q J Nucl Med 2003;47:77–84.
[132] Yang QM, Bando E, Kawamura T, et al. The diagnostic value of PET-CT for peritoneal dissemination of abdominal malignancies. Gan To Kagaku Ryoho 2006;33(12):1817–21.
[133] Sironi S, essa C, Mangili G, et al. Integrated FDG PET/CT in patients with persistent ovarian cancer: correlation with histologic findings. Radiology 2004;233:433–40.
[134] Bristow RE, del Carmen MG, Pannu HK, et al. Clinically occult recurrent ovarian cancer: patient selection for secondary cytoreductive surgery using combined PET/CT. Gynecol Oncol 2003;90:519–28.
[135] Havrilesky LJ, Kulasingam SL, Matchar DB, et al. FDG-PET for management of cervical and ovarian cancer. Gynecol Oncol 2005;97:183–91.
[136] Cho SM, Ha HK, Byun JY, et al. Usefulness of FDG PET for assessment of early recurrent epithelial ovarian cancer. AJR Am J Roentgenol 2002;179:391–5.
[137] Nakamoto Y, Safa T, Ishimori T, et al. Clinical value of positron emission tomography with FDG for recurrent ovarian cancer. AJR Am J Roentgenol 2001;176:1449–54.
[138] Rose PG, Faulhaber P, Miraldi F, et al. Positive emission tomography for evaluating a complete clinical response in patients with ovarian or peritoneal carcinoma: correlation with second-look laparotomy. Gynecol Oncol 2001;82:17–21.

ELSEVIER
SAUNDERS

Surg Oncol Clin N Am
16 (2007) 493–506

SURGICAL
ONCOLOGY CLINICS
OF NORTH AMERICA

Hepatectomy for Resectable Colorectal Cancer Metastases—Indicators of Prognosis, Definition of Resectability, Techniques and Outcomes

Renato Lupinacci, MD, Christophe Penna, MD, Bernard Nordlinger, MD*

Hôpital Ambroise-Paré, Service de Chirurgie Digestive, 9 av Charles De Gaulle, 92100 Boulogne Billancourt, France

Hepatic metastases are present in 15% to 25% of patients at the time of diagnosis of colorectal cancer [1], and another 25% to 50% will develop liver metastases within 3 years, following resection of the primary tumor [2].

Hepatic resection for colorectal liver metastases has become the standard of care, and currently remains the only potentially curative therapy. Complete surgical resection of isolated or multiple hepatic metastases has been associated with a 25% to 50% 5-year survival. Although there are no randomized trials comparing resection and chemotherapy in patients with potentially resectable liver metastases, several retrospective studies have reviewed the outcome of patients treated nonsurgically for potentially resectable liver lesions. Those studies strongly suggested a survival advantage for patients undergoing curative hepatic resections [3,4].

Following the conventional indications for resection, only a minority of patients with colorectal liver metastases are amenable to surgery; however, all these criteria have been challenged by different groups over the past decade leading to a more aggressive approach in the management of colorectal liver metastases.

Definition of resectability, patient's selection

The decision and the extent of surgical resection for liver metastasis are based on the patient's condition, extent of the disease, and liver function.

* Corresponding author.
E-mail address: bernard.nordlinger@apr.ap-hop-paris.fr (B. Nordlinger).

1055-3207/07/$ - see front matter © 2007 Elsevier Inc. All rights reserved.
doi:10.1016/j.soc.2007.04.014 **_surgonc.theclinics.com_**

Surgical resection can be discussed if the patient is suitable for a general anesthesia and if there is no nonresectable extrahepatic disease. Liver metastases will be considered as resectable if all liver deposits can be removed with clear margins leaving a remnant liver parenchyma accounting for at least 25% of nontumorous liver along with its arterial/portal inflow and hepatic vein outflow. In summary, liver metastases are nonresectable if there is invasion of the two main portal pedicles, if there is an invasion of one portal pedicle and the controlateral hepatic vein, if the three major hepatic veins are invaded, or if the total removal of liver deposits will leave less than 25% of functional liver.

Resectable lesions are usually divided into two subtypes. Liver metastases that can be resected with an anatomical resection removing less than four segments and leaving more than 40% of healthy liver parenchyma are referred to as type I resectability. Resections of more than four segments (major hepatectomy), which can be complex and hazardous because of the close relationship of lesions to major hepatic vessels or biliary pedicles, are referred as type II resectability.

Patients

Operative risk assessment to determine if the patient is suitable for general anesthesia and potentially hemorrhagic surgery is similar to other major abdominal procedures. Particular attention should be directed to pulmonary and cardiac status, because clamping maneuvers of the hepatic pedicle and the vena cava may be necessary during resection.

Liver function

When underlying liver parenchyma is normal, up to six anatomical segments or 75% of the liver volume can be resected without inducing postoperative liver failure. The remnant liver volume following planned hepatectomy can be measured on CT scan with volumetric reconstruction. The functional capacity of the liver can be assessed by the Child-Pugh classification, hepatic biological blood tests, and in some cases by the indocyanin green test. Liver metastases rarely develop in cirrhotic liver [5] but following recent development of more efficient chemotherapy regimens and targeted agents, an increased number of patients may present with damaged livers as a result of chemotherapy given before liver resection (neoadjuvant therapy). Because of the specific liver toxicity of some of the chemotherapy agents used in these newer regimens, the enthusiasm over potential positive effects of neoadjuvant chemotherapy has been damped somewhat by the liver toxicity seen after preoperative chemotherapy. Preoperative chemotherapy has been associated with specific pathologic changes of the liver parenchyma with potential deleterious effects on the postoperative liver function and ability of the patient to recover from surgery [5–12]. Two main types of chemotherapy-associated liver injuries have been reported: vascular changes and chemotherapy-associated steatohepatitis (CASH). The vascular changes include sinusoidal dilation with erythrocytic congestion, occasionally accompanied by perisinusoidal fibrosis and fibrotic venous occlusion, which can result in sinusoidal obstruction syndrome mimicking veno-occlusive disease [6]. CASH is defined as the association of severe steatosis, lobular inflammation, and ballooning of hepatocytes and may progress toward liver fibrosis [6]. These changes can increase the risk of perioperative bleeding or postoperative liver insufficiency. We [9] and others [10–12] have shown that prolonged systemic chemotherapy with either CPT-11 or oxaliplatin can increase postoperative morbidity after major liver resections. Preoperative liver biopsy has been suggested in patients who have received prolonged systemic chemotherapy to evaluate the degree of chemotherapy-induced liver injury [5]. The validity of such an approach is uncertain because of the problems with intra- and interobserver variations in the evaluation of CASH [6] and the heterogeneity of the observed histologic changes associated with chemotherapy. Therefore, it is very difficult to deny a patient with resectable metastases surgical therapy based on biopsy results of the uninvolved liver alone.

Control of other metastatic sites

Adequate control of the site of the primary tumor (anastomotic recurrence or locoregional spread) as well as the absence of a new colonic cancer should be demonstrated, usually by CT scan and colonoscopy. Thoracic CT scan is performed to rule out nonresectable pulmonary metastases. PET scan, if available, may prove to be useful to detect extrahepatic recurrences at any site with a single examination, but its efficacy in this setting is not yet established.

Preoperative assessment of the hepatic involvement

An accurate localization of all hepatic lesions and their relationship to major hepatic vessels and biliary pedicles is essential to plan an adequate type of resection. Transabdominal ultrasound has a good (85% to 95%) specificity for the diagnoses of hepatic metastases [13–15], but its sensitivity for the detection of lesions smaller than 1 cm remains low. Contrast-enhanced ultrasonography has a higher sensitivity and specificity for detecting small metastases and is helpful for the differential diagnosis of doubtful lesions. In a recent prospective trial of 100 patients who had liver resection, contrast-enhanced ultrasonography improved the sensitivity for detecting liver metastases from 56% with standard ultrasonography to 84%. The contrast agent was particularly helpful for the detection of nodular metastases smaller than 1 cm, after adjuvant chemotherapy, for near-surface lesions, and for lesions situated around the ligamentum teres. Abdominal CT scan with intravenous contrast infusion has good sensitivity (75% to 85%) and excellent specificity (85% to 97%) [16]. It allows 3-dimensional reconstruction, which helps to analyze the relationship between liver metastases and vasculo-biliary pedicles and facilitates calculation of the liver volume that will remain in place after resection. MRI also has very good sensitivity and specificity, is less invasive than CT scan, and uses low-toxicity contrast agents [16].

Hepatic biopsy

In the unusual situation of diagnostic uncertainty, a percutaneous biopsy may be necessary. However, a recent study [17] found needle-track deposits in 19% after biopsy of suspected colorectal liver metastases. This cannot be justified in patients with potentially resectable disease.

Intraoperative assessment

Several reports suggest that laparoscopic exploration, including laparoscopic ultrasound, can avoid an unnecessary laparotomy in approximately one third of patients considered resectable by preoperative evaluation [18].

During laparotomy, careful exploration of the abdominal cavity is performed. If lymph nodes or peritoneal deposits are found, specimens should be taken for frozen sections. The presence of metastatic lymph nodes in the porta hepatis or the celiac region worsens the prognosis. They should not be considered as an absolute contraindication to liver resection if they can be completely removed with a type I hepatectomy. Five-year recurrence-free survival has been reported in such cases. However, a type II hepatectomy should not be performed in the presence of metastatic nodes.

Intraoperative ultrasonography is a mandatory part of a planned hepatic metastasectomy because of its ability to detect small intraparenchymal lesions and thus modify the initially planned operation. Its sensitivity approaches 100%. Several studies have shown that intraoperative ultrasonography may give additional information in 30% to 89% of patients and change therapeutic plans in 10% to 42% [19]. It is invaluable for guidance of fine-needle biopsies and the precise mapping of the anatomical relationship between metastases and main hepatic vessels.

Following a complete preoperative assessment, only 10% to 15% of patients with liver metastases are candidates for surgical resection. New treatment modalities, including systemic or intra-arterial hepatic chemotherapy, biotherapies, portal vein embolization, radiofrequency ablation or cryotherapy, and staged hepatectomies, have substantially increased the number of patients amenable to resection.

Techniques

Types of surgery

Anatomically, the liver can be divided into eight segments (I to VIII). Each segment is vascularized by a portal pedicle. Liver resection can be divided into two groups: anatomical resections removing one or several segments, and atypical or wedge resections removing a portion of liver parenchyma surrounding a hepatic lesion. Resections removing three or more continuous segments are defined as major resections. Four types of anatomic liver resections are commonly performed: left lateral lobectomy (segments II, III); right hepatectomy (segments V, VI, VII, VIII); left hepatectomy (segments II, III, IV); and extended right hepatectomy, also called right lobectomy (segments IV, V, VI, VII, VIII). Other types of anatomical resections can be performed: extended left hepatectomy or left trisegmentectomy (segments II, III, IV, V, VIII); central hepatectomy (segments IV, V, VIII); or bisegmentectomies (V-VI, VII-VIII, VI-VII) [17,20,21].

Selecting the type of resection

The goal of oncological surgery for liver metastases is to remove all the metastatic sites with macroscopically free margins, ideally 1 cm. The extent of liver resection (anatomic/major versus nonanatomic/limited) is not by itself a prognostic factor [22]. The type of liver resection depends on the size, number, and location of the metastases, their relationship to main vascular and biliary pedicles, and the volume of liver parenchyma that can be left in place after surgery. Small metastases located near the liver capsule can be removed by wedge resections; larger lesions often require major resections.

In some cases the surgeon must choose between performing several wedge resections or a major liver resection that includes all deposits. The first solution preserves a larger portion of healthy liver parenchyma but increases the risk of postoperative hemorrhage and in some cases may increase the incidence of hepatic recurrence. On the other hand, a major liver resection allows for safer margin control and decreases the risk of postoperative hemorrhage on the liver cut surface. However, a larger portion of normal liver parenchyma is removed increasing the risk of postoperative hepatic failure. Theoretically, this also increases the risk of promoting tumor growth of dormant liver metastases by the same mechanisms involved in liver regeneration.

Lesions that have disappeared after neoadjuvant treatment

There is still uncertainty concerning the timing, type, and extent of resection needed after a complete clinical response, ie, when all or some of the liver metastases have disappeared after neoadjuvant chemotherapy. The major question for the surgeon is whether to resect the site in the liver that is corresponding to the metastasis that has become undetectable. This is particularly important when this scenario may allow a smaller resection with a lower risk than originally planned. In a recent study [23], we have shown that in 80% of cases (of liver metastases that are considered as disappeared on preoperative imaging techniques), microscopic cancer persists after disappearance of a liver metastasis, either by pre- or intraoperative imaging. This supports resection of all sites of initial metastatic disease. Finding the site of a metastasis that has become undetectable after preoperative chemotherapy can be a challenging technical problem. The surgeon is faced with the necessity to identify the precise site of the former metastasis and resect sufficient liver parenchyma to achieve an adequate margin, without the ability to palpate the tumor or rely on intraoperative ultrasound. Thus the inherent risk of neoadjuvant chemotherapy to render some patients marginally operable that presented initially with identifiable and resectable liver metastases. In patients deemed resectable, it is therefore paramount to include the hepatic surgeon in the clinical decision process before initiation of preoperative chemotherapy. Close imaging surveillance of the response to chemotherapy is necessary to make sure that surgical resection is performed before complete disappearance of the metastatic foci. This can only be accomplished by a multimodality team approach and will ensure the maximum oncologic benefit for the patient.

Timing of liver and intestinal surgery for synchronous metastases

Synchronous hepatic metastases are found in 15% to 20% of patients undergoing an operation for colorectal cancer [24]. Resection of primary tumor and liver metastases can be either synchronous or delayed. In most cases it seems preferable to delay the hepatic resection [25,26]. The abdominal wall incision is usually different for the colorectal procedure. The possibility of peritoneal contamination during bowel resection can favor the infection of a perihepatic or subphrenic fluid collection. Likewise, hemodynamic changes and portal hypertension subsequent to vascular clamping during liver resection can be detrimental to the viability of the bowel anastomosis. In a large multicentric study [26], the postoperative morbidity was significantly increased when bowel and liver resections were performed simultaneously (6.1% versus 2.4%). However, others have reported one-stage procedures without added morbidity and no difference in 5-year survival in selected cases [27,28]. The most common and safest approach is to remove simultaneously metastases if they require a minor hepatectomy and are accessible through the same incision. In all other cases, the liver resection is postponed and realized 2 to 4 months later. During this period, systemic chemotherapy can be administered.

Operative technique

Blood loss during liver resection constitutes the primary determinant and independent risk factor of postoperative outcome [29]. Refinements of vascular occlusion techniques, use of low central venous pressure anesthesia, and application of innovative technologies for parenchymal trans-section have significantly improved the safety of hepatic resection.

The most common approach to minimize blood loss is to perform the Pringle maneuver (interruption of vascular inflow by compression of the hepatoduodenal ligament). The use of hepatic pedicle clamping is efficient in hemorrhage control but induces ischemia and portal hypertension, which can be deleterious, especially in cases with simultaneous gastrointestinal surgical procedures. An alternative method involves unilobar vascular inflow control. Preservation of normal flow to the contralateral lobe reduces warm ischemia to zero and minimizes reperfusion injury.

The exposure of the liver to short duration of ischemia-reperfusion before resection, the so-called ischemic preconditioning, seems to protect the liver against subsequent prolonged ischemia. Clavien and colleagues [30] showed significantly reduced serum transaminase levels after ischemic preconditioning in a prospective randomized study of 100 patients undergoing liver resection. The multivariate analysis showed an increased benefit of ischemic preconditioning in younger patients, in patients with longer duration of inflow occlusion (up to 60 minutes), in patients with steatosis, and in cases of less then 50% resected liver volumes.

For complex hepatic resections, particularly central hepatectomies and en bloc resections of the inferior vena cava, total vascular exclusion is mandatory [31]. The principal advantage of this technique is the prevention of profuse hemorrhage or air embolism. Despite careful hemodynamic monitoring and fluid expansion, total vascular isolation is not tolerated in 10% to 15% of patients. The choice of the clamping method is based on the distance to main vascular pedicles, the quantity of liver parenchyma, and the expertise of the surgeon and the anesthesiologist. Vascular pedicles can either be divided in the liver during the transection of the parenchyma or in the porta hepatis during preliminary dissection.

The parenchymal trans-section may be done with Kelly forceps or using more refined techniques such as water-jet and ultrasonic dissection without any noticeable difference in perioperative bleeding or morbidity. Once located, vessels and bile ducts are controlled according to their size by metal clips, ligation, or staples. Hemostasis of the cut liver surface is secured either by suture ligation, application of fibrin tissue-adhesive sealant, or argon beam coagulation. Recent development of innovative devices includes the TissueLink dissecting sealer (TissueLink Medical Inc, Dover, NH) that combines saline and radiofrequency energy. With this technique, liver parenchyma is precoagulated and small vessels and bile ducts occluded by heat-induced collagen shrinking before transection. The subdiaphragmatic space is generally drained after major resections. However, drainage catheters for liver resection have not been validated in randomized trials [32].

Unlike other abdominal surgeries, laparoscopic liver resections have been slow to gain wide acceptance because of technical difficulties and considerations of oncologic adequacy. Recent reports have shown the feasibility of laparoscopic resection even for major hepatectomies [33,34]. A recent study of 37 patients subjected to laparoscopic hepatic resection for colorectal cancer metastases demonstrated very acceptable 3-year overall and disease-free survival rates of 87% and 51% respectively [35].

Outcomes

Postoperative complications

In-hospital mortality varies from 0% to 5% and is strongly influenced by perioperative blood loss, preoperative liver function, and extent of liver resection. Postoperative complications are observed in 13% to 39% of patients [26,36–38]. Morbidity after hepatic resection is usually a result of transient liver failure, hemorrhage, subphrenic abscesses, or biliary fistula (Table 1). The mean hospital stay after liver surgery averages 10 to 15 days in the absence of complication.

Long-term results

Liver resection of colorectal metastases is associated with 3-, 5-, and 10-year survival rates of around 40% to 74%, 25% to 58%, and 22% to 38%, respectively [26,38–45] (Table 2). Improvement in survival is due not only to refinements in surgical technique and perioperative management, but also to better selection of patients for resection based on prognostic factors.

Indicators of prognosis

To improve prognosis and assist in appropriate patient selection for surgery and for postoperative adjuvant treatment, numerous studies have

Table 1
Complications of liver resection

Liver-related complications	
Perihepatic fluid collection or abscess	5%–10%
Bile leak	3%
Liver failure	1%–5%
Hemorrhage	1%–2%
Infections	
Wound	1%–3%
Intra-abdominal sepsis	1%–3%
General complications	
Pleural effusion	2%–5%
Pneumonia	2%–5%
Deep vein thrombosis–pulmonary embolism	1%–2%
Cardiac failure, myocardial infarction	1%

Data from Refs. [26,36,37,40].

Table 2
Results of surgical resection of liver metastases from colorectal cancer

First author, year	N	Operative mortality, %	Post-operative morbidity	Survival 1 y, %	3 y, %	5 y, %	10 y, %
Nordlinge, 1987 [39]	80	5	13	—	40	25	—
Scheele, 1991 [38]	207	5	22	—	41	31	—
Doci, 1991 [36]	100	5	39	—	—	30	—
AFC[a], 1992 [26]	1818	2	24	—	41	26	—
Scheele, 1995 [40]	469	4	—	83	—	33	—
Jamison, 1997 [41]	280	4	—	84	—	27	—
Fong, 1999 [42]	1001	3	—	—	—	38	22
Minagawa, 2000 [43]	235	0	—	—	51	38	38
Tanaka, 2004 [44]	193	1	26	69	46	43	—
Pawlik[a], 2005 [45]	557	1	—	97	74	58	—

Abbreviation: –, data not available in the study.
[a] Multicenter trials.

looked at factors influencing survival. They are summarized in Table 3. The interval between colorectal and hepatic surgery, the number of hepatic tumors (usually $\geq$ 4), the size of the hepatic tumor (usually $\geq$ 5 cm), preoperative CEA level, and the stage of the primary colorectal cancer are considered the most important preoperative predictors of outcome. Patient sex, site of the primary tumor, and involvement of one or both lobes do not seem to influence outcome. The stage of the primary tumor is associated with 5-year survival rate: 70% for stage I or II compared with 33% in stage III colorectal cancers [26]. Many authors include factors such as surgical margin and hepatic lymph node involvement in their assessment of survival risks. In a retrospective study with over 1500 patients, 5-year survival was 30% when margin was superior to 1 cm, 15% when it was less than 1 cm, and 0% with a positive margin [26]. A free margin of at least 1 cm has been proposed as best practice to avoid local to recurrence but a recent multicenter study has shown that smaller margins do not adversely affect survival [26]. Based on these more recent results a predicted resection margin of less than 1 cm may not be a contraindication to curative resection. The importance of hepatic lymph node involvement has been recently investigated in a prospective study with 156 patients. Five-year survival in the lymph-node positive group was poor (5%) [46]. The type of resection does not seem to influence the prognosis provided that a clear margin is obtained. Blood transfusions have been reported to adversely affect outcome but this may reflect the surgical difficulties faced with large and numerous lesions.

Using uni- and multivariate analysis, simple prognostic scoring systems have been proposed to predict oncologic outcome in patients undergoing metastatic liver resections [42,47,48]. One of these scoring systems was developed from a retrospective series of 1568 patients with resected liver metastases [26]. Two- and 5-year survival rates were 64% and 28%,

Table 3
Predictive factors associated with tumor recurrence and survival following surgical resection of liver metastases

First author, year	No. of patients	Sex	Site of primary tumor	Type of resection	Pre-op CEA level	Disease-free interval	Age	Tumor size	Stage of the primary	Synchronous/ Metachroncus	Number of metastases	Tumor-free margin	Incomplete tumor removal	Lymph node metastases
Doci, 1991 [36]	100	no	no	no	no	—	no	—	yes	no	no	—	—	—
Scheele, 1995 [40]	469	no	no	yes	no	—	no	yes	yes	yes	no	yes	—	—
Nordlinger, 1996[a] [47]	1568	no	no	no	yes	yes	yes	yes	yes	yes	yes	yes	yes	—
Jamison, 1997 [41]	280	—	—	—	—	—	—	no	no	—	no	no	—	yes
Fong, 1999 [42]	1001	no	—	—	yes	yes	no	no	no	—	yes	—	—	—
Minagawa, 2000 [43]	235	no	no	no	no	no	no	no	yes	no	yes	No	—	yes
Tanaka, 2004 [44]	193	no	no	no	no	—	no	no	no	yes	yes	yes	—	—
Sasaki, 2005 [48]	103	no	no	no	yes	yes	no	no	no	—	yes	—	—	—
Pawlik, 2005[a] [45]	557	no	no	no	yes	no	no	yes	no	no	yes	yes	—	—

Abbreviations: no, not a prognostic factor; yes, prognostic factor; –, not tested.
[a] Multicenter trials.

respectively, and were affected by age, size of the largest metastasis, CEA level, stage of the primary tumor, disease-free interval, number of liver nodules, and resection margin greater or less than 1 cm. Assigning 1 point to each factor, the population was divided into three risk groups with 2-year survival rates as follows: 0–2 points = 79%, 3–4 points = 60%, 5–7 points = 43% [26].

Repeat liver resections

Despite hepatic resections with curative intent in well-selected patients, up to 60% subsequently develop recurrent liver metastases. Of these, approximately 20% to 30% present with recurrent colorectal liver metastases isolated to the liver and are potentially amenable to further hepatic resection. Postoperative mortality and morbidity do not differ from those reported after a first resection and the mean survival approaches 2 years. In a series of 146 patients with intrahepatic recurrence treated by repeat liver resection, the actuarial survival rates were 78% at 1 year, 30% at 3 years, 16% at 5 and 10 years, and thus comparable to the survival rates observed following primary liver resection [49]. A more recent comparative series showed a greater median blood loss during repeat resection (450 mL versus 350 mL) but very impressive actuarial 1-, 3-, and 5-year survival rates of 94%, 68%, and 44%, respectively, compared with 89.3%, 51.7%, and 29.5% following single hepatectomy [50]. Hepatic recurrences without extrahepatic relapse should therefore be regarded as oncologically similar to metastatic disease at initial presentation and resected whenever possible.

Summary

The field of surgery for liver metastases is evolving rapidly. The proportion of patients viewed as amenable to resection is increasing with surgeons becoming more aggressive and systemic therapy more effective. Resection should be considered in the absence of nonresectable extrahepatic disease, when all liver metastases can be resected with clear margins and more than 20% of healthy liver parenchyma remains. Following a complete preoperative work-up combining multiple imaging techniques, currently more than 20% of all patients are candidates for liver resection. This number is likely to increase with further refinement in surgical technique and systemic therapy. The choice between anatomical or wedge resection depends on the number and the location of the metastases. Surgical resection is associated with a very low mortality and an overall 5-year survival approaching 40%. Best candidates for resection are those with stage I or II colorectal cancer, less than 4 hepatic lesions and none greater than 5 cm in diameter, without evidence of extra-hepatic disease, a CEA level less than 5 ng/mL, and a disease-free interval of at least 2 years. Perioperative chemotherapy with or without biotherapies, in situ ablation techniques, portal vein embolization, and staged hepatectomy have extended the indications without lessening the results of liver resection for colorectal metastases.

References

[1] Fong Y, Kemeny N, Paty P, et al. Treatment of colorectal cancer: hepatic metastasis. Semin Surg Oncol 1996;12:219–52.
[2] Steele GJ, Ravikumar TS. Resection of hepatic metastases from colorectal metastases: biologic perspectives. Ann Surg 1989;210:127–38.
[3] Scheele J, Stangl R, Altendorf-Hofmann A. Hepatic metastases from colorectal carcinoma: impact of surgical resection on the natural history. Br J Surg 1990;77:1241–6.
[4] Adson MA, van Heerden JA, Adson MH, et al. Resection of hepatic metastases from colorectal cancer. Arch Surg 1984;119:647–51.
[5] Bilchik AJ, Postone G, Curley SA, et al. Neoadjuvant chemotherapy for metastatic colon cancer: a cautionary note. J Clin Oncol 2005;23:9073–8.
[6] Rubbia-Brandt L, Audard V, Sartoretti P, et al. Severe hepatic sinusoidal obstruction associated with oxaliplatin-based chemotherapy in patients with metastatic colorectal cancer. Ann Oncol 2004;15:460–6.
[7] Kooby DA, Fong Y, Suriawinata A, et al. Impact of steatosis on perioperative outcome following hepatic resection. J Gastrointest Surg 2003;7:1034–44.
[8] Fernandez FG, Ritter J, Goodwin JW, et al. Effect of steatohepatitis associated with irinotecan or oxaliplatin pretreatment on resectability of hepatic colorectal metastases. J Am Coll Surg 2005;200:845–53.
[9] Karoui M, Penna C, Amin-Hashem M, et al. Influence of preoperative chemotherapy on the risk of major hepatectomy for colorectal liver metastases. Ann Surg 2006;243:1–7.
[10] Vauthey JN, Pawlik TM, Ribero D, et al. Chemotherapy regimen predicts steatohepatitis and an increase in 90-day mortality after surgery for hepatic colorectal metastases. J Clin Oncol 2006;24:2065–72.
[11] Parikh AA, Gentner B, Wu TT, et al. Perioperative complications in patients undergoing major liver resection with or without neoadjuvant chemotherapy. J Gastrointest Surg 2003;7:1082–8.
[12] Aloia Aloia T, Sebagh M, Plasse M, et al. Liver histology and surgical outcomes after preoperative chemotherapy with fluorouracil plus oxaliplatin in colorectal cancer liver metastases. J Clin Oncol 2006;24:4983–90.
[13] Scholmerich J, Volk BA, Gerok W. Value and limitations of abdominal ultrasound in tumor staging—liver metastasis and lymphoma. Eur J Radiol 1987;7:243–5.
[14] Hagspiel KD, Neidl KF, Eichenberger AC, et al. Detection of liver metastases: comparison of superparamagnetic iron oxide-enhanced and unenhanced MR imaging at 1.5T with dynamic CT, intraoperative US and percutaneous US. Radiology 1995;196:471–8.
[15] Konopke R, Kersting S, Bergert H, et al. Contrast-enhanced ultrasonography to detect liver metastases: a prospective trial to compare transcutaneous unenhanced and contrast-enhanced ultrasonography in patients undergoing laparotomy. Int J Colorectal Dis 2007; 22:201–7.
[16] Zerhouni EA, Rutter C, Hamilton SR, et al. CT and MR imaging in the staging of colorectal carcinoma: report of the Radiology Diagnostic Oncology Group II. Radiology 1996;200: 443–51.
[17] Starzl TE, Iwatsuki S, Shaw B. Left hepatic trisegmentectomy. Surg Gynecol Obstet 1982; 155:21–7.
[18] Rahusen FD, Cuesta MA, Borgstein PJ, et al. Selection of patients for resection of colorectal metastases to the liver using diagnostic laparoscopy and laparoscopic ultrasonography. Ann Surg 1999;230:31–7.

[19] Bloed W, van Leeuwen MS, Borel Rinks IH. Role of intraoperative ultrasound of the liver with improved preoperative hepatic imaging. Eur J Surg 2000;166:691–5.
[20] Bismuth H, Houssin D, Castaing D. Major and minor segmentectomies "réglées" in liver surgery. World J Surg 1982;6:10–24.
[21] Starzl TE, Bell RH, Beart RW, et al. Hepatic trisegmentectomy and other liver resections. Surg Gynecol Obstet 1975;141:429–37.
[22] Kokudo N, Tada K, Seki M, et al. Anatomical major resections versus nonanatomical limited resections for liver metastases from colorectal carcinoma. Am J Surg 2001;181:153–9.
[23] Benoist S, Brouquet A, Penna C, et al. Complete response of colorectal liver metastases after chemotherapy: does it mean cure? J Clin Oncol 2006;24:3939–45.
[24] Bengtsson G, Carlsson G, Hafstrom L, et al. Natural history of patients with untreated liver metastases from colorectal cancer. Am J Surg 1981;141:586–9.
[25] Lambert LA, Colacchio TA, Barth RJ Jr. Interval hepatic resection of colorectal metastases improves patient selection. Arch Surg 2000;135:473–80.
[26] Nordlinger B, Jaeck D, Guiguet M, et al. Surgical resection of hepatic metastases. Multicentric retrospective study by the French Association of Surgery. In: Nordlinger B, Jaeck D, editors. Treatment of hepatic metastases of colorectal cancer. Paris: Springer-Verlag; 1992. p. 129–46.
[27] Tanaka K, Shimada H, Matsuo K, et al. Outcome after simultaneous colorectal and hepatic resection for colorectal cancer with synchronous metastases. Surgery 2004;136:650–9.
[28] Weber JC, Bachellier P, Oussoultzoglou E, et al. Simultaneous resection of colorectal primary tumour and synchronous liver metastases. Br J Surg 2003;90:956–62.
[29] Jarnagin WR, Gonen M, Fong Y, et al. Improvement in perioperative outcome after hepatic resection: analysis of 1,803 consecutive cases over the past decade. Ann Surg 2002;236:397–407.
[30] Clavien PA, Selzner M, Rudiger HA, et al. A prospective randomized study in 100 consecutive patients undergoing major liver resection with versus without ischemic preconditioning. Ann Surg 2003;238:843–52.
[31] Delva E, Camus Y, Nordlinger B, et al. Vascular occlusion for liver resection. Operative management and tolerance to hepatic ischemia: 142 cases. Ann Surg 1989;209:211–8.
[32] Belghiti J, Kabbej M, Sauvanet A, et al. Drainage after elective hepatic resection. A randomized trial. Ann Surg 1993;218:748–53.
[33] Gigot JF, Glineur D, Santiago Azagra J, et al. Laparoscopic liver resection for malignant liver tumors: preliminary results of a multicenter European study. Ann Surg 2002;236:753–62.
[34] Cherqui D, Husson E, Hammoud R, et al. Laparoscopic liver resections: a feasibility study in 30 patients. Ann Surg 2000;232:753–62.
[35] Vibert E, Pernicerni T, Levard H, et al. Laparoscopic liver resection. Br J Surg 2006;93:67–72.
[36] Doci R, German L, Bigmani P, et al. One hundred patients with hepatic metastases from colorectal cancer treated by resection: analysis of prognostic determinant. Br J Surg 1991;78:797–801.
[37] Fong Y, Cohen AM, Fortner JG, et al. Liver resection for colorectal metastases. J Clin Oncol 1997;15:938–46.
[38] Scheele J, Stangl R, Altendorf-Hofmann A, et al. Indicators of prognosis after hepatic resection for colorectal secondaries. Surgery 1991;110:13–29.
[39] Nordlinger B, Quilichini MA, Parc R, et al. Hepatic resection for colorectal liver metastases. Influence on survival of preoperative factors and surgery for recurrence in 80 patients. Ann Surg 1987;205:256–63.
[40] Scheele J, Stang R, Altendorf-Hofmann A, et al. Resection of colorectal liver metastases. World J Surg 1995;19:59–71.
[41] Jamison RL, Donohue JH, Nagorney DM, et al. Hepatic resections for metastatic colorectal cancer. Results in cure for some patients. Arch Surg 1997;132:505–11.

[42] Fong Y, Fortner J, Sun RL, et al. Clinical score for predicting recurrence after hepatic resection for metastatic colorectal cancer: analysis of 1001 consecutive cases. Ann Surg 1999;230: 309–18.
[43] Minagawa M, Makuuchi M, Torzilli G, et al. Extension of the frontiers of surgical indications in the treatment of liver metastases from colorectal cancer. Ann Surg 2000;231:487–99.
[44] Tanaka K, Shimada H, Ohta M, et al. Procedures of choice for resection of primary and recurrent liver metastases from colorectal câncer. World J Surg 2004;28:482–7.
[45] Pawlik T, Scoggins CR, Zorzi D, et al. Effect of surgical margin status on survival and site of recurrence after hepatic resection for colorectal metastases. Ann Surg 2005;241:715–24.
[46] Laurent C, Sa Cunha A, Rullier E, et al. Impact of microscopic hepatic lymph node involvement on survival after resection of colorectal liver metastases. J Am Coll Surg 2004;198: 884–91.
[47] Nordlinger B, Guiguet M, Vaillant JC, et al. Surgical resection of colorectal carcinoma metastases to the liver. A prognostic scoring system to improve case selection, based on 1568 patients. Cancer 1996;77:1254–62.
[48] Sasaki A, Iwashita Y, Shibata K, et al. Analysis of preoperative prognostic factors for long-term survival after hepatic resection of liver metastasis of colorectal carcinoma. J Gastrointest Surg 2005;9:374–80.
[49] Lange JF, Leese T, Castaing D, et al. Repeat hepatectomy for recurrent malignant tumors of the liver. Surg Gynecol Obstet 1989;169:119–26.
[50] Shaw IM, Rees M, Welsh FKS, et al. Repeat hepatic resection for recurrent colorectal liver metastases is associated with favourable long-term survival. Br J Surg 2006;93:457–64.

ELSEVIER
SAUNDERS

Surg Oncol Clin N Am
16 (2007) 507–523

SURGICAL
ONCOLOGY CLINICS
OF NORTH AMERICA

Hepatectomy for Colorectal Metastases in the Presence of Extrahepatic Disease

Daniel Jaeck, MD, PhD, FRCS*,
Elie Oussoultzoglou, MD, Edoardo Rosso, MD

Centre de Chirurgie Viscérale et de Transplantation, Hôpital de Hautepierre, Hôpitaux Universitaires de Strasbourg, Université Louis Pasteur, Avenue Molière, Strasbourg 67200, France

Liver resection is considered the standard treatment for colorectal liver metastases (CLM). Only 10% to 20% of patients who have hepatic CLM, however, are eligible for resection [1–3]. In recent years efforts have been made to improve the rate of resection for CLM [4–10]. Today the availability of more efficient chemotherapy, the innovation in surgical strategies (two-stage hepatectomy resection, portal vein embolization, radiofrequency ablation), and multimodality treatment approaches have increased the number of patients considered for liver resection and frequently include patients deemed unresectable not long ago [2–11]. As a result surgeons in many hepatobiliary centers are more likely to resect patients who have CLM in the presence of extrahepatic disease discovered during preoperative staging or during laparotomy. The adequacy of this approach remains a matter of debate. In the early 1990s the presence of abdominal extrahepatic disease at the time of hepatectomy was considered an absolute contraindication for liver resection, mainly because of low reported 5-year survival rates in these patients, ranging from 0% and 12% [1,12]. In this article the authors focus on hepatectomy for CLM in the presence of intra-abdominal extrahepatic disease. The results reported in the literature are reviewed, and the indications and contraindications for hepatectomy in patients who have CLM with extrahepatic disease are discussed in light of the available evidence.

* Corresponding author.
E-mail address: daniel.jaeck@chru-strasbourg.fr (D. Jaeck).

1055-3207/07/$ - see front matter © 2007 Elsevier Inc. All rights reserved.
doi:10.1016/j.soc.2007.04.010

Incidence and distribution of intra-abdominal extrahepatic disease

Intra-abdominal extrahepatic disease is defined as any metastasis outside the liver except for direct locoregional invasion of other structures by CLM (ie, diaphragmatic invasion). Intra-abdominal extrahepatic metastases include local recurrence of the primary tumor, visceral metastases (eg, adrenal glands, pancreas, ovary), abdominal wall metastases, and lymph node metastases (retroperitoneal and hepatic pedicle). Colorectal metastases have been described in all intra-abdominal and retroperitoneal organs. Only peritoneal carcinomatosis and hepatic pedicle lymph node metastases, however, are frequent occurrences. Peritoneal carcinomatosis is discovered in 7% to 20% of patients undergoing liver resection for CLM [1–3,13–15]. Microscopic or macroscopic hepatic pedicle lymph node metastases are detected in 3% to 33% of patients undergoing hepatic resection for CLM [1,2, 16–33]. All other metastatic sites, such as the spleen, the adrenal glands, the ovary, the brain, and the pancreas, are uncommon.

The concept of curative resection and the rationale for colorectal liver metastases resection in the presence of extrahepatic disease

Nearly 50% of all patients who undergo a potentially curative resection of colorectal cancer die from metastatic disease within 5 years after resection of the colorectal tumor. Most of the early deaths occur among patients presenting with more advanced disease [34]. The current definition of curative resection takes into consideration the macroscopic and microscopic status of the resection margins, the number and involvement of lymph nodes in the specimen, and the presence of any macroscopic residual disease. This definition does not include the presence or absence of minimal occult residual disease. Several recent studies have shown that micrometastases and circulating tumor cells in blood, lymph nodes, and bone marrow can be detected in 13% to 89% of patients subjected to a curative resection for colorectal cancer [34–38]. Even if the prognostic significance of minimal occult residual disease is not yet fully understood, this underscores the possibility that the conventional staging methods for colorectal cancer may be imprecise [34]. It is likely that in metastatic colorectal cancer an apparent complete surgical resection according to the traditional staging criteria is not equal to the eradication of all tumor cells present in the host.

What are the consequences for current surgical practice? With this premise in most cases surgical resection for metastatic colorectal cancer would represent a form of cytoreductive surgery, a necessary but not sufficient step in the curative multimodality treatment of these patients. Because of the presence of minimal occult disease, the authors surmise that in certain patients "curative" surgery for advanced locoregional colorectal cancer (disease confined to liver and primary site only) can be viewed as equivalent to "cytoreductive" surgery for metastatic disease extending beyond the liver (but limited to the abdominal cavity). This constitutes the authors' rationale for performing liver resection in selected patients who have extrahepatic intra-abdominal metastatic colorectal cancer.

Hepatectomy for colorectal liver metastases in the presence of peritoneal carcinomatosis

In contrast to lymphatic and hematogenous dissemination, colorectal peritoneal carcinomatosis should be regarded as a locoregional extension of the malignant process rather than a manifestation of systemic disease [14,15,39]. In fact, in 25% of the patients no other tumor localization can be found [15]. Moreover, it has been shown that colorectal peritoneal carcinomatosis is caused by either full-thickness invasion of the bowel wall by invasive cancer or by iatrogenic seeding during surgery [40]. Both are locoregional mechanisms of tumor dissemination. A combination of cytoreductive surgery and adjuvant hyperthermic intraperitoneal chemotherapy has been the most effective treatment, with reported 5-year survival rates ranging from 7% to 26% [41–43]. Most of the studies, however, either include only patients who have isolated colorectal peritoneal carcinomatosis or they do not separately analyze results after resection of liver metastases and peritoneal carcinomatosis.

In 2003 the Institute Gustave Roussy group reported their experience with intra-abdominal extrahepatic metastases [44]. Between January 1987 and January 2001, 111 patients who had CLM and intra-abdominal extrahepatic metastases underwent radical resection. The 5-year survival rate was 29%. In the multivariate analysis worst survival was associated with incomplete resection, more than five liver metastases, preoperative chemotherapy, or the discovery of intra-abdominal extrahepatic metastases at the time of laparotomy. In this analysis, however, different types of intra-abdominal extrahepatic metastases were lumped together.

Presently only two institutions have reported their experience in patients who have CLM and concomitant peritoneal carcinomatosis [13,39]. Carmignani and colleagues [39] reported a series of 27 patients who had synchronous colorectal peritoneal carcinomatosis and hematogenous metastasis from colorectal cancer. Of these, 20 patients presented with CLM and 14 were subjected to a curative resection. Median survival time after complete cytoreductive surgery was 20.6 months compared with only 9 months after incomplete cytoreductive surgery. Postoperative morbidity and mortality rates were 14.8% and 0%, respectively. Perioperative chemotherapy was administered in 17 of 27 patients. The investigators concluded that in young patients who had good performance status and who presented with colorectal peritoneal carcinomatosis and distant metastases (mostly liver), cytoreductive surgery with intra-peritoneal chemotherapy is beneficial.

In the second study Elias and colleagues [13] demonstrated 3-year overall and disease-free survival rates of 41.5% and 23%, respectively, among 24 patients who underwent simultaneous resection of CLM and peritoneal carcinomatosis with curative intent. Surgery was combined with intraperitoneal chemotherapy. The mortality rate was 4% and the morbidity rate was 58%. The investigators concluded that the indications for such extended operations should be limited to young patients who have a good performance status, a response to neoadjuvant chemotherapy, no more than two CLM, and a moderate volume of peritoneal carcinomatosis [13,45].

Both studies reported similar results from a well-selected population of patients and are the first to show the effectiveness of multimodality therapy in these patients [13,39]. They also report significant morbidity caused by the combination of intraperitoneal chemotherapy and extensive surgery necessary to obtain a complete cytoreduction. One has to consider the retrospective nature of these studies, the small number of patients, the varying degree of treatment protocols, and the lack of control groups, ie, systemic chemotherapy alone. Several questions remain unanswered: (1) Is intraperitoneal chemotherapy necessary for these patients? (2) How can morbidity be reduced? And (3) What is their quality of life after treatment?

By consensus evidence is not sufficient to declare resection of low-volume peritoneal carcinomatosis in patients who have colorectal cancer as standard therapy [46]. Furthermore, evidence is also insufficient to advocate simultaneous resection of CLM and peritoneal carcinomatosis outside clinical trials. More recent reports, however, demonstrate an advantage of such cytoreductive surgery compared with nonsurgical therapy in metastatic colorectal cancer [13,39,43,47]. In the absence of a proven survival benefit from nonsurgical therapy one is left with evidence suggesting a benefit for surgical cytoreduction with or without intraperitoneal chemotherapy in patients who have colorectal metastases to liver and peritoneal carcinomatosis [13,39,43,47]. These patients should be selected for age, good performance status, response to preoperative chemotherapy, low-volume disease, and the ability to perform complete cytoreductive surgery. This approach should only be contemplated by an experienced hepatobiliary treatment team facile in hepatobiliary surgery and intraperitoneal chemotherapy. For this reason it remains confined to specialized centers with multidisciplinary teams.

Hilar lymph node metastases

Definition and perioperative assessment

Involvement of regional lymph nodes represents locoregional spread from CLM and therefore is considered as lymphatic re-metastases from liver secondaries, not from the primary tumor [30,48,49]. These lymph node metastases can be microscopic or macroscopic in nature and are diagnosed preoperatively by imaging or are discovered at the time of laparotomy

[2,16,17,19,21,23–25,28–32]. Some investigators report that hepatic pedicle lymph node dissection should include a minimum of three to four lymph nodes to obtain reliable staging information [31,32]. A recent study examines the value of perioperative detection of hepatic pedicle lymph nodes by imaging or by intraoperative evaluation [33]. The investigators found only 1 patient who had hepatic pedicle lymph node metastases among 48 patients presenting with negative preoperative CT and PET scans. They concluded that routine sampling of hepatic pedicle lymph nodes is not helpful in patients who have no evidence of lymph node involvement on preoperative imaging. Routine perioperative lymph node assessment in patients who have CLM to guide operative decision-making therefore remains questionable.

Results of colorectal liver metastases resection in patients who have hepatic pedicle lymph node metastases

Currently major hepatic resection and extended lymphadenectomy constitutes the standard surgical approach for hilar cholangiocarcinomas or gallbladder cancer [50–53]. Selected patients who have hilar cholangiocarcinomas and locoregional metastatic peripancreatic lymph nodes may benefit from radical locoregional resection, including major hepatectomy and pancreaticoduodenectomy [54].Whether or not lymph node dissection benefits patients who have colorectal cancer liver metastases, however, is still a matter of debate. The prognostic significance of perihepatic lymph node involvement in colorectal cancer has been examined by several investigators (Table 1) [1,17,18,20,23,25–27,55]. Only two studies reported significant 5-year survival in patients who had perihepatic metastatic lymph node involvement [1,26]. Most did not show a significant survival benefit. Based on this evidence it was concluded that resection of metastatic hepatic pedicle lymph nodes does not improve the poor prognosis in these patients and therefore represents a contraindication for CLM resection [1,17,18,20,22,23,25,27,55–57].This conclusion, however, is based on retrospective studies with heterogeneous patient populations in which CLM were associated either with microscopic or macroscopic hepatic pedicle lymph node metastases or other extrahepatic metastases. Whether or not microscopic hepatic pedicle lymph node dissection improves survival is the subject of two recent prospective nonrandomized studies in patients presenting with CLM [30,32]. Laurent and colleagues [32] reported a 3-year survival rate of 27% in patients who had microscopically involved hepatic lymph nodes, whereas the authors' group evaluated prospectively whether resection of involved hepatic pedicle lymph node could improve the outcome in patients who have CLM [30]. The overall survival rate was significantly lower among patients who had lymph node metastases compared with those who did not, making lymph node involvement the most significant prognostic factor. The survival rate was significantly higher when lymph node involvement was limited to the hepatoduodenal ligament and

Table 1
Prognostic significance of hepatic pedicle lymph node involvement on overall survival

Reference	Number of patients	Number of patients who had hepatic pedicle lymph node involvement (%)	Hepatic pedicle lymph node involvement: 3-year survival rate (%) Yes	3-year survival rate (%) No	5-year survival rate (%) Yes	5-year survival rate (%) No
Ekberg et al 1986 [17]	31	8 (26)	—	—	0	18
Chang et al 1987 [18]	24	8 (33)	—	—	0	20
Nordlinger et al 1992 [1]	1256	100 (8)	12	44	12	28
Rosen et al 1992 [20]	40	9 (22)	11	54	0	37
Yasui and Kato 1993 [55]	52	7 (13)	—	—	0	31
Beckurts et al 1997 [23]	126	35 (28)	3	48	0	22
Iwatsuki et al 1999 [25]	305	9 (3)	11	50	0	33
Kokudo et al 1999 [27]	78	9 (12)	0	—	0	—
Nakamura et al 1999 [26]	43	7 (16)	—	—	42	43

the retropancreatic area (proximal, area 1) compared with patients who had lymph node involvement along the common hepatic artery and around the celiac axis (distal, area 2; Fig. 1). Specifically the 3-year survival rate in patients who had hepatoduodenal and retropancreatic lymph node metastases (proximal) was 38% compared with 0% survival rate at 1-year in patients who had common hepatic artery and celiac axis lymph node metastases (distal; Fig. 2). Although 3-year survival for patients who had no lymph node metastases was highest at 62%, the documented 38% 3-year survival rate for lymph node-positive patients was higher than expected (Figs. 2 and 3), particularly because it was achieved without increased mortality and morbidity. The authors' study also revealed several factors predicting hepatic pedicle lymph node metastases: (1) the presence of more than three liver metastases, (2) liver metastases located in segment 4 and/or segment 5, (3) the presence of a resectable peritoneal deposit, and (4) poorly differentiated histology of liver metastases [30].

Both prospective studies demonstrated substantial 3-year survival and low mortality and morbidity after resection of involved proximal lymph nodes in patients who had CLM. They stand in contrast to previously published outcomes for patients who had lymph node-positive CLM. It is

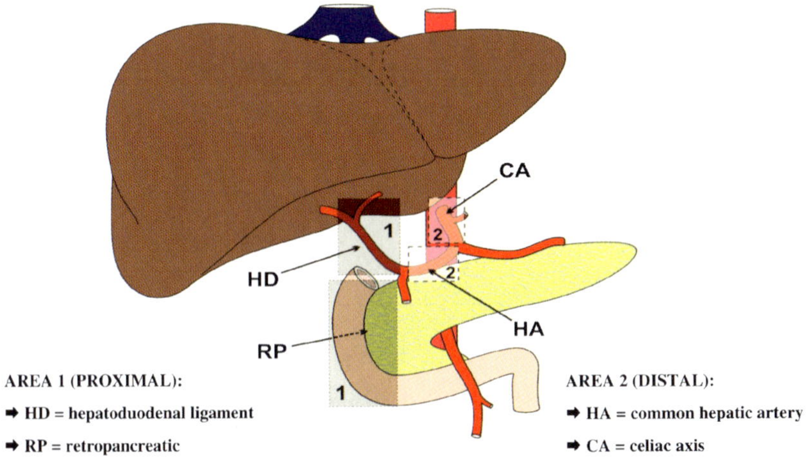

Fig. 1. Schematic representation of the main groups of hepatic pedicle lymph nodes subdivided into two areas. Area1 (proximal) includes the hepatoduodenal ligament and retropancreatic lymph nodes. Area 2 (distal) includes common hepatic artery and celiac axis lymph nodes.

important to point out that none of the patients in these two series had macroscopic lymph node metastases and that the data on chemotherapy treatments was inconsistent. The authors caution to extend the conclusion made from these two studies to patients who have macroscopic lymph node metastases detected by palpation or preoperative imaging. In the absence of perioperative suspicion of hepatic pedicle lymph nodes metastases, however, a lymphadenectomy at the time of CLM resection is recommended and may convey a survival benefit to those patients who have microscopic

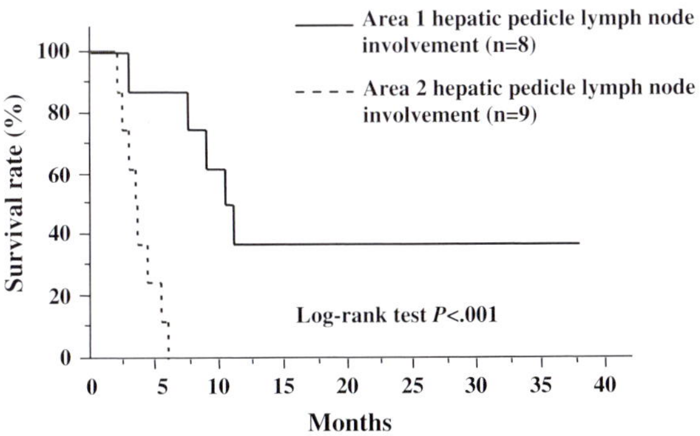

Fig. 2. Survival after hepatectomy for colorectal liver metastases in patients who have metastatic involvement of hepatic pedicle lymph nodes according to the involved area (area 1 proximal versus area 2 distal). The survival rate is significantly higher in patients who have area 1 hepatic pedicle lymph node involvement compared with area 2 hepatic pedicle lymph node involvement (3-year survival of 38% versus 1-year survival of 0%, respectively).

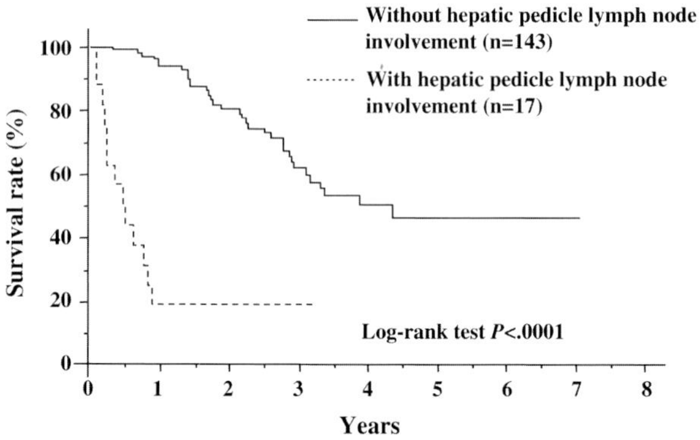

Fig. 3. Survival after hepatectomy for colorectal liver metastases according to status of hepatic pedicle lymph node involvement. The 3-year survival rates in patients with and without involvement of the hepatic pedicle lymph nodes were 19% versus 62%, respectively.

lymph nodes metastases. This recommendation is particularly relevant in high-risk patients who have more than three metastases, lesions located in segments 4 and 5, solitary resectable peritoneal deposit, and poorly differentiated liver metastases (Tables 2 and 3) [30].

Advantages and side effects of lymphadenectomy

Several hypothetical advantages of hepatic pedicle lymph node dissection in patients who have CLM can be discussed. First, the assessment of hepatic

Table 2
Univariate analysis of factors associated with hepatic pedicle lymph node involvement

Variables	With hepatic pedicle involvement (n = 17)	Without hepatic pedicle involvement (n = 143)	*P* value
Number of CLM			
1–3	5	91	.007
>3	12	52	
CLM location in segment 4 or 5			
Absent	3	78	.004
Present	14	65	
Differentiation grade of CLM			
Well-differentiated	1	31	.005
Moderately differentiated	7	85	
Poorly differentiated	9	27	
Resectable solitary peritoneal tumor			
Absent	10	130	.0002
Present	7	13	

Values are number of patients.

Abbreviation: CLM, colorectal liver metastases.

Data from Jaeck D, Nakano H, Bachellier P, et al. Significance of hepatic pedicle lymph node involvement in patients with colorectal liver metastases: a prospective study. Ann Surg Oncol 2002;9(5):430–8.

Table 3
Multivariate analysis of prognostic factors for overall survival

		95% confidence interval		
Variables	Relative risk	Lower	Upper	*P* value
Hepatic pedicle lymph node involvement present (versus absent)	15.1	6.5	34.9	<.0001
Resectable solitary peritoneal tumor present (versus absent)	3.5	1.6	7.5	.002
Number of CLM 4 or more (versus 1 to 3)	2.5	1.2	5.2	.014
Synchronous or metachronous CLM synchronous (versus metachronous)	1.9	1	3.4	.048
Distribution of liver metastases bilobar (versus unilobar)	1.3	1.6	3.1	.190

Abbreviation: CLM, colorectal liver metastases.

Data from Jaeck D, Nakano H, Bachellier P, et al. Significance of hepatic pedicle lymph node involvement in patients with colorectal liver metastases: a prospective study. Ann Surg Oncol 2002;9(5):430–8.

pedicle lymph nodes in patients who have CLM provides a more accurate prognosis, and second, it provides a more appropriate selection for postoperative chemotherapy, particularly in the absence of other prognostic factors [1,17,18,20,22,23,25–27,30–33,58]. Third, a complete lymph node dissection can prevent obstructive jaundice in cases of disease progression in the hepatic pedicle lymph nodes [27,59]. Fourth, in the context of multi-institutional clinical trials, the assessment of hepatic pedicle lymph nodes allows for a more accurate stratification. Fifth, and most important, in selected patients presenting with limited hepatic pedicle lymph node metastases, resection can result in long-term survival [26,30–32].The role of lymph node dissection, however, remains unresolved in patients who have macroscopic involvement. In this setting, a planned biliary drainage (hepaticojejunostomy) or a gastrojejunostomy may be indicated to prevent biliary and gastric obstructions.

Adverse effects related to hepatic lymph node dissection such as vascular or biliary injuries are described. Severe adhesions around the hepatoduodenal ligament can lead to difficulties in subsequent laparotomies for recurrent liver metastases and may compromise the safety of a scheduled repeat hepatectomy. If one plans a two-stage hepatectomy, it is therefore recommended to postpone the hepatic pedicle lymph node dissection until the time of the second-stage hepatectomy [4,7,60]. Hepatic lymph node dissection can be performed safely without mortality and with low morbidity [22,30–33].

Radical versus "cherry picking" lymphadenectomy

Most surgeons would not embrace routine radical hepatic pedicle lymph node dissection in patients presenting with CLM. Few surgeons prefer lymph node sampling. Currently the recommendation for routine radical lymphadenectomy is not evidence-based. The major argument in favor of a routine radical lymphadenectomy, however, is to avoid tumor spread from primary or secondary liver tumors through lymphatic pathways that include: (1) drainage through the hepatic hilum and retropancreatic area and along the common hepatic artery and celiac axis; (2) along the falciform ligament, the diaphragm, and the mediastinum; (3) through the esophageal hiatus, the caval foramen, and the mediastinum; (4) through the lesser omentum and the paracardiac area; and (5) along the phrenic artery and celiac axis [48,61,62]. A correlation between tumor location in particular liver segments and the pathways of lymph node dissemination has been demonstrated with the possibility of skip metastases and overlapping of metastatic routes [30,48]. In the authors' prospective study, six of nine patients presented with "skip" metastases to area 2 lymph nodes, ie, area 1 lymph nodes were not involved [30].

Radical lymph node dissection may also prevent late complication by gross lymphatic tumor burden. As reported by Kokudo and colleagues [27] recurrent lymph node metastases occurred in three of nine patients after previous sampling for positive hepatic pedicle lymph nodes. These three patients developed biliary obstruction by metastatic lymphadenopathy and required drainage procedures. Others have reported similar findings with recurrent lymph node metastases [55].

Routine regional lymphadenectomy has become standard treatment in patients who have extrahepatic bile duct cancers [50–54] and may show benefit in selected patients who have pancreatic cancer [63]. For patients who have CLM, however, the benefit of a radical lymphadenectomy remains controversial. Currently the lack of clinical trial results calls into question routine radical hepatic pedicle lymphadenectomy during surgical management of CLM [46]. Particularly the presence of positive lymph nodes in the para-aortic or celiac zone is associated with poor prognosis [30–32]. These conclusions, however, are based on series of patients who did not receive optimal chemotherapy before or after surgical resection. The concept begs to be tested in clinical trials on optimally selected patients subjected to complete cytoreductive surgery and treated with current, more effective systemic therapy.

Extrahepatic and extra-abdominal metastases

Colorectal pulmonary metastases

Among patients who undergo curative resection for colorectal cancer 10% to 20% develop pulmonary metastases. Of those, 10% show isolated pulmonary lesions [64–66]. Five-year survival rates ranging from 24% to 62% after resection of synchronous or metachronous pulmonary metastases from colorectal cancer have been reported [67–72]. Such favorable outcomes were achieved with simultaneous or sequential resections and after repeat pulmonary metastasectomies [73,74]. Whether to resect lung and liver metastases simultaneously or sequentially should be decided case by case. Simultaneous resections are appropriate for healthy patients who have limited hepatic or pulmonary disease mainly located in the right lung. On the other hand, sequential resection is the preferable approach for complex cases. The most difficult metastasis should be resected first, independent of its location in the lung or liver. Several helpful prognostic factors have been reported. They include Union of International Cancer Committees stage of the primary tumor, pre-thoracotomy carcinoembryonic antigen level, mediastinal lymph node status, number and size of lung metastases, laterality of lung metastases, intraoperative blood transfusion requirement, resection margins, type of lung resection, and disease-free interval after colorectal tumor resection [67–72,74,75]. The role and timing of chemotherapy are still a matter of debate.

Other rare extrahepatic extrapulmonary colorectal metastases

Long-term survival following resection of rare extrahepatic metastases (adrenal, spleen, brain) has been demonstrated, mostly from case reports or short series [76–79]. Long-term outcome after resection of metastases in these locations is unknown. Liver resection in the presence of these rare extrahepatic metastases should only be attempted if a complete resection of all known disease can be achieved.

Neoadjuvant and adjuvant therapy

Neoadjuvant chemotherapy

There is evidence from two systematic reviews that chemotherapy for metastatic colorectal cancer can improve survival and should be considered in all patients not suitable for surgery [80,81].The timing and indications for chemotherapy in patients who have colorectal hepatic and extrahepatic metastases, however, are less well established. These patients can be divided into those presenting with initially resectable disease and those with unresectable lesions.

The role of preoperative chemotherapy in patients who have resectable metastases is still under investigation. The results of a prospective trial conducted by the European Organisation for Research and Treatment of Cancer group should be known by the end of 2007.

There is evidence to support the use of neoadjuvant chemotherapy in patients who have initially unresectable CLM. In fact, up to 16% of the patients became resectable after traditional chemotherapy, and this rate can be improved by using newer chemotherapeutic regimens and targeted therapies [82–84]. Long-term survival in these patients has been reported [85].

Two of the major concerns regarding chemotherapy are the deleterious effects on liver function, particularly by Oxaliplatin-based regimens, and the risk for progression. Systemic chemotherapy in patients who have peritoneal carcinomatosis is not effective because of its limited penetration and diffusion into the peritoneal cavity. The current evidence suggests that cytoreductive surgery combined with perioperative intraperitoneal chemotherapy may improve overall survival in these patients.

Adjuvant chemotherapy

The aim of the postoperative adjuvant therapy is to reduce the risk for recurrence. It is an accepted treatment component in patients who received preoperative chemotherapy to make their CLM resectable. Moreover, even for patients who have initially resectable disease, adjuvant chemotherapy may be of benefit because of the high failure rate observed with surgery alone. Despite these theoretic advantages, most trials evaluating adjuvant chemotherapy have been inconclusive. Currently the National Surgical Adjuvant Breast and Bowel Project C0-9 randomized trial is evaluating the benefit of combining regional hepatic arterial chemotherapy and systemic chemotherapy after CLM resection and ablation.

The significance of the location of extrahepatic metastases

In a prospective study, Elias and colleagues [86] recently challenged the assumption that the site of extrahepatic colorectal metastases influences the prognosis in patients undergoing metastasectomy. Eighty-four patients were treated with hepatectomy for CLM combined with resection of miscellaneous extrahepatic metastases. The overall 5-year survival rate was 32%. In a multivariate analysis, the investigators showed that the total number of metastases (intrahepatic or extrahepatic) had a greater prognostic impact than the location of the metastases. These results seem to suggest that once a colorectal primary tumor becomes metastatic, the prognosis is determined by the ability to achieve optimal cytoreduction and not by the disease localization. Based on these findings patients who have CLM may be divided into two main groups: (1) the surgical group, including all patients in whom known metastatic disease can be completely resected irrespective of location, and (2) the palliative group, in which surgical cytoreduction cannot be achieved. Based on this premise extensive and aggressive surgical therapy should be offered to patients in whom a complete metastasectomy is likely to be successful.

Summary

In selected patients who have CLM and limited extrahepatic disease, either hepatic pedicle lymph node involvement or resectable carcinomatosis, complete metastasectomy and lymphadenectomy can be recommended based on its curative potential and low associated mortality and morbidity. Patients who have poor prognostic factors may still benefit from hepatic resection. The authors recommend to proceed with surgery when it is technically feasible according to the rules of safe hepatic surgery and to use adjuvant chemotherapy to consolidate the benefit of a potentially curative resection.

References

[1] Nordlinger B, Jaeck D, Guiguet M, et al. Surgical resection of hepatic metastases. Multicentric retrospective study by the French Association of Surgery. In: Nordlinger B, Jaeck D, editors. Treatment of hepatic metastases of colorectal cancer. Paris: Springer-Verlag; 1992. p. 129–46.

[2] Minagawa M, Makuuchi M, Torzilli G, et al. Extension of the frontiers of surgical indications in the treatment of liver metastases from colorectal cancer: long-term results. Ann Surg 2000;231(4):487–99.

[3] Fong Y, Fortner J, Sun RL, et al. Clinical score for predicting recurrence after hepatic resection for metastatic colorectal cancer: analysis of 1001 consecutive cases. Ann Surg 1999; 230(3):309–18 [discussion: 318–21].

[4] Adam R, Laurent A, Azoulay D, et al. Two-stage hepatectomy: a planned strategy to treat irresectable liver tumors. Ann Surg 2000;232(6):777–85.

[5] Jaeck D. The significance of hepatic pedicle lymph nodes metastases in surgical management of colorectal liver metastases and of other liver malignancies. Ann Surg Oncol 2003;10(9): 1007–11.

[6] Adam R, Pascal G, Azoulay D, et al. Liver resection for colorectal metastases: the third hepatectomy. Ann Surg 2003;238(6):871–83 [discussion: 883–4].

[7] Jaeck D, Oussoultzoglou E, Rosso E, et al. A two-stage hepatectomy procedure combined with portal vein embolization to achieve curative resection for initially unresectable multiple and bilobar colorectal liver metastases. Ann Surg 2004;240(6):1037–49 [discussion: 1049–51].

[8] Abdalla EK, Vauthey JN, Ellis LM, et al. Recurrence and outcomes following hepatic resection, radiofrequency ablation, and combined resection/ablation for colorectal liver metastases. Ann Surg 2004;239(6):818–25 [discussion: 825–7].

[9] Adam R, Delvart V, Pascal G, et al. Rescue surgery for unresectable colorectal liver metastases downstaged by chemotherapy: a model to predict long-term survival. Ann Surg 2004; 240(4):644–57 [discussion: 657–8].

[10] Simmonds PC, Primrose JN, Colquitt JL, et al. Surgical resection of hepatic metastases from colorectal cancer: a systematic review of published studies. Br J Cancer 2006;94(7):982–99.

[11] Leonard GD, Brenner B, Kemeny NE. Neoadjuvant chemotherapy before liver resection for patients with unresectable liver metastases from colorectal carcinoma. J Clin Oncol 2005; 23(9):2038–48.

[12] Hughes KS, Simon R, Songhorabodi S, et al. Resection of the liver for colorectal carcinoma metastases: a multi-institutional study of patterns of recurrence. Surgery 1986;100(2):278–84.

[13] Elias D, Benizri E, Pocard M, et al. Treatment of synchronous peritoneal carcinomatosis and liver metastases from colorectal cancer. Eur J Surg Oncol 2006;32(6):632–6.

[14] Sugarbaker PH. Colorectal carcinomatosis: a new oncologic frontier. Curr Opin Oncol 2005; 17(4):397–9.

[15] Koppe MJ, Boerman OC, Oyen WJ, et al. Peritoneal carcinomatosis of colorectal origin: incidence and current treatment strategies. Ann Surg 2006;243(2):212–22.

[16] Fortner JG, Silva JS, Golbey RB, et al. Multivariate analysis of a personal series of 247 consecutive patients with liver metastases from colorectal cancer. I. Treatment by hepatic resection. Ann Surg 1984;199(3):306–16.

[17] Ekberg H, Tranberg KG, Andersson R, et al. Determinants of survival in liver resection for colorectal secondaries. Br J Surg 1986;73(9):727–31.
[18] Chang AE, Schneider PD, Sugarbaker PH, et al. A prospective randomized trial of regional versus systemic continuous 5-fluorodeoxyuridine chemotherapy in the treatment of colorectal liver metastases. Ann Surg 1987;206(6):685–93.
[19] Hughes KS, Rosenstein RB, Songhorabodi S, et al. Resection of the liver for colorectal carcinoma metastases. A multi-institutional study of long-term survivors. Dis Colon Rectum 1988;31(1):1–4.
[20] Rosen CB, Nagorney DM, Taswell HF, et al. Perioperative blood transfusion and determinants of survival after liver resection for metastatic colorectal carcinoma. Ann Surg 1992; 216(4):493–504 [discussion: 504–5].
[21] Gayowski TJ, Iwatsuki S, Madariaga JR, et al. Experience in hepatic resection for metastatic colorectal cancer: analysis of clinical and pathologic risk factors. Surgery 1994;116(4): 703–10 [discussion 710–1].
[22] Elias D, Saric J, Jaeck D, et al. Prospective study of microscopic lymph node involvement of the hepatic pedicle during curative hepatectomy for colorectal metastases. Br J Surg 1996; 83(7):942–5.
[23] Beckurts KT, Holscher AH, Thorban S, et al. Significance of lymph node involvement at the hepatic hilum in the resection of colorectal liver metastases. Br J Surg 1997;84(8):1081–4.
[24] Ohlsson B, Stenram U, Tranberg KG. Resection of colorectal liver metastases: 25-year experience. World J Surg 1998;22(3):268–76 [discussion 276–7].
[25] Iwatsuki S, Dvorchik I, Madariaga JR, et al. Hepatic resection for metastatic colorectal adenocarcinoma: a proposal of a prognostic scoring system. J Am Coll Surg 1999;189(3):291–9.
[26] Nakamura S, Suzuki S, Konno H. Resection of hepatic metastases of colorectal carcinoma: 20 years' experience. J Hepatobiliary Pancreat Surg 1999;6(1):16–22.
[27] Kokudo N, Sato T, Seki M, et al. Hepatic lymph node involvement in resected cases of liver metastases from colorectal cancer. Dis Colon Rectum 1999;42(10):1285–90 [discussion: 1290–1].
[28] Harms J, Obst T, Thorban S, et al. The role of surgery in the treatment of liver metastases for colorectal cancer patients. Hepatogastroenterology 1999;46(28):2321–8.
[29] Ambiru S, Miyazaki M, Isono T, et al. Hepatic resection for colorectal metastases: analysis of prognostic factors. Dis Colon Rectum 1999;42(5):632–9.
[30] Jaeck D, Nakano H, Bachellier P, et al. Significance of hepatic pedicle lymph node involvement in patients with colorectal liver metastases: a prospective study. Ann Surg Oncol 2002; 9(5):430–8.
[31] Ercolani G, Grazi GL, Ravaioli M, et al. The role of lymphadenectomy for liver tumors: further considerations on the appropriateness of treatment strategy. Ann Surg 2004;239(2): 202–9.
[32] Laurent C, Sa Cunha A, Rullier E, et al. Impact of microscopic hepatic lymph node involvement on survival after resection of colorectal liver metastasis. J Am Coll Surg 2004;198(6): 884–91.
[33] Grobmyer SR, Wang L, Gonen M, et al. Perihepatic lymph node assessment in patients undergoing partial hepatectomy for malignancy. Ann Surg 2006;244(2):260–4.
[34] Tsavellas G, Patel H, Allen-Mersh TG. Detection and clinical significance of occult tumour cells in colorectal cancer. Br J Surg 2001;88(10):1307–20.
[35] Lindemann F, Schlimok G, Dirschedl P, et al. Prognostic significance of micrometastatic tumour cells in bone marrow of colorectal cancer patients. Lancet 1992;340(8821):685–9.
[36] Oberg A, Stenling R, Tavelin B, et al. Are lymph node micrometastases of any clinical significance in Dukes Stages A and B colorectal cancer? Dis Colon Rectum 1998;41(10): 1244–9.
[37] Weitz J, Koch M, Kienle P, et al. Detection of hematogenic tumor cell dissemination in patients undergoing resection of liver metastases of colorectal cancer. Ann Surg 2000; 232(1):66–72.

[38] Koch M, Kienle P, Hinz U, et al. Detection of hematogenous tumor cell dissemination predicts tumor relapse in patients undergoing surgical resection of colorectal liver metastases. Ann Surg 2005;241(2):199–205.
[39] Carmignani CP, Ortega-Perez G, Sugarbaker PH. The management of synchronous peritoneal carcinomatosis and hematogenous metastasis from colorectal cancer. Eur J Surg Oncol 2004;30(4):391–8.
[40] Moran BJ, Cecil TD. The etiology, clinical presentation, and management of pseudomyxoma peritonei. Surg Oncol Clin N Am 2003;12(3):585–603.
[41] Elias D, Blot F, El Otmany A, et al. Curative treatment of peritoneal carcinomatosis arising from colorectal cancer by complete resection and intraperitoneal chemotherapy. Cancer 2001;92(1):71–6.
[42] Verwaal VJ, van Ruth S, de Bree E, et al. Randomized trial of cytoreduction and hyperthermic intraperitoneal chemotherapy versus systemic chemotherapy and palliative surgery in patients with peritoneal carcinomatosis of colorectal cancer. J Clin Oncol 2003;21(20): 3737–43.
[43] Yan TD, Black D, Savady R, et al. Systematic review on the efficacy of cytoreductive surgery combined with perioperative intraperitoneal chemotherapy for peritoneal carcinomatosis from colorectal carcinoma. J Clin Oncol 2006;24(24):4011–9.
[44] Elias D, Ouellet JF, Bellon N, et al. Extrahepatic disease does not contraindicate hepatectomy for colorectal liver metastases. Br J Surg 2003;90(5):567–74.
[45] Begossi G, Gonzalez-Moreno S, Ortega-Perez G, et al. Cytoreduction and intraperitoneal chemotherapy for the management of peritoneal carcinomatosis, sarcomatosis and mesothelioma. Eur J Surg Oncol 2002;28(1):80–7.
[46] Abdalla EK, Adam R, Bilchik AJ, et al. Improving resectablety of hepatic colorectal metastases: expert consensus statement. Ann Surg Oncol 2006;13(10):1271–80.
[47] Jayne DG, Fook S, Loi C, et al. Peritoneal carcinomatosis from colorectal cancer. Br J Surg 2002;89(12):1545–50.
[48] August DA, Sugarbaker PH, Schneider PD. Lymphatic dissemination of hepatic metastases. Implications for the follow-up and treatment of patients with colorectal cancer. Cancer 1985; 55(7):1490–4.
[49] August DA. Metastases from metastasis. N J Med 1996;93(7):10.
[50] Kitagawa Y, Nagino M, Kamiya J, et al. Lymph node metastasis from hilar cholangiocarcinoma: audit of 110 patients who underwent regional and paraaortic node dissection. Ann Surg 2001;233(3):385–92.
[51] Lin HT, Liu GJ, Wu D, et al. Metastasis of primary gallbladder carcinoma in lymph node and liver. World J Gastroenterol 2005;11(5):748–51.
[52] Shimada H, Endo I, Togo S, et al. The role of lymph node dissection in the treatment of gallbladder carcinoma. Cancer 1997;79(5):892–9.
[53] Kondo S, Nimura Y, Hayakawa N, et al. Regional and para-aortic lymphadenectomy in radical surgery for advanced gallbladder carcinoma. Br J Surg 2000;87(4):418–22.
[54] Araida T, Yoshikawa T, Azuma T, et al. Indications for pancreatoduodenectomy in patients undergoing lymphadenectomy for advanced gallbladder carcinoma. J Hepatobiliary Pancreat Surg 2004;11(1):45–9.
[55] Yasui K, Kato T. A significance and indication of anatomical major hepatic resection of the liver metastases from colorectal cancer [in Japanese]. Shoukaki Geka 1993;16: 1693–9.
[56] Nakamura S, Yokoi Y, Suzuki S, et al. Results of extensive surgery for liver metastases in colorectal carcinoma. Br J Surg 1992;79(1):35–8.
[57] Holm A, Bradley E, Aldrete JS. Hepatic resection of metastasis from colorectal carcinoma. Morbidity, mortality, and pattern of recurrence. Ann Surg 1989;209(4): 428–34.
[58] Elias DM, Ouellet JF. Incidence, distribution, and significance of hilar lymph node metastases in hepatic colorectal metastases. Surg Oncol Clin N Am 2003;12(1):221–9.

[59] Ishizaki N, Hamada N, Kadono J, et al. Obstructive jaundice caused by lymphatic remetastasis from the hepatic metastasis of rectosigmoid cancer. J Hepatobiliary Pancreat Surg 2001;8(5):469–72.
[60] Jaeck D, Bachellier P, Nakano H, et al. One- or two-stage hepatectomy combined with portal vein embolization for initially nonresectable colorectal liver metastases. Am J Surg 2003; 185(3):221–9.
[61] Trutmann M, Sasse D. The lymphatics of the liver. Anat Embryol (Berl) 1994;190(3):201–9.
[62] Ito M, Mishima Y, Sato T. An anatomical study of the lymphatic drainage of the gallbladder. Surg Radiol Anat 1991;13(2):89–104.
[63] Sierzega M, Popiela T, Kulig J, et al. The ratio of metastatic/resected lymph nodes is an independent prognostic factor in patients with node-positive pancreatic head cancer. Pancreas 2006;33(3):240–5.
[64] Brister SJ, de Varennes B, Gordon PH, et al. Contemporary operative management of pulmonary metastases of colorectal origin. Dis Colon Rectum 1988;31(10):786–92.
[65] McCormack PM, Burt ME, Bains MS, et al. Lung resection for colorectal metastases. 10-year results. Arch Surg 1992;127(12):1403–6.
[66] Shirouzu K, Isomoto H, Hayashi A, et al. Surgical treatment for patients with pulmonary metastases after resection of primary colorectal carcinoma. Cancer 1995;76(3):393–8.
[67] Inoue M, Ohta M, Iuchi K, et al. Benefits of surgery for patients with pulmonary metastases from colorectal carcinoma. Ann Thorac Surg 2004;78(1):238–44.
[68] Lee WS, Yun SH, Chun HK, et al. Pulmonary resection for metastases from colorectal cancer: prognostic factors and survival. Int J Colorectal Dis 2006 [Epub ahead of print].
[69] Saito Y, Omiya H, Kohno K, et al. Pulmonary metastasectomy for 165 patients with colorectal carcinoma: a prognostic assessment. J Thorac Cardiovasc Surg 2002;124(5):1007–13.
[70] Watanabe I, Arai T, Ono M, et al. Prognostic factors in resection of pulmonary metastasis from colorectal cancer. Br J Surg 2003;90(11):1436–40.
[71] Yedibela S, Klein P, Feuchter K, et al. Surgical management of pulmonary metastases from colorectal cancer in 153 patients. Ann Surg Oncol 2006;13(11):1538–44.
[72] Pfannschmidt J, Klode J, Muley T, et al. Nodal involvement at the time of pulmonary metastasectomy: experiences in 245 patients. Ann Thorac Surg 2006;81(2):448–54.
[73] Mineo TC, Ambrogi V, Tonini G, et al. Long-term results after resection of simultaneous and sequential lung and liver metastases from colorectal carcinoma. J Am Coll Surg 2003; 197(3):386–91.
[74] Ogata Y, Matono K, Hayashi A, et al. Repeat pulmonary resection for isolated recurrent lung metastases yields results comparable to those after first pulmonary resection in colorectal cancer. World J Surg 2005;29(3):363–8.
[75] Ercan S, Nichols FC 3rd, Trastek VF, et al. Prognostic significance of lymph node metastasis found during pulmonary metastasectomy for extrapulmonary carcinoma. Ann Thorac Surg 2004;77(5):1786–91.
[76] Murakami S, Terakado M, Hashimoto T, et al. Adrenal metastasis from rectal cancer: report of a case. Surg Today 2003;33(2):126–30.
[77] Cante D, Girelli G, La Porta MR, et al. Late brain metastases from colorectal cancer: a case report and review of the literature. Tumori 2005;91(3):280–2.
[78] Kanjo T, Albertini M, Weber S. Long-term disease-free survival after adrenalectomy for isolated colorectal metastases. Asian J Surg 2006;29(4):291–3.
[79] Gencosmanoglu R, Aker F, Kir G, et al. Isolated metachronous splenic metastasis from synchronous colon cancer. World J Surg Oncol 2006 [Epub ahead of print].
[80] Simmonds PC. Palliative chemotherapy for advanced colorectal cancer: systematic review and meta-analysis. Colorectal Cancer Collaborative Group. BMJ 2000;321(7260):531–5.
[81] Jonker DJ, Maroun JA, Kocha W. Survival benefit of chemotherapy in metastatic colorectal cancer: a meta-analysis of randomized controlled trials. Br J Cancer 2000;82(11):1789–94.
[82] Adam R, Avisar E, Ariche A, et al. Five-year survival following hepatic resection after neoadjuvant therapy for nonresectable colorectal. Ann Surg Oncol 2001;8(4):347–53.

[83] Bismuth H, Adam R, Levi F, et al. Resection of nonresectable liver metastases from colorectal cancer after neoadjuvant chemotherapy. Ann Surg 1996;224(4):509–20 [discussion: 520–2].
[84] Adam R, Huguet E, Azoulay D, et al. Hepatic resection after down-staging of unresectable hepatic colorectal metastases. Surg Oncol Clin N Am 2003;12(1):211–20.
[85] Tanaka K, Adam R, Shimada H, et al. Role of neoadjuvant chemotherapy in the treatment of multiple colorectal metastases to the liver. Br J Surg 2003;90(8):963–9.
[86] Elias D, Liberale G, Vernerey D, et al. Hepatic and extrahepatic colorectal metastases: when resectable, their localization does not matter, but their total number has a prognostic effect. Ann Surg Oncol 2005;12(11):900–9.

ELSEVIER
SAUNDERS

Surg Oncol Clin N Am
16 (2007) 525–536

SURGICAL
ONCOLOGY CLINICS
OF NORTH AMERICA

Two-stage Hepatectomy Approach for Initially Unresectable Colorectal Hepatic Metastases

René Adam, MD, PhD[a,d,e,*], Rafael Miller, MD[a,b], Marcos Pitombo, MD[a], Dennis A. Wicherts, MD[a,c], Robbert J. de Haas, MD[a,c], Georgia Bitsakou, MD[a], Thomas Aloia, MD[a]

[a] *AP-HP Hôpital Paul Brousse, Centre Hépato-Biliaire, 12 Avenue Paul Vaillant Couturier, 94804 Villejuif, France*

[b] *Department of Surgery, Kaplan Medical Center Rehovot and Hebrew University Jerusalem, Israel*

[c] *Department of Surgery, University Medical Center Utrecht, Utrecht, The Netherlands*

[d] *Université Paris-Sud, UMR-S 785, Villejuif, France*

[e] *Inserm, Unité 785, Villejuif, France*

Liver metastases occur in up to 70% of patients with colorectal cancer (CRC). Approximately 25% of these patients present with synchronous metastases and an additional 35% to 45% develop metachronous metastases during the course of their disease, mostly within 3 years [1,2]. The median survival time for untreated patients ranges from 6 to 18 months with no documented long-term survival [3].

In the last decade, survival of these patients has been improved by modern chemotherapy protocols, including oxaliplatin and irinotecan, with reports of median survival reaching 20 months or more and objective tumor regression in 40% to 50% of patients [4–6].

Hepatic resection is currently accepted as the most effective and only curative treatment for colorectal liver metastases. Improvements in preoperative assessment, operative technique, and perioperative care have resulted in better short-term outcomes, with experienced centers reporting in-hospital mortality rates of <5%, even after major resections. In the current

* Corresponding author. AP-HP Hôpital Paul Brousse, Centre Hépato-Biliaire, 12 Avenue Paul Vaillant Couturier, 94804 Villejuif, France.

E-mail address: rene.adam@pbr.aphp.fr (R. Adam).

1055-3207/07/$ - see front matter © 2007 Elsevier Inc. All rights reserved.
doi:10.1016/j.soc.2007.04.016

literature, 5-year survival for patients undergoing complete (R0) resections ranges from 15% to 67%, with median 5-year survival rates of 30% to 35% [7]. However, most patients with CRC liver metastases have unresectable disease at the time of diagnosis. Based on the current resectability criteria, only 15% to 25% of newly diagnosed patients are eligible for surgery [8].

Given the number of patients who present with extensive bilateral and multinodular metastatic liver disease and who are deemed unresectable and thus incurable by standard criteria, surgeons and oncologists have been searching for ways to make resection possible and improve outcome in these patients.

Management of unresectable disease

The main cause of unresectability of CRC liver metastases is the inability to remove all the malignant lesions with safe margins while retaining at least 30% of the functional liver parenchyma, thus avoiding severe postoperative liver insufficiency. Many studies have recently revisited other relative contraindications to surgery, such as wide extent of disease, unfavorable location, large number and size of metastases, inability to achieve adequate resection margins, and presence of extrahepatic disease. Some reports suggest that bilobar distribution of metastases per se has no impact on overall survival [9,10]. The same conclusions have been drawn regarding number and size of metastases and resection margins [8–12]. However, each of these factors plays an important role in surgical decision-making, since such factors determine both feasibility of resection and long-term results.

Currently, a multidisciplinary approach is the best strategy for addressing the problem of unresectability. Some of the important components of this approach include assessment of liver function [13], modern imaging to characterize the malignant lesions and define their relationship to important anatomical structures, precise volumetric studies of the liver, advanced surgical techniques and approaches, portal vein embolization, multistage hepatectomy, local ablation therapy, and perioperative systemic and hepatic artery chemotherapy [14]. This armamentarium, when used in close cooperation within a multidisciplinary team for each individual case, increases the number of patients amenable to potentially curative operative treatment, even if they are initially considered unresectable.

Surgical strategies in unresectable disease

The management of unresectable colorectal liver metastases represents an example of a clinical task for which a multidisciplinary approach is fundamentally the only successful strategy. The goal is to achieve resection in a maximum number of patients by means of careful selection, optimal radiological assessment, downstaging chemotherapy, and application of specific surgical techniques.

The main cause of the unresectability of CRC liver metastases is technical. That is, resection under oncological principles would sacrifice >70% of functional liver parenchyma with consequent risk of postoperative liver failure. In our experience, multinodularity represents the most frequent cause of technical unresectability.

Based on our clinical experience, we have developed a set of strategic surgical approaches to multinodular metastatic disease, depending on the number, size, and location of the metastases (Fig. 1) [15]:

Patients with unilobar multinodular metastases requiring resection of more than 60% to 70% of total functional liver parenchyma should undergo preoperative portal vein embolization (PVE). Following PVE, the induced hypertrophy of the future remnant liver allows for a curative resection while minimizing the risk of postoperative hepatic insufficiency (see *a* in Fig. 1).

Patients with bilobar multinodular metastases for which a planned resection would leave no more than three nodules and none larger than 3 cm in the remnant liver are preferentially treated with a multimodal approach consisting of hepatic resection combined with radiofrequency ablation or cryotherapy of the unresectable nodules (see *b* in Fig. 1).

Patients with bilobar multinodular metastases for which a planned resection would leave more than three nodules or any nodule larger than 3 cm in the remnant liver are candidates for a two-stage hepatectomy (see *c* in Fig. 1).

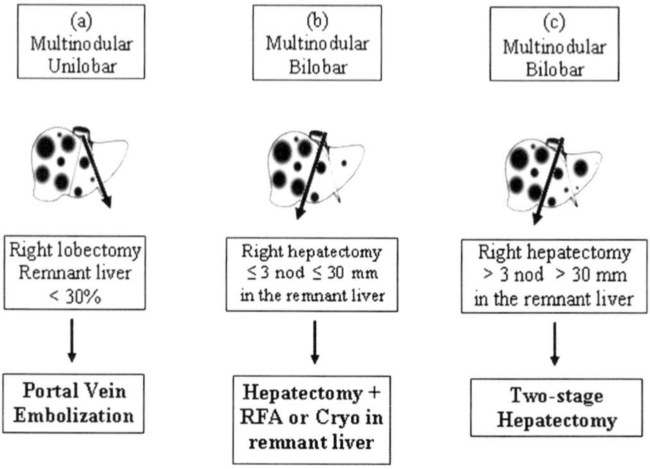

Fig. 1. Strategy for primary unresectable multinodular liver metastases depending on size, number, and location of metastases. Cryo, cryotherapy; nod, nodules; RFA, radiofrequency ablation. (*Adapted from* Adam R, Lucidi V, Bismuth H. Hepatic colorectal metastases: methods of improving resectability. Surg Clin North Am 2004;84:667; with permission.)

Two-stage hepatectomy

Principles

Two-stage hepatectomy has been developed as a surgical strategy for extremely difficult cases of bilobar multinodular metastatic liver disease. This strategy is applied when it is impossible to resect all malignant lesions in a single procedure.

The main principle of this approach is sequential resection by a two-staged hepatectomy. Its goal is to achieve a complete metastasectomy in those cases in which a complete resection with a single hepatectomy would have left a remnant postresection liver too small for patient survival.

The objective of the first hepatectomy is to render the final future remnant liver free of disease so that the second liver resection becomes feasible and potentially curative. The success of this method relies on liver regeneration between the two interventions, allowing the second hepatectomy to be performed with a lower risk of serious complications, including postoperative liver failure.

The decision to embark on a two-stage strategy is taken either before or during the first hepatectomy. This approach, in principle, excludes repeat hepatectomy for recurrent disease and is different from the "two-step liver surgery" described previously, in which microwave ablation of lesions (but not resection) in the less-involved hemiliver combined with portal vein ligation of the contralateral lobe precedes a second operation for resection of the more extensively involved lobe [16].

The role of preoperative chemotherapy

Patients selected for treatment by two-stage hepatectomy are highly selected and usually beyond the common accepted indications for treatment of liver metastases. They typically have multinodular bilobar liver metastases not amenable to standard curative resection or other nonresectional surgical therapies. In our reports on this technique [17] and in reports by Jaeck and colleagues [18], all patients had bilobar disease with a median lesion size of 37 mm and 60 mm, respectively, and a median number of seven metastases (range: 2–23). Shimada and colleagues [19] applied two-stage hepatectomy only to patients with more than five liver lesions. In our updated data (R. Adam unpublished data, 2007), all patients had on average nine bilobar metastases with a mean size of 42 mm for the largest lesion.

Because of the extent and perceived unresectability of the metastatic disease in patients considered for the two-stage approach, most are treated with chemotherapy before resection. We have previously reported on 1104 patients treated with preoperative chemotherapy for CRC liver metastases thought unresectable at initial presentation [20]. Multinodularity or extrahepatic disease was the main cause of initial unresectability. Chemotherapy consisted of oxaliplatin- and irinotecan-based chronomodulated regimens. After an average of 10 courses of chemotherapy, 13% of the patients (n=138) demonstrated an adequate response and underwent hepatic resection, 75% of which were major hepatectomies and 93% considered potentially curative. Overall survival was 33% at 5 years and 23% at 10 years and disease-free survival was 17% at 10 years, despite high recurrence rates of 80% after a mean follow-up of 49 months. This study established the concept of "downstaging" by preoperative chemotherapy in patients with initially unresectable CRC liver metastases. Subsequently, we were able to show that the response to preoperative chemotherapy in these patients is a critical determinant of postresection outcome [21]. In a retrospective analysis of 131 consecutive patients treated with metastasectomy after preoperative chemotherapy, tumor progression during chemotherapy was associated with poor outcome, almost equal to that observed in nonresected patients with 5-year overall survival of only 8%. Conversely, patients who stabilized or showed objective responses clearly benefited from resection with overall 5-year survival rates of 30% and 37%, respectively.

Likewise, in the series of two-stage hepatectomies reported by Jaeck and colleagues [18], stabilization of the malignant process was observed in at least 27 of the 33 patients after preoperative chemotherapy. In our first report on two-staged hepatectomy, all but 1 of 13 patients received preoperative chemotherapy with 6 patients showing partial response [17]. An updated report showed no evidence of disease progression before surgery in 26 of 30 patients treated with preoperative chemotherapy. These results underscore the importance of a multimodality approach in patients eligible for a two-stage hepatectomy.

The role of chemotherapy between the two hepatectomies in a two-stage approach still has to be clarified. Its effectiveness with regard to survival, perioperative morbidity, and mortality has not yet been elucidated. The rationale behind systemic or local chemotherapy treatment between hepatectomies is to halt tumor progression, as growth factors involved in the hypertrophy of the remnant liver have been shown to stimulate tumor growth after resection [22,23] and portal vein embolization [24]. Conversely, chemotherapy may also inhibit crucial liver regeneration after the first operation and thus jeopardize the ability to perform the second-stage operation [17].

Despite these caveats, we generally treat these patients with chemotherapy between liver resections, beginning with the same protocol that was used before the first hepatectomy. We prefer to delay chemotherapy administration for 3 to 4 weeks after the first hepatectomy to allow for maximal early liver regeneration, while minimizing the chance for tumor progression. In the current update of our series, 24 patients out of 31 received on average 4.5 cycles of chemotherapy between the two hepatectomies. Only 1 patient had evidence of disease progression before the second-stage operation.

In summary, preoperative chemotherapy plays an indispensable role in the concept of two-stage hepatectomy for CRC liver metastases, both in enabling resection by appropriate "downstaging" in many patients and by assisting in the selection of those patients most likely to benefit from resection.

Technical aspects: which side first?

Two-stage hepatectomies can be done in several ways. One approach begins with the resection of metastases located in the right liver. In this scenario, several large lesions or multiple smaller metastases occupy the right liver whereas tumor burden in the left liver is much less extensive (Fig. 2) [18]. Performing a right hepatectomy first allows removal of the main tumor burden. Subsequent resection of the remaining left-sided metastases is delayed until the left-liver sufficiently regenerates. This approach involves a more extensive first operation, resulting in a more difficult dissection at the second stage due to adhesions of the cut liver surface to the diaphragm and right colon. More importantly, this approach exposes the remaining liver metastases to high levels of growth factors, with the potential for the left-liver metastases to grow more quickly than the nontumoral hepatic parenchyma.

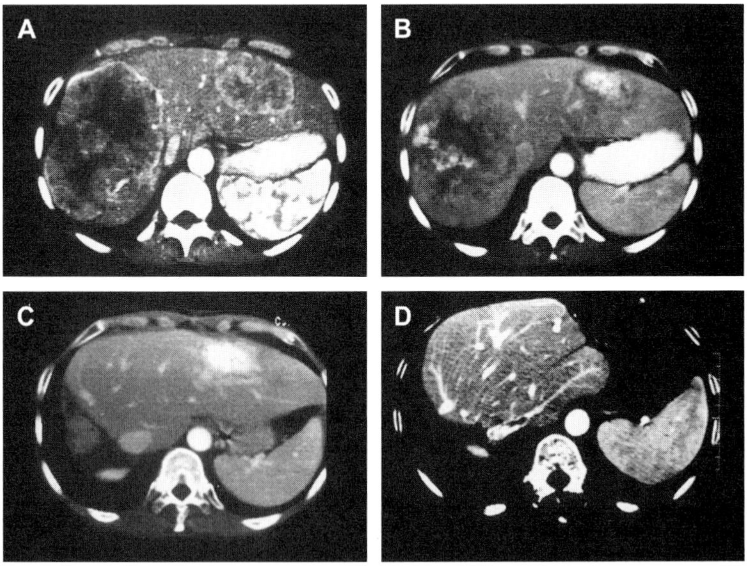

Fig. 2. Comparative abdominal CT of a patient treated by preoperative chemotherapy and two-stage hepatectomy. (*A*) Before chemotherapy. (*B*) Just before first-stage hepatectomy. (*C*) After the first stage (right hepatectomy). (*D*) After the second stage (left lobectomy). Only segments 1 and 4 remain. (*From* Adam R, Laurent A, Azoulay D, et al. Two-stage hepatectomy: a planned strategy to treat irresectable liver tumors. Ann Surg 2000;232:781; with permission.)

A different approach combines the first-stage resection of the left-sided metastases with a right PVE. Following left-liver regeneration, the second-stage operation achieves complete tumor "clearance" by resection of the right hemiliver [18,25]. This approach has the advantage of limiting the extent of dissection near the hepatic pedicle at the first stage, facilitating the second-stage resection. However, this procedure is only applicable for a small tumor burden of the left liver with limited first-stage resection to leave a sufficient future liver remnant.

This latter strategy was routinely used in the series reported by Jaeck and colleagues [18]. The first stage included a nonanatomical resection of three or fewer left-sided liver metastases with or without local ablation of additional metastases. Right PVE was performed shortly after the first hepatectomy by means of interventional radiology. After sufficient left-sided liver regeneration, a major right hepatectomy was performed, completing the removal of all metastatic nodules. Our preference is to embolize the right portal vein at the time of the first hepatectomy by a combination of right portal ligature and absolute alcohol injection. This prevents (1) backflow of alcohol into the common and left portal vein and (2) cavernous transformation of the ligated portal system [26].

In our review of 31 patients selected for a two-stage hepatectomy, 23 patients (74%) underwent a left-sided resection in the first stage. In 20 of these patients, right PVE was added. In 8 patients (26%), the first stage consisted of a right-sided hepatectomy. Operations on most of these patients took place during the initial study period when we chose to resect first the largest area of tumor burden, most often in the right lobe. A comparison of both operative strategies demonstrated no statistically significant differences in complication rates, operative times, or amount of blood loss.

Our initial concept for two-staged hepatectomies was based on the general oncological principle of removing as much malignant disease as possible at the first-stage procedure. Since in most patients the majority of the tumor burden is located in the right liver, the first-stage procedure usually required a right hepatectomy. However, this also meant that the future liver remnant—usually the left lobe—was subjected to growth stimulation after right PVE while still harboring tumor tissue. With increased experience and the realization that PVE-induced liver regeneration can lead to preferential tumor proliferation [24], our approach changed to first clearing the future liver remnant from all metastatic disease before subjecting it to the hypertrophic stimulus of contralateral PVE. Since the future remnant liver in almost all cases represents the left lobe of the liver, we now perform a partial hepatectomy for complete metastasectomy of the left lobe first. Local ablation is used only when resection alone does not allow complete tumor clearance without jeopardizing the integrity of the future liver remnant. In the same setting, the right portal vein is embolized to stimulate hypertrophy of the left lobe in anticipation of a second-stage right hepatectomy. This is currently our preferred approach for two-staged hepatectomies for CRC metastases.

When the clinical situation does not permit this strategy, it is advisable to select the site where the resection appears technically most challenging for the first-stage operation. In practice, two-stage hepatectomy should be tailored to the distribution of tumor burden in each patient.

In summary, we propose the following decision guidelines for two-stage hepatectomies:

Do not leave tumor in the future remnant liver at the first operation.

If resection alone cannot remove all the metastases from the future remnant liver, use local nonresectional techniques (eg, radiofrequency ablation) for tumor destruction to avoid tumor progression while the remnant liver hypertrophies.

At the first operation, avoid dissection of the hepatic pedicle and mobilization of the liver lobe that is to be resected at the second stage.

Portal vein embolization

PVE should be considered if there is a risk of insufficient remnant liver volume after the second operation. In patients with a liver compromised by high-dose chemotherapy, a larger residual volume of up to 40% may be required [27]. The optimal time interval necessary to induce maximum hypertrophy after PVE has not been established. De Baere and colleagues [28] have reported that 29 of their 31 patients reached adequate hypertrophy in 4 to 5 weeks after embolization. The embolization procedure itself does not add significant morbidity and may itself provide a 5-year survival benefit [29]. Published series report a 46% to 100% use of PVE in two-stage hepatectomies [17–19]. In 2004, Shimada and colleagues [19] described their surgical management for multiple bilobar hepatic metastases in 12 patients treated by two-stage hepatectomy. In 10 of these patients (83%), PVE was used in combination with resection at the first stage. Jaeck and colleagues [18] used the procedure in all patients subjected to two-stage resections. In our series, 23 of 31 patients (74%) underwent PVE.

Surgical and oncologic outcomes

Success rates of the two-stage approach depend on careful patient selection and judicious use of preoperative chemotherapy. PVE and chemotherapy after the first operation may further increase the completion rate of two-stage hepatectomies. The second (curative) hepatectomy should only be performed after reassessment of liver volume by imaging to exclude disease progression and confirm a sufficiently large liver remnant.

Recent studies have reported a completion rate for the second stage of 76% to 100% using this highly selective approach (Table 1) [17–19,25,30]. In our experience, 31 of 45 patients (69%) scheduled to undergo a two-staged hepatectomy were able to complete the treatment. Considering the extent of hepatic metastatic disease in these patients, published surgical

Table 1
Reported outcomes following two-stage hepatectomy for colorectal cancer liver metastases

Investigator	Total no. of patients	No. of two-stage completed patients	Success rate (%)	Mortality rate (%)	Morbidity rate (%)	Survival: Median (mo)	Survival: 3 years	Survival: 5 years
Adam, 2000 [17]	16	13	81	15[a]	45[a]	31	35	NA
Jaeck, 2004 [18]	33	25	76	0	56[a]	NA	54	NA
Shimada, 2004 [19]	12	12	100	0	NA	NA	NA	NA
Togo, 2005 [28]	11	11	100	0	18[a]	18	45	NA
Present series (2007)[b]	45	31	69	6.5[a]	48[a]	35	47	28

Abbreviation: NA, not available.
[a] After second operation.
[b] Unpublished data.

and oncologic outcomes are very encouraging (see Table 1). Shimada and colleagues [19] reported a mean survival time of 25.5 months after two-stage hepatectomy for CRC metastases with a median follow-up period of 36.2 months (range: 1–134 months). The cumulative 5-year survival for all the patients with five or more metastases was 40.2% [19]. Jaeck and colleagues [18] reported a 3-year survival rate of 54.4% with a median follow-up interval of 12 months (range: 4–76 months). Sixteen patients (64%) developed recurrences. There were no postoperative deaths and morbidity rates were 15.1% after the first-stage hepatectomy and 56.0% after the second-stage hepatectomy. The investigators attributed their favorable results to careful patient selection, a "test of time" of 2 to 3 months before resection, and the use of systemic chemotherapy between the two surgical stages to control residual disease.

Togo and colleagues [30] reported on 11 patients treated with a two-stage approach and found a 3-year survival rate of 45% with a median survival of 18 months. Liver recurrences occurred in 6 patients (55%). This group had no operative mortality and only two cases of complications after the second procedure. These two studies demonstrate the higher morbidity rates associated with the second-stage procedure, but mortality rates are low and similar to those observed with single-stage procedures. Our own study included 31 patients who completed all phases of the planned treatment. Actuarial 3-year and 5-year overall survivals were 47% and 28%, respectively, with median survival of 35 months at a mean follow-up of 34 (± 29) months. Fifteen patients (48.4%) experienced liver recurrences. Of these, 7 underwent an additional liver resection and 1 patient had two additional resections for recurrent liver metastases after two-stage hepatectomy. Twelve patients (39%)

are alive at last follow-up and 5 of them are free of disease. Fourteen patients (45%) have developed extrahepatic recurrence, predominantly in the lung. The general complication rate was 6.5% for the first and 22.6% for the second operation. The rate of liver-specific complications, such as perihepatic collections, ascites, and liver insufficiency, was 12.9% and 48.4% for the first- and second-stage, respectively. We observed two deaths within 60 days after the second operation for a mortality rate of 6.5%. Operative time, vascular clamping time, intraoperative blood loss, and length of hospital stay were each greater in the second stage than in the first, indicating the second operation as more complex than the first.

Summary

Two-stage hepatectomy is an infrequently used, but important and potentially curative surgical strategy for highly selected CRC patients with multinodular bilobar liver metastases. Systemic chemotherapy given in close collaboration with medical oncologists in a multidisciplinary setting is an integral part of this treatment strategy. Despite its complexity, two-stage hepatectomies can be successful in 70% to 100% of patients. Those who complete the treatment experience a durable benefit with 3-year survivals above 35%. Morbidity rates are high, particularly after the second-stage hepatectomy, but mortality is relatively low.

Major improvements in chemotherapy response rates, the ability to safely perform radical multistage hepatectomies and the dismal prognosis of unresected patients with extensive hepatic-only metastases warrant an aggressive oncosurgical strategy in all patients with CRC liver metastases. For selected patients who respond to systemic chemotherapy and can sustain extensive surgical procedures, two-stage hepatectomy may provide a chance at long-term disease-free and overall survival.

References

[1] Bengston G, Carlsson G, Hafström L, et al. Natural history of patients with untreated liver metastases from colorectal cancer. Am J Surg 1981;141:586–9.

[2] Jaeck D, Bachellier P, Guiguet M, et al. Long-term survival following resection of colorectal metastases. Br J Surg 1997;84:977–80.

[3] Wagner JS, Adson MA, Van Heerden JA, et al. The natural history of hepatic metastases from colorectal cancer. Ann Surg 1984;199:502–8.

[4] de Gramont A, Figer A, Seymour M, et al. Leucovorin and fluorouracil with or without oxaliplatin as first-line treatment in advanced colorectal cancer. J Clin Oncol 2000; 18:2938–47.

[5] Douillard JY, Cunningham D, Roth AD, et al. Irinotecan combined with fluorouracil compared with fluorouracil alone as first-line treatment for metastatic colorectal cancer: a multicentre randomized trial. Lancet 2000;355:1041–7.

[6] Saltz LB, Cox JV, Blanke C, et al. Irinotecan plus fluorouracil and leucovorin for metastatic colorectal cancer. Irinotecan Study Group. N Engl J Med 2000;343:905–14.
[7] Simmonds PC, Primrose JN, Colquitt JL, et al. Surgical resection of hepatic metastases from colorectal cancer: a systematic review of published studies. Br J Cancer 2006;94:982–99.
[8] Minagawa M, Makuuchi M, Torzilli G, et al. Extension of the frontiers of surgical treatment of liver metastases from colorectal cancer: long-term results. Ann Surg 2000;231: 487–99.
[9] Nordlinger B, Guiguet M, Vaillant JC, et al. Surgical resection of colorectal cacinoma metastases to the liver. A prognostic scoring system to improve case selection, based on 1568 patients. Association Francaise de Chirurgie. Cancer 1996;77:1253–62.
[10] Scheele J, Stangl R, Altendorf-Hofman A, et al. Indicators of prognosis after hepatic resection for colorectal secondaries. Surgery 1991;110:13–29.
[11] Elias D, Cavalcanti A, Sabourin JC, et al. Resection of liver metastases from colorectal cancer: the real impact of surgical margin. Eur J Surg Oncol 1998;24:174–9.
[12] Kokudo N, Miki Y, Sugai S, et al. Genetic and histological assessment of surgical margins in resected liver metastases from colorectal carcinoma: minimum surgical margins for successful resection. Arch Surg 2002;137:833–40.
[13] Yamanaka N, Okamoto E, Kuwata E, et al. A multiple regression equation for prediction of posthepatectomy liver failure. Ann Surg 1984;200:658–63.
[14] Shimada H, Tanaka K, Matsua K, et al. Treatment for multiple bilobar liver metastases of colorectal cancer. Langenbecks Arch Surg 2006;391:130–42.
[15] Adam R, Lucidi V, Bismuth H. Hepatic colorectal metastases: methods of improving resectability. Surg Clin North Am 2004;84:659–71.
[16] Lygidakis NJ, Singh G, Bardaxoglou E, et al. Two-stage liver surgery for advanced liver metastases synchronous with colorectal tumor. Hepatogastroenterology 2004;51:413–8.
[17] Adam R, Laurent A, Azoulay D, et al. Two-stage hepatectomy: a planed strategy to treat irresectable liver tumors. Ann surg 2000;232:777–85.
[18] Jaeck D, Oussoultzoglou E, Rosso E, et al. A two-stage hepatectomy procedure combined with portal vein embolization to achieve curative resection for initially unresectable multiple and bilobar colorectal liver metastases. Ann Surg 2004;240:1037–51.
[19] Shimada H, Tanaka K, Masui H, et al. Results of surgical treatment for multiple (≥5 nodules) bi-lobar hepatic metastases from colorectal cancer. Langenbecks Arch Surg 2004;389: 114–21.
[20] Adam R, Delvart V, Pascal G, et al. Rescue surgery for unresectable colorectal metastases downstaged by chemotherapy. Ann Surg 2004;240:644–58.
[21] Adam R, Pascal G, Castaing D, et al. Tumor progression while on chemotherapy: a contraindication to liver resection for multiple colorectal metastases? Ann Surg 2004;240(6): 1052–61 [discussion: 1061–4].
[22] Slooter GD, Marquet RJ, Jeekel J, et al. Tumor growth stimulation after partial hepatectomy can be reduced by treatment with tumor necrosis factor alpha. Br J Surg 1995;82: 129–32.
[23] Picardo A, Karpoff HM, Ng B, et al. Partial hepatectomy accelerates local tumor growth: potential role of cytokine activation. Surgery 1998;124:57–64.
[24] Elias D, de Baere T, Roche A, et al. During liver regeneration following right portal embolization the growth rate of liver metastases is more rapid than that of the liver parenchyma. Br J Surg 1999;86:784–8.
[25] Garcea G, Polemonivi N, O'Leary E, et al. Two-stage liver resection and chemotherapy for bilobar colorectal liver metastases. Eur J Surg Oncol 2004;30:759–64.
[26] Azoulay D, Castaing D, Krissat J, et al. Percutaneous portal vein embolization increases the feasibility and safety of major liver resection for hepatocellular carcinoma in injured liver. Ann Surg 2000;232(5):665–72.
[27] Fusai G, Davidson BR. Strategies to increase the resectability of liver metastases from colorectal cancer. Dig Surg 2003;20:481–96.

[28] De Baere T, Roche A, Elias D, et al. Preoperative portal vein embolization for extension of hepatectomy indications. Hepatology 1996;24:1386–91.
[29] Elias D, Ouellet JF, de Baere T, et al. Preoperative selective portal vein embolization before hepatectomy: long-term results and impact on survival. Surgery 2002;131:294–9.
[30] Togo S, Nagano Y, Masui H, et al. Two-stage hepatectomy for multiple bilobular liver metastases from colorectal cancer. Hepatogastroenterology 2005;52:913–9.

ELSEVIER
SAUNDERS

Surg Oncol Clin N Am
16 (2007) 537–556

SURGICAL
ONCOLOGY CLINICS
OF NORTH AMERICA

The Role of Chemotherapy in the Curative Treatment of Patients with Liver Metastases from Colorectal Cancer

Lawrence Leichman, MD, FACP

Aptium Oncology, Comprehensive Cancer at Desert Regional Medical Center, 1180 N. Indian Canyon Drive, Suite E218, Palm Springs, CA 92264, USA

New therapeutic paradigms for the treatment of colorectal liver metastases (CRLM) have brought medical and surgical oncologists into new, complex, and largely uncharted territory. Already in many centers the shift in approach from considering these patients as candidates for palliative treatment to candidates for potentially curative treatments has had a major impact on clinical practice and treatment for patients with CRLM. Undoubtedly, in the near future, these changes will carry over to affect the way *all* solid tumor oncology is practiced.

It is only within the past decade that treatment for patients with colorectal cancers has advanced beyond single-agent 5-fluorouracil (5-FU), its modifiers such as leucovorin (LV), and related scheduling debates. The successful introduction of new systemic therapies including the camptothecan, irinotecan [1]; the platinum compound, oxaliplatin [2]; new schedules for combination of the 5-fluorouracil-based therapies with irinotecan and oxaliplatin [3,4]; the oral fluorinated pyrimidine, capecitabine [5]; the monoclonal antibodies against epidermal growth factor receptor (EGFR) cetuximab [6]; and the vascular endothelial growth factor (VEGF) receptor bevacizumab [7] has extended the median survival for patients with disseminated colorectal cancer to approximately 2 years. With evidence showing improved survival for patients with isolated CRLM treated with hepatic arterial therapy [8], medical oncologists now have an array of systemic and regional therapies available for the treatment of CRLM. Indeed, it is now more likely than not that treatment directed against gross and/or microscopic CRLM will produce a response [9]. Technical improvements, including portal vein embolization [10], improved hemostasis

E-mail address: lleichman@aptiumoncology.com

1055-3207/07/$ - see front matter © 2007 Elsevier Inc. All rights reserved.
doi:10.1016/j.soc.2007.04.003

[11], intraoperative ultrasonography [12], and staged hepatic resections [13], as well the enlarging pool of well-trained surgical oncologists permit more frequent, more extensive and safer attempts at potential surgical cure of these patients that only a few years ago would have been candidates only for palliative or experimental chemotherapy.

Therapy with curative or palliative intent for patients with CRLM, which in the past used to be prescribed by either the surgeon or the medical oncologist, now require interdisciplinary consultations with the additional advice from radiologists, pathologists, and hepatologists. Moreover, definitions of "neoadjuvant therapy," "therapy for curative intent," and "palliative therapy" that were once clearly defined and understood by all clinicians have become blurred. Thus, with a shifting landscape of new curative possibilities for patients with CRLM, even the descriptive terminology needs to be revisited and clarified.

Scope of the problem

Worldwide there will be over a million new patients diagnosed with colorectal cancer. Although tumors are being diagnosed earlier with the advent of screening colonoscopies, over half a million deaths will be recorded this year due to disseminated colorectal cancer [14,15]. Approximately 50% of those diagnosed will develop liver metastases some time during the course of their battle with colorectal cancer. In absolute numbers, close to 120,000 patients will be diagnosed with colorectal cancer metastases confined to the liver [16]. Until recently, only 10% to 20% of these patients had the potential for a curative resection and the cure rate for those fortunate enough to undergo resection approximated 30% [17]. Even if advances in therapy could increase the number of patients with curable CRLM by only 20%, an additional 24,000 lives per year could be saved worldwide.

Although the risks of aggressive therapy for patients with CRLM are substantial, because the goal is *cure* and not palliation, the stakes for patients and clinicians are high. In the absence of a large body of class I evidence for the role of chemotherapy either before or after liver resection for patients with CRLM, it is essential for clinicians to convey the risk/benefit ratio to patients as accurately as possible using currently available data. The goals of this chapter are to elucidate the evidence regarding the benefits of chemotherapy and surgery for patients with curable CRLM and to balance the described benefits against the risks incurred by adding chemotherapy either before or after potentially curative surgery.

Postoperative therapy: chemotherapy after R0 resection of colorectal liver metastases

Without systemic or regional chemotherapy, approximately 75% of colorectal cancer patients who have had successful resection of liver metastases will develop recurrences within 2 years. Fifty percent of these recurrences will recur within the liver [18,19]. Because postoperative adjuvant chemotherapy for patients with stage III colorectal cancer has become standard worldwide practice, it is a logical assumption that systemic or regional therapy following surgery for CRLM will lead to an improvement in survival or, at the very least, to a decrease in the rate of liver recurrences following surgery. Logic not withstanding, there have been only a few randomized studies to guide postoperative therapy for CRLM.

The dual blood supply to the liver has particularly useful implications in liver- directed regional chemotherapy because established liver metastases greater than 2 mm in diameter derive their blood supply from the hepatic artery, while normal liver cells derive their blood supply from the portal vein [20]. It is, of course, probable that at the very earliest stages of metastatic tumor growth in the liver, the blood supply that matters most to the incipient hepatic tumor remains the portal system. Hepatic arterial infusion (HAI) therapy directs chemotherapy preferentially against the tumor, allowing normal liver perfusion by the portal vein system.

Randomized trials comparing hepatic arterial infusion (HAI) therapy with single-agent floxuridine (FUDR) for unresectable liver metastases against single-agent systemic, ie, intravenous, 5-fluorouracil (5-FU), have found response rates ranging from 42% to 62% for HAI therapy versus 10% to 21% for systemic therapy [8,21,22]. Despite these high response rates obtained by HAI FUDR for patients with established CRLM, most North American and European medical oncologists do not use HAI therapies as first-line treatments. This is partly because of lack of training and/or clinical experience, as HAI therapy is generally performed only in centers that have developed a special interest and expertise in this treatment method. Moreover, the filling of implanted pumps requires special training and the hepatic toxicities produced by direct hepatic arterial infusion of FUDR and 5-FU can be idiosyncratic to the patient in terms of timing and severity. Although the first-pass extraction of FUDR is far greater than 5-FU (about 70% first-pass extraction for 5-FU versus 95% for FUDR) [23], 5-FU can be advantageous because it is more readily available and less expensive than FUDR. Also, because it is not entirely cleared by the liver, the patient will derive a greater systemic effect from 5-FU than from FUDR.

This review will outline the results of eight trials reported in peer-reviewed journals in which patients, following R0 resection for CRLM, were randomized to receive a form of chemotherapy as HAI, hepatic arterial bolus, systemic, or combinations of hepatic arterial and systemic treatments.

Trials with "no-treatment controls" (observation)

Lorenz and colleagues [24] prospectively randomized 226 patients from 26 centers across Germany and Switzerland to HAI 5-FU 1000 mg^2/day for 5 days with intraarterial LV 200 mg/m^2 for 5 days cycled every 28 days versus a no-therapy control arm. To be eligible for this trial, patients could have a maximum of six completely resectable liver metastases without extrahepatic or primary residual disease. Most patients were randomized during their surgical procedure. The investigators chose survival as their primary end point; accrual to the trial was predicated on the hypothesis that treatment would improve survival by 50%; their accrual goal was 374 patients. The systemic effect of HAI 5-FU is appreciated in the author's report that 57.6% of patients treated developed stomatitis (11.8% grades three and four) and 55.4% developed nausea and vomiting (8.4% grades three and four). With at least 18 months of follow-up, 33.3% of the patients who received intraarterial 5-FU and LV had liver recurrence versus 36.7% of those in the control arm ($P = .715$). Most striking is their report that median survival for the HAI group was 34.5 months versus 40.8 months for the group who received no treatment after resection of CRLM. In viewing the confidence interval of hazard ratios for treatment by HAI versus no treatment, the authors concluded that, at best, the risk of death might be reduced by 15% and, at worst, the risk of death is doubled with HAI 5-FU and LV. Thus, with 108 patients randomized to postoperative adjuvant therapy and 111 patients randomized to observation after resection, the trial was closed [24].

As part of a cohort of 91 patients with CRLM surgically treated at the City of Hope over a 53-month period, Wagman and colleagues [25] randomized 22 patients with solitary CRLM who underwent an R0 resection to observation after resection (n = 12) or HAI FUDR 0.1 to 0.3 mg/kg over 2 weeks with a 2-week rest for 1 year (n = 10). These investigators reported that the time to failure for the HAI group was 30.7 months versus 8.7 months for the group undergoing observation after R0 resection for CRLM ($P = .03$). The differences in median overall survival for the two groups, 28.3 months for observation versus 37.3 months for the HAI therapy, were not statistically significant ($P = .66$).

Lygidakis and colleagues [26] randomized 40 patients with CLRM (20 to therapy, 20 to observation). In the treatment arm following surgical resection, patients received therapy splenic arterial injections of interleukin (IL)-2 18 $\times$ 10^6 U daily and γ interferon (γIFN) 100 μg daily for 5 consecutive days. At the completion of the intrasplenic arterial therapy, patients received the same doses of IL-2 and γIFN into the hepatic artery. Fifteen days later, chemotherapy with 5-FU 10 mg/kg, mitomycin-c 0.4 mg/kg, carboplatin 1.5 mg/kg, and farmorubicin 1 mg/kg were administered. All intraarterial therapy was administered with an emulsion of lipiodol and urographin. Treatments were administered every 3 months for the first year, every 4 months for the second year, and every 6 months for the third year. Although a median or mean follow-up time was not reported, none of the patients in the treated cohort had developed recurrences, while eight of the observed patients had developed intrahepatic recurrences ($P < .001$).

The mean survival for the treatment arm was 20 months versus 11 months for the observation arm ($P = .001$).

A trial conducted in Germany by Rudroff and colleagues [27] used hepatic arterial 5-FU and mitomycin-c. Mitomycin-c (8 mg/m^2) was administered as intraarterial bolus on day 1 while 5-FU 800 mg/m^2 was administered as a 4-hour infusion days 1 to 5. Four courses of intraarterial therapy were administered every 4 weeks. This small trial included only 14 treated patients and 16 no-treatment controls. All randomized patients had synchronous liver metastases and positive lymph nodes at the time of primary tumor resection. Although the investigators reported that initial tumor relapse appeared to be "shifted toward extrahepatic sites," no significant difference in either 5-year survival or long-term disease-free status was found between the treatment and control arms.

A National Cancer Institute (NCI)-sponsored Intergroup trial prospectively randomized patients who had one to three surgical resectable CRLM to receive systemic continuous-infusion 5-FU 200 mg/m^2 daily for 14 days followed by FUDR 0.1 mg/kg/day for 14 days with dose escalations up to 0.2 mg/kg/day for 14 days (for those without hepatic toxicity) versus an observation group. In this trial patients were preoperatively randomized; therefore, patients randomized to the control arm (no treatment) did not undergo placement of a hepatic arterial catheter. Patients were excluded from final analysis if intraoperative findings noted more than three hepatic metastases, extrahepatic cancer, an R0 resection could not be accomplished, or if the patient had no evidence of hepatic metastases at the time of surgery. The accrual goal of 109 patients was based on the hypothesis that combined systemic and intrahepatic therapy after successful resection for CRLM would improve median time to recurrence by 100% [28].

Although the accrual goal was met with 56 patients randomized into the control arm without postoperative treatment and 53 patients randomized to the combined systemic and intrahepatic regional therapy arm, 29 patients were excluded from final analysis (11 in the treatment arm and 18 in the control arm) based on the ineligibility criteria noted above. An additional 6 patients did not receive protocol-designated therapy and were also excluded from final analysis. Assessments for this trial were made on 75 patients from 34 different institutions: 45 in the control arm and 30 in the treatment arm. Of 30 patients who were to receive chemotherapy, only 20 patients (66%) received the four planned cycles of hepatic infusion therapy [28].

At a median follow-up of 51 months, 35 of 45 patients (77.8%) randomized to the observation arm had developed recurrences versus 16 of 30 patients (53%) in the treatment arm. The 4-year recurrence-free rate was 46% for the observation group and 25% for the treated group ($P = .04$). The 4-year liver-free recurrence rate was 67% for the treated cohort and 43% for observation alone ($P = .03$). The majority of patients (68.6%) had their first recurrence in the liver. In the multivariate analysis, the only statistically significant factor for liver recurrence was treatment (odds ratio = 3.15; $P = .02$). While the median survival was over a year longer for those patients who received postoperative therapy (63.7 months versus 49.4 months), this did not translate into a statistically significant difference ((log rank $P = .60$) [28].

Hepatic arterial infusion versus systemic therapy

A trial reported by Tono and colleagues [29] from Japan randomized 19 patients after R0 resection for CRLM to receive either six cycles of HAI 5-FU 500 mg total dose/over 24 hours with the next cycle beginning after a 3-day rest (9 patients) or oral 5-FU 200 mg/day for 2 years (10 patients). The median disease-free interval for the HAI patients compared with orally treated patients was 62.6 months versus 13.8 months, respectively ($P = .045$). Median overall survival for the HAI patients was 62.6 months versus 39.9 months for the patients treated with oral 5-FU ($P = .26$). Those given 5-FU by HAI had a median disease-free interval after surgery of 62.6 months versus 13.8 months for those who were observed without therapy ($P = .045$).

Lygidakis [30], in a follow-up to his smaller chemo-immunotherapy plus lipiodol study discussed above, reported another single-institution trial. Between 1991 and 2000, 143 patients with surgically resected CRLM were randomized to receive *systemic* therapy with intravenous bolus 5-FU 750 mg/m^2 bolus and LV 400 mg/m^2 days 1 to 5, mitomycin-c 20 mg/m^2 day 1, and intravenous IL-2 18 $\times$ 10^6 IU days 6 to 15, or a combination of *intraarterial plus systemic therapy*. Those patients randomized to the combination treatment received the same total dose of 5-FU/LV and mitomycin-c splitting the total dose in half between hepatic artery infusion and systemic infusion. In the group randomized to intraarterial therapy, the entire dose of IL-2 was administered into the hepatic artery. This unique trial treated patients intermittently for 6 years. For the first 2 years, patients were treated every 2 months; for the third and fourth years, patients were treated every 3 months; and for the fifth and sixth years, patients were treated every 4 months.

Because randomization took place immediately after completion of surgery, a total of 21 patients were dropped from analysis after randomization due to postoperative death (5 patients) or discontinuation of therapy (16 patients). Those randomized to intrahepatic therapy had the intraarterial catheter placed into the gastroduodenal artery and attached to a subcutaneous abdominal wall infusion port. The aim of this study was to compare overall survival, disease-free survival, and the incidence of intra- or extrahepatic recurrence between patients assigned to HAI plus immunotherapy versus those assigned to systemic therapy plus immunotherapy. At the time of manuscript submission, median follow-up time was 79 months. The median survival for the group randomized to receive hepatic plus systemic therapy was 79 months versus 66 months for the group that received only systemic therapy ($P = .05$ Gehan's Wilcoxon test and $P = .04$ log rank test). During the first 2-year period, 34% of patients receiving HAI therapy versus 52% of the patients receiving only systemic therapy developed either intrahepatic or extrahepatic disease recurrences ($P < .002$) [30].

Hepatic arterial infusion plus systemic therapy versus systemic therapy

In the only published trial testing HAI plus systemic therapy against systemic therapy alone, investigators at Memorial Sloan Kettering Cancer Center (MSKCC) intraoperatively randomized 156 patients after CRLM resection: 76 patients were in the combined HAI/systemic arm; 82 were in the systemic arm. In the combined arm, systemic LV 200 mg/m^2 was given followed by 5-FU 325 mg/m^2 daily for 5 days; 2 weeks later, patients received HAI FUDR 0.25 mg/kg/day for 14 days with dexamethasone 20 mg; a total of six treatment cycles were planned. In the systemic arm, 82 patients were randomized to receive six cycles of LV 200 mg/m^2 before 5-FU 370 mg/m^2 daily for 5 days with LV 200 mg/m^2 before each dose of 5-FU. Accrual was based on the hypothesis that HAI therapy following resection of CRLM would result in a 20% improvement of survival rates and hepatic-only recurrence rates at 2 years of follow-up [31].

The majority of patients in each arm had more than 2 metastatic deposits. Indeed, 24% in each arm had more than 4 metastatic lesions resected. After 2 years, the *hepatic-free-recurrence rate* for the cohort randomized to systemic plus HAI versus the cohort randomized to systemic therapy alone was 90% versus 60% ($P < .001$). In their first report of this trial, the overall progression-free survival (PFS) was 57% in the group randomized to systemic and HAI therapy versus 42% in the group randomized to systemic therapy ($P = .07$). At 2 years, the risk ratio for death was 2.34 among patients treated with systemic therapy alone versus those who received systemic and HAI therapy (95% confidence interval [CI] 1.10 to 2.98; $P = .027$) [31]. In 2005, Kemeny and Gonen reported an updated PFS in a letter to the editor of the *New England Journal of Medicine* [32]. Now, with a median follow-up of 10.3 years, overall PFS was 31.3 months for the systemic plus HAI cohort versus 17.2 months for the systemic cohort ($P = .02$). The difference in median survival was not statistically significant (68.4 months for the combined group versus 58.8 months for the systemic monotherapy group; $P = .10$) [32].

Postoperative systemic therapy

Portier and colleagues [33] recently reported a French/Swiss multicenter collaborative group trial in which patients with CRLM who completed an R0 liver resection were randomized to receive either *systemic* chemotherapy or observation. In this trial, 173 patients from 47 hospitals were randomized a median of 19.5 days after their operation to observation (n = 87) versus treatment with LV 200 mg/m^2 daily × 5 followed by 5-FU bolus

400 mg/m^2 daily × 5 every 28 days for six cycles (n = 86). Accrual was set to show a predicted 20% absolute difference in the 2-year disease-free survival in favor of those receiving postoperative chemotherapy.

With a median follow-up of 87.4 months, 52 recurrences were found in the treated group versus 55 in the group observed without 5-FU and LV. Almost all patients received second-line chemotherapy after recurrence. The median disease-free survival was 24.4 months for the treated patients and 17.6 months for the group assigned to observation. The 2- and 5-year disease-free survival rates for treated patients were 50.4% and 33.5% versus 38.1% and 26.7% for observed patients. The multivariate analysis found a statistically significant positive effect for systemic chemotherapy on disease-free survival (odds ratio for recurrence or death 0.6; 95% CI: 0.46 to 0.96, $P = .028$). Median survival was 62.1 months for the treated patients and 46.4 months for the observed patients. Two and 5-year overall survival estimates for the treated group was 81.1% and 51.1% versus 82% and 41.9% in the control group. The multivariate analysis indicated that the odds ratio for death in the treated group was 0.73 (95% CI 0.48 to 1.10) but the difference did not reach statistical significance ($P = .13$) [33]. By the time these results were published, the assigned systemic chemotherapy was described as "suboptimal" by the investigators.

Table 1 summarizes the postoperative randomized trials testing chemotherapy for patients who completed R0 resections of their CRLM.

Summary: postoperative chemotherapy for patients with colorectal liver metastases

Through the efforts of investigators with long-standing interest and expertise in HAI therapy, two prospectively randomized trials have been performed in North America. Both trials used HAI FUDR; both used systemic 5-FU/LV in conjunction with HAI therapy. The study conducted at MSKCC included more patients than the NCI Intergroup trial and it included a systemic therapy control arm. After a 10-year follow-up, the MSKCC investigators demonstrated a statistically significant improvement in disease-free survival derived from the combination therapy versus systemic therapy alone. Although the NCI Intergroup had a no-treatment control arm, their trial accrued poorly and many patients entered into the trial were not counted in the final analysis. In their smaller trial, with an observation arm, the NCI investigators reported that treatment did not result in a statistically improved disease-free or a statistically improved overall survival. However, the improvement of the *2-year disease-free interval for liver progression* after HAI plus systemic therapy was statistically significant. In the only large randomized trial using systemic therapy after R0 resection for CRLM, the investigators reported a statistically significant improvement in disease-free, but not overall survival. Ironically, the positive HAI trials and the systemic therapy trial used what would now be considered suboptimal systemic chemotherapy. These were designed and well

Table 1
Randomized trials for patients with R0 resection of colorectal liver metastases

First Author/Year/Group or nationality/Ref no.	Total no. of patients	Arms Tx versus control	Median liver-disease-free survival (mos) Tx versus control	RFS (%) or median DFS (mos) or median TTF (mos) Tx versus control	Median overall survival (mos) Tx versus control
Lorenz/1998/Germany and Switzerland [24]	226	HAI 5-FU + mitomycin-c versus Observation	Not stated	14.2 versus 13.2	34.5 versus 40.8 (P = .15)
Wagman/1990/City of Hope (United States) [25]	22	FUDR versus Observation	Not stated	30.7 versus 8.7 (P = .02)	37.3 versus 28.3 (P = .66)
Lygidakis/1995/Greece [26]	40	HA and SA IL-2 + γIFN + bolus chemotherapy with lipiodol versus Observation	Not stated	Not stated	20 versus 11 (P = .001)
Rudroff/1999/Germany [27]	30	HA 5-FU (4 h) and mitomycin-c (bolus) versus Observation	Not stated	Not stated in months. P value noted as "not significant"	Not stated in months. P value noted as "not significant"
Kemeny MM/2001/ United States [28]	109	CI 5-FU 200 mg/m2 daily × 14 + HAI FUDR 0.1–0.3 mg/kg daily × 14 versus Observation	At 4 y: 43% versus 67% (P = .03)	RFS at 4 y 46% versus 25% (P = .04)	63.7 versus 49 (P = .19)
Tono/2000/Japan [29]	19	5-FU HAI 500 mg total dose over 24 h × 96 h for 6 cycles versus oral 5-FU 200 mg daily × 2 years	Not stated	62.6 versus 13.8 (P = .045)	62.6 versus 39.9 (P = .26)
Lygidakis/2001/Greece [30]	143	HA 5-FU/LV/mitomycin-c + IL-2 versus IV 5-FU/LV/mitomycin-c + IL2	Not stated	At 2 y: 34% versus 52% (P = .002)	79 versus 66 (P = .05)
Kemeny N/1999/ MSKCC [31]	156	IV bolus 5FU 325 mg/m^2 plus LV 200 mg/m^2 + HAI FUDR 0.25 mg/kg/d x 14 + dexamethasone versus IV bolus 5-FU 370 mg/m^2 IV q daily × 5 + LV 200 mg/m^2 q daily × 5	At 2 yrs: 90 versus 60 (P = .001)	31.3 versus 17.2 (P = .02)	68.4 versus 58.8 (P = .10)
Portier/2006/ French-Swiss [33]	173	Bolus 5-FU 400 mg/m2 q d × 5 + LV 200 mg/m^2 q d × 5 versus Observation	Not stated	24.4 versus 17.6 (P = .028)	62.1 versus 46.4 (P = 0.13)

Abbreviations: CI, continuous infusion; DFS, disease-free survival; γIFN, γ interferon; 5-FU, 5-fluorouracil; FUDR, floxuridine; HA, hepatic arterial; HAI, hepatic arterial infusion; IL, interleukin; IV, intravenous; LV, leucovorin; MSKCC, Memorial Sloan Kettering Cancer Center; RFS, relapse-free survival; SA, splenic arterial; TTF, time to failure; Tx, treatment.

under way before the era of irinotecan, oxaliplatin, or targeted agents. Unlike the positive North American HAI infusion trials, the positive trials conducted by Lygidakis and his colleagues use intraarterial 5-FU and mitomycin plus IL-2. Although the trial reported by Lorenz and colleagues using HAI 5-FU was did not support the use of HAI chemotherapy following an R0 resection for CRLM, postoperative combination of hepatic-arterial (with FUDR) and systemic therapy (5-FU-based) for patients with CRLM who have had R0 liver resections is supportable. Thus, for surgeons and medical oncologists who are comfortable with the insertion and use of current arterial pump technology, HAI using FUDR plus dexamethasone *with* systemic therapy following R0 resection of CRLM can be recommended. The complex 6-year treatment program using the addition of IL-2 as reported by Lygidakis and colleagues is not likely to gain traction in the United States. Nevertheless, the data are sufficiently provocative to warrant verification by a collaborative effort.

Before leaving this subject, a caveat: we do not know if the addition of irinotecan and oxaliplatin (both of which can cause liver toxicity, see below) to the systemic component of therapy will add or take away from the results already reported. Despite recommendations toward routine postoperative systemic therapy for patients with CRLM who have had an R0 resection, adding systemic FOLFOX or CAPOX or systemic FOLFIRI to patients with regenerating livers should be done with great care. To address this issue and to further analyze the contribution of HAI therapy following R0 resection of CRLM, a multi-institutional randomized controlled trial of combined regional (FUDR)/systemic (capecitabine and oxaliplatin) versus systemic alone therapy after complete resection of CRLM using capecitabine and oxaliplatin and modern surgical approaches is currently under way in the United States (NSABP CO-9).

Chemotherapy before liver resection for patients with colorectal liver metastases

Despite dramatic improvements in operative techniques that allow for expanding the number of patients with CRLM who may have potentially curative surgery [34], only 10% to 25% of patients with CRLM have tumors that can be removed with an R0 resection [35,36]. In an era with multiple agents effective against disseminated colorectal cancer, the question of whether combination chemotherapy with classic cytotoxics in addition to agents targeted against epidermal growth factor receptor (EGFR) and vascular endothelial growth factor (VEGF) can increase the number of patients who can undergo curative resection begs an answer.

Before exploring the current literature on this subject, it is worthwhile to review terminology that, in the area of liver resection for CRLM, has become blurred. In general, when solid tumor medical, surgical, and radiation oncologists refer to "neoadjuvant therapy" before surgery, they are referring to treatments that are administered before potentially curative surgery. A patient receiving neoadjuvant cancer therapy before surgery has a tumor that can be resected for cure (R0 resection) without the administration of chemotherapy (breast cancer) or chemotherapy plus radiation (esophageal and rectal cancers). Preoperative treatment designed to administer cytotoxic or targeted therapy to patients who can undergo an R0 resection for CRLM is appropriately termed, "neoadjuvant therapy" [37]. In this setting, preoperative therapy is designed to attack *occult* metastatic cancer at the earliest time point and to decrease, even eliminate the *clinically visible* cancer, from the surgical field.

Unfortunately, most patients with CRLM do not have tumors that lend themselves to an R0 resection. Therefore, the breakthrough being sought by administering systemic or regional chemotherapy to patients with CRLM is to render the inoperable patient operable for cure. This rationale is therefore different from the "neoadjuvant" approach. It would be more appropriate if investigators referred to cytotoxic treatment that is designed to improve respectability rates as "preoperative chemotherapy for liver metastases" or "combined modality therapy for liver metastases" rather than "neoadjuvant" therapy. In these situations, both components of treatment, chemotherapy *and* surgery, are necessary to cure the patient; neither modality has curative potential alone. This is well illustrated in the publication by Capussotti and colleagues [38], in which the investigators note that in a prospective study of 150 patients undergoing surgery for CRLM, the recurrence rate for 34 patients who needed preoperative chemotherapy before resection was 94%, versus 66% for those who were resectable without preoperative chemotherapy. In addition to the lack of clarity regarding the goals of preoperative therapy for patients with CRLM, the lack of uniformity in the definitions of resectability for cure have hampered efforts to reproducibly define successful preoperative chemotherapy or to identify appropriate patients for true neoadjuvant chemotherapy [39].

Systemic chemotherapy before surgery for patients with colorectal liver metastases

As early as 2001, studies by Fowler and colleagues [40] and Shankar and colleagues [41] indicated that systemic chemotherapy could render patients with initially unresectable CRLM resectable for cure. In a report on the sequential administration of FOLFIRI and FOLFOX6 for patients with disseminated colorectal cancers, Tournigand and colleagues [42] demonstrated that 10 patients (9%) who received FOLFIRI first and 24 patients (22%) who received FOLFOX6 first could have resection of what appeared to be unresectable liver metastases before treatment. Indeed, the authors reported a median overall survival of 47 months for these "down-staged" patients who underwent an R0 resection following treatment with either FOLFIRI or FOLFOX6.

In a far larger retrospective review, Bismuth and colleagues [36] reported on 434 patients with CRLM. In this series, 330 patients were declared unresectable for cure because of the size, the number, and the location of their liver lesions or because of extrahepatic disease. These patients were treated with chronomodulated oxaliplatin/5-FU/LV. Following treatment it was determined that 53 (16%) could undergo liver resection. No mortality following surgery was reported, but 14 patients (26%) had significant complications such as fluid retention and sepsis. Of note, the 5-year survival rate for the patients rendered resectable after chemotherapy was 40%. In updating this series, Adam and colleagues [43] reported outcomes for 701 patients with unresectable CRLM treated with combination chemotherapy. Of these, 95 patients (13.6%) responded and were deemed resectable for cure. The 5-year survival for the resectable patients was 34%. Giachetti and colleagues [44], reviewed data on 389 patients with CRLM enrolled in six different clinical trials. They identified 151 patients unresectable because of tumor size (>5 cm), tumor number (>4), and poor location. They observed a 59% response rate for these patients with treatment consisting of oxaliplatin and 5-FU/LV. In all, 77 patients were surgically explored. Of these, 58 patients had a resection for cure with a median survival of 48 months. It is apparent that these published median survival figures are very similar to those reported for patients who are resected for cure without undergoing preoperative chemotherapy. They also suggest that many of these down-staged patients are being cured by the combination of chemotherapy and surgery.

In a prospective study, Alberts and colleagues [45] reported on a North Central Cancer Treatment Group phase II study that enrolled patients with CRLM deemed "not optimally resectable" by surgeons considered experts in this field. Patients were treated with biweekly oxaliplatin 85 mg/m^2 followed sequentially by LV 200 mg/m^2, bolus 5-FU 400 mg/m^2, and then continuous infusion 600 mg/m^2 over 22 hours on day 1. These same doses of 5-FU were repeated on day 2 without oxaliplatin (FOLFOX4). In this trial, 44 patients were assessable; 25 patients (60%) showed reduction of tumor. After a median of 6 months of chemotherapy, of 17 patients surgically explored, 15 patients (36%) underwent successful R0 resection. Two patients underwent incomplete resections. Eleven of the 17 patients who underwent surgery recurred (8 in the liver) at a median follow-up of 22 months. Median survival for the entire group was 26 months; the median survival for those undergoing surgery was 31 months [45].

A prospective evaluation of 40 patients with CRLM who could not undergo an R0 resection was reported by Pozzo and colleagues [46]. In this trial, 40 patients were treated with irinotecan 180 mg/m^2 on day 1, LV 200 mg/m^2 and 5-FU 400 mg/m^2 IV bolus on days 1 and 2, and 5-FU 1200 mg/m^2 as a continuous 48-hour infusion starting day 1. Treatment was repeated every 2 weeks (FOLFIRI). Response was assessed every 12 weeks (six cycles). Of the 16 patients taken to surgery, 14 had an objective response. Thirteen patients underwent liver resection with curative intent. The median disease-free survival in the operated patients was 14.3 months.

The authors noted that their treatment had the greatest effect on those whose tumors were considered unresectable secondary to size (> 5 cm) [46].

Targeted agents

Inclusion of bevacizumab as first-line therapy for patients with disseminated colorectal cancer has been an important addition to treatment [7]. It is safe to state that most patients in the United States who present with CRLM receive first- or second-line therapy with bevacizumab in combination with either oxaliplatin-based or irinotecan-based chemotherapy. However, by hitting its intended target, VEGF-A, bevacizumab may inhibit wound healing. Bevacizumab binds to vascular endothelial growth factor receptor 1 (VEGFR1) and vascular endothelial growth factor receptor 2 (VEGFR2). VEGFR1 and VEGFR2 have roles in liver regeneration [47,48]. Also, in comparison to standard chemotherapeutic agents, the half-life of bevacizumab of approximately 20 days (range 11 to 50 days) is relatively long [49]. Thus, optimal timing of surgery for patients with CRLM after bevacizumab administration is still unknown. This is made more relevant because pooled data have confirmed the increased incidence of complications in patients undergoing surgery while receiving bevacizumab-containing regimens for metastatic colorectal cancer [50].

Although the appropriate integration of bevacizumab into preoperative chemotherapeutic regimens for patients with CRLM or its use in combination therapy after successful surgery needs further clarification by prospective study, emerging data suggest that it *can* be safely used in these settings. A letter to the editor by Gruenberger and colleagues [51] gave preliminary details on nine patients with CRLM deemed suboptimal for surgical resection. These patients were treated with capecitabine 3500 $mg/m^2/d$ on days 1 through 7 plus oxaliplatin 85 mg/m^2 and bevacizumab 5 mg/kg on day 1 of the 2-week cycle (XELOX plus bevacizumab). Patients received five cycles of XELOX plus bevacizumab and six cycles of XELOX without bevacizumab. Eight of nine patients underwent liver resection 5 weeks after their last dose of bevacizumab. Patients resumed the XELOX plus bevacizumab 5 weeks after surgery. There was no reported increase in mortality or morbidity. In another preliminary report, investigators at MSKCC retrospectively identified 16 patients with CRLM who received bevacizumab before hepatic resection and 16 patients who received bevacizumab after hepatic resection [52]. In each case, bevacizumab was administered with cytotoxic chemotherapy. The median time from the last dose of bevacizumab before surgery was 6.9 weeks. The median time from surgery to the first dose of bevacizumab was 7.4 weeks. Perioperative complications were observed in 40.6% of their patients. However, the investigators reported no statistical difference in the perioperative morbidity with a set of matched controls who did not receive bevacizumab. The MKSCC investigators concluded that bevacizumab, administered before or after surgery for patients with CRLM, does not significantly increase the risk of the surgical morbidity. While Ellis and colleagues suggest a window of 8 to 12 weeks from bevacizumab before surgery [47], the investigators from MSKCC advocate a window of between 6 to 8 weeks from the last dose of bevacizumab [52] and the Gruenberger and colleagues report suggests safety after 5 weeks [51].

Although there is no theoretical reason to believe that treatment with an EGFR inhibitor such as cetuximab will hamper wound healing or increase the surgical risk for patients with CRLM, there is even less data available for cetuximab than for bevacizumab. The phase II ACROBAT study using FOLFOX plus cetuximab has been published only as an abstract. This trial demonstrated a response rate of 72%. Of 42 assessable patients, 8 patients were able to undergo liver resection. However, details on the perioperative outcome and treatment complications were not provided [53].

Preoperative hepatic arterial infusion therapy

Neoadjuvant or preoperative HAI with FUDR or 5-FU for patients with CRLM does maximizes drug exposure to the liver. It also exposes the liver to direct toxicity before an operation whose outcome may depend on liver regeneration. Thus, HAI therapy before surgery for patients with CRLM has both theoretical advantages and distinct theoretical risks. Just as with systemic chemotherapy before surgery for patients with CRLM, there are few trials that were designed to detect the resectability rate for those patients with apparently unresectable liver metastases. In a review of this subject, Leonard and colleagues identified eight published trials that include 967 patients. From this mixture of patients, 72 (7.4%) underwent what is described as a "complete resection" of liver metastases [39]. In a series from MSKCC, 44 patients with unresectable CRLM were treated with HAI FUDR and dexamethasone plus oxaliplatin-based systemic chemotherapy. Nine patients (20%) were taken to surgery after this treatment and had a complete resection of their metastatic liver tumors. While the median survival for patients who could not undergo resection was 24 months, median survival for those resected had not been reached by the time of publication [54].

Hepatic toxicities associated with preoperative chemotherapy

The intrahepatic toxicities of HAI are well known. Chemical hepatitis and sclerosing cholangitis have been reported and are appreciated by those who regularly administer HAI therapy [55]. Although chemical hepatitis with transaminasemia is generally reversible, sclerosing cholangitis may become a chronic problem, outlasting the cancer, especially for patients treated with HAI after complete liver resection. Thus, the question of when to operate on the liver for the patient who is receiving HAI as preoperative therapy is very relevant to the potential surgical morbidity and mortality.

Recently, experienced investigators have called attention to the fact that newer, effective combination chemotherapies for patients with disseminated colorectal cancer have direct hepatic toxicities [56]. Oxaliplatin can cause elevations of liver-associated alkaline phosphatase and transaminases [57]. It can also cause sinusoidal obstruction and fibrotic venular occlusion [58]. These vascular alterations lead to a characteristic bluish discoloration of the liver associated with edema and spongiform consistency similar to that seen with early cirrhosis. This "blue liver syndrome" increases the risk for operative bleeding and decreases hepatic functional reserve [56]. Steatohepatitis, a form of nonalcoholic fatty liver disease (NAFLD), appears to be more closely associated with irinotecan-based therapies [59]. NAFLD is actually the earlier phase of nonalcoholic steatohepatitis, a condition associated with inflammation and hepatocyte ballooning [60]. In a report on 465 patients who underwent liver resections for CRLM, Vauthey and colleagues [61] reported a statistically significant 90-day mortality for those patients with chemotherapy-induced steatohepatitis. In this report, the association of irinotecan-based therapy and steatohepatitis was well documented [61]. 5-FU and LV have been linked to hepatic steatosis, not steatohepatitis, in over 45% of patients [62]. Although hepatic steatosis has not been implicated in surgical complications as severe as those seen with steatohepatitis [56], hepatic steatosis has been found to be an independent predictor for infection following liver resections for patients with CRLM [62].

Important questions are raised by the known hepatic toxicities of the preoperative regimens. Is there an optimal length of time that preoperative therapy can be given safely before surgery? Is there a danger to the patient by continuing with the same regimen after surgery (even though successful before surgery) if hepatic toxicity to the normal liver is recognized at the time of surgery? Is there an increased risk for patients receiving both irinotecan and oxaliplatin in combination with 5-FU?

Preoperative treatment recommendations

Existing information does not allow recommendation of one form of systemic therapy over another. Moreover, despite the toxicities and complexities involved with HAI therapy, those centers familiar with preoperative HAI therapy appear to be able to treat patients with CRLM with very low toxicity rates. Regardless, considerations of hepatic toxicity due to chemotherapy have led to current recommendations that the duration of preoperative therapy for liver metastases should last only until liver lesions regress to the point that an operation is likely to be curative. Finally, known liver toxicity associated with current chemotherapy combinations provides a good reason why, in the absence of class I clinical evidence to the contrary, patients with CRLM who are initially resectable for cure should go to surgery immediately without neoadjuvant chemotherapy. Conversely, preoperative chemotherapy should be reserved for those patients with CRLM whose tumors cannot be surgically cured unless chemotherapy successfully produces a response.

The new paradigm

The treatment of patients with metastatic cancer to the liver is no longer in the province of one discipline. Postoperatively, after successful liver resection for patients with CRLM, the medical oncologist will be called upon to discuss and treat the patient with either HAI therapy or systemic therapy. With response rates for disseminated colorectal cancer treated with currently available systemic agents exceeding 50% and overall median survival approaching 2 years, a small percentage of patients who were deemed incurable just a decade ago are undoubtedly being cured today. While it has long been appreciated that patients with liver-only or lung-only colorectal cancer metastases can be cured with surgery, there are now reports of long-term survival for those patients with liver metastases *and* lung metastases or liver metastases *and* peritoneal recurrences [63,64]. The patients in these reports have been treated aggressively with combination chemotherapy and surgery. As noted at the outset of this chapter, these patients do not represent a large portion of individual practices, but the stakes are so high in terms of the potential for cure, that multidisciplinary teams have to be established for the modern treatment of disseminated colorectal cancers. At the very least, these teams must include medical, surgical, and radiation oncologists and ideally each team should also include pathologists, radiologists, gastroenterologists, and hepatologists.

The importance of the multidisciplinary team was recently pointed out by Benoist and colleagues [65] They noted that radiographic complete responses in the liver after systemic chemotherapy usually demonstrated residual viable cancer by pathologic analysis of the surgical specimen. They laid the scientific foundation for the practice of resecting *all* metastatic colorectal cancer in the liver regardless of radiographic response. The determination of adequate margins, the histology of the non-tumor-involved liver, and the response to chemotherapy (complete or partial) all require the assistance of the pathologist reviewing the surgical specimen. The amount of normal liver that must be left for the patient to survive the postoperative period is an area that must be addressed by the surgeon together with qualified radiologists, gastroenterologists, and hepatologists. With this in mind, the multidisciplinary team for the patient with disseminated colorectal cancer is not a distant concept or a concept that is viable only at large centers: it is necessary, right now, in all venues where patients with disseminated colorectal cancer are being treated.

References

[1] Cunningham D, Pyrhonen S, James RD, et al. Randomized trial of irinotecan plus supportive care versus supportive care alone after fluorouracil failure for patients with metastatic colorectal cancer. Lancet 1998;352:1413–8.
[2] Andre T, Bensmaine MA, Louviet C, et al. Multicenter phase II study of bimonthly high-dose leucovorin, fluorouracil infusion and oxaliplatin for metastatic colorectal cancer resistant to the same leucovorin and fluorouracil regimen. J Clin Oncol 1999;17:3560–8.
[3] Goldberg RM, Sargent DJ, Morton RF, et al. A randomized controlled trial of fluorouracil plus leucovorin, irinotecan and oxaliplatin combinations in patients with previously untreated metastatic colorectal cancer. J Clin Oncol 2004;22:23–30.
[4] Hebbar M, Tournigand C, Lledo G, et al. Phase II trial alternating FOLFOX-6 and FOLFIRI regimens in second-line therapy of patients with metastatic colorectal cancer (FIRE-FOX study). Cancer Invest 2006;24:154–9.
[5] Hoff PM, Ansari R, Batist G, et al. Comparison of oral capecitabine versus intravenous fluorouracil plus leucovorin as first-line treatment in 605 patients with metastatic colorectal cancer: results of a randomized phase III study. J Clin Oncol 2001;19:2282–92.
[6] Saltz L, Meropol NJ, Loehrer PJ, et al. Phase II trial of cetuximab in patients with refractory colorectal cancer that expresses the epidermal growth factor receptor. J Clin Oncol 2004;22:1201–8.
[7] Hurwitz H, Fehrenbacher L, Novotny W, et al. Bevacizumab plus irinotecan, fluorouracil and leucovorin for metastatic colorectal cancer. N Engl J Med 2004;350:2335–42.
[8] Kemeny NE, Niedzwiecki D, Hollis DR, et al. Hepatic arterial infusion versus systemic theapy for hepatic metastases from colorectal cancer: a randomized trial of efficacy, quality of life, and molecular markers (CALGB 9481). J Clin Oncol 2006;24:1395–403.
[9] Gorlick R, Metzger R, Danenberg KD, et al. Higher levels of thymidylate synthase gene expression are observed in pulmonary as compared with hepatic metastases in colorectal adenocarcinoma. J Clin Oncol 1998;16:1465–9.
[10] Azoulay D, Castgaing D, Smail A, et al. Resection of nonresectable liver metastases from colorectal cancer after percutaneous portal vein embolization. Ann Surg 2000;231:480–6.
[11] Chen H, Merchant NB, Didolkar MS. Hepatic resection using intermittent vascular inflow occlusion and low central venous pressure anesthesia improves morbidity and mortality. J Gastrointest Surg 2000;4:162–7.
[12] Makuuchi M, Hasegawa H, Ymazaki S, et al. Ultrasonically guided subsegmentectomy. Surg Gynecol Obstet 1985;161:346–50.
[13] Adam R, Laurent A, Azoulay D, et al. Two-stage hepatectomy: a planned strategy to treat irresectable liver tumors. Ann Surg 2000;232:777–85.
[14] Ferlay J, Bray F, Pisani P, et al. GLOBCAN 2002. Cancer incidence, mortality and prevalence worldwide. IARC CancerBase No. 5. version 2.0. Lyon (France): IARC Press; 2004. Available at: http://www-depdb.iarc.fr/globocan/GLOBOframe.htm.
[15] Jemal A, Tiwari RC, Murray T, et al. Cancer statistics, 2004. CA Cancer J Clin 2004;54:8–29.
[16] Scheele J, Stangl R, Altendorf-Hofmann A, et al. Resection of colorectal liver metastases. World J Surg 1995;19:59–71.
[17] Biasco G, Derenzini GL, Grazi G, et al. Treatment of hepatic metastases from colorectal cancer: many doubts, some certainties. Cancer Treat Rev 2006;32:214–28.
[18] Fortner JG. Recurrence of colorectal cancer after hepatic resection. Am J Surg 155: 378–382.
[19] Fong Y, Cohen AM, Fortner JG, et al. Liver resection for colorectal metastases. J Clin Oncol 1997;15:938–46.
[20] Ackerman NB. The blood supply of experimental liver metastases IV. Changes in vascularity with increasing tumor growth. Surgery 1974;75:589–96.
[21] Hohn DC, Stagg RJ, Friedman MA, et al. A randomized trial of continuous intravenous versus hepatic intraarterial floxuridine in patients with colorectal cancer metastatic to the liver: The Northern California Oncology Group trial. J Clin Oncol 1989;7:1646–54.

[22] Rougier P, Laplanche A, Huguier M, et al. Hepatic arterial infusion of floxuridine in patients with liver metastases from colorectal carcinoma: long-term results of a prospective randomized trial. J Clin Oncol 1992;10:1112–8.
[23] Ensminger WD, Gyves JW. Clinical pharmacology of hepatic arterial chemotherapy. Semin Oncol 1983;10:176–82.
[24] Lorenz M, Muller HH, Schramm H, et al. Randomized trial of surgery versus surgery followed by adjuvant hepatic areterial infusion with 5-fluorouracil and folinic acid for liver metastases of colorectal cancer. Ann Surg 1998;228:756–62.
[25] Wagman LD, Kemeny MM, Leong L, et al. A prospective, randomized evaluation of the treatment of colorectal cancer metastatic to the liver. J Clin Oncol 1990;11:1885–93.
[26] Lygidakis NJ, Ziras N, Parissis J. Resection versus resection combined with adjuvant pre-and postoperative chemotherapy-immunotherapy for metastatic colorectal liver cancer: a new look at an old problem. Hepatogastroenterology 1995;42:155–61.
[27] Rudroff C, Altendorf-Hoffmann A, Stangle R, et al. Prospective randomized trial on adjuvant hepatic-artery infusion chemotherapy afer R0 resection of colorectal liver metastases. Langenbecks Arch Surg 1999;384:243–9.
[28] Kemeny MM, Sudeshna A, Gray B, et al. Combined-modality treatment for resectable metastatic colorectal carcinoma to the liver: surgical resection of hepatic metastases in combination with continuous infusion of chemotherapy—An intergroup study. J Clin Oncol 2002;20:1499–505.
[29] Tono T, Hasuike Y, Ohzato H, et al. Limited but definite efficacy of prophylactic hepatic arterial infusion chemotherapy after curative resection of colorectal liver metastases: a randomized study. Cancer 2000;88:1549–56.
[30] Lygidakis NJ, Sgourakis G, Vlachos L, et al. Metastatic liver disease of colorectal origin: the value of locoregional immunochemotherapy combined with systemic chemotherapy following liver resection. Results of a prospective randomized study. Hepatogastroenterology 2001;48:1685–91.
[31] Kemeny N, Huang Y, Cohen A, et al. Hepatic arterial infusion of chemotherapy after resection of hepatic metastases from colorectal cancer. N Engl J Med 1999;341:2031–48.
[32] Kemeny N, Gonen M. Hepatic arterial infusion after liver resection. N Engl J Med 2005;352:734–5 [letter to the editor].
[33] Portier G, Elias D, Bouche O, et al. Multicenter randomized trial of adjuvant fluorouracil and folinic acid compared with surgery alone after resection of colorectal liver metastases: FFCD ACHBTH AURC 9002 Trial. J Clin Oncol 2006;24:4976–82.
[34] Khatri VP, Petrelli NJ, Belghiti J. Extending the frontiers of surgical therapy for hepatic colorectal metastases: Is there a limit? J Clin Oncol 2006;23:8490–9.
[35] Steele GJ, Ravikumar TS. Resection of hepatic metastases from colorectal metastases: biologic perspectives. Ann Surg 1989;210:127–38.
[36] Bismuth H, Adam R, Levi F, et al. Resection of nonresectable liver metastases after neoadjuvant chemotherapy. Ann Surg 1996;224:509–22.
[37] Wein A, Riedel C, Bruckl W, et al. Neoadjuvant treatment with weekly high-dose 5-fluorouracil as 24-hour infusion, folinic acid and oxaliplatin in patients with primary resectable liver metastases of colorectal cancer. Oncology 2003;64:131–8.
[38] Capussotti L, Muratore A, Mulas MM, et al. Neoadjuvant chemotherapy and resection initially irresectable colorectal liver metastases. Br J Surg 2006;93:1001–6.
[39] Leonard GD, Brenner B, Kemeny NE. Neoadjuvant chemotherapy before liver resection for patients with unresectable liver metastases from colorectal cancer. J Clin Oncol 2005;23:2038–48.
[40] Fowler WC, Eisenberg BL, Hoffman JP. Hepatic resection following systemic chemotherapy for metastatic colorectal carcinoma. J Am Surg Oncol 2004;51:122–5.
[41] Shankar A, Leonard P, Renaut AJ, et al. Neo-adjuvant therapy improves resectability rates for colorectal liver metastases. Ann R Coll Surg Engl 2001;83:85–8.

[42] Tournigand C, Thiery A, Achille E, et al. FOLFIRI followed by FOLFOX6 or the reverse sequence in advanced colorectal cancer: a randomized GERCOR Study. J Clin Oncol 2004;22:229–37.
[43] Adam R, Avisar E, Ariche A, et al. Five-year survival following hepatic resection after neoadjuvant therapy for nonresectable colorectal liver metastases. Ann Surg Oncol 2001;10: 663–9.
[44] Giachetti S, Itzhaki M, Gruia G, et al. Long-term survival of patients with unresectable colorectal liver metastases following infusional chemotherapy with 5-fluorouracil, leucovorin, oxaliplatin and surgery. Ann Surg Oncol 1999;8:347–53.
[45] Alberts SR, Hovrath WL, Sternfeld WC, et al. Oxaliplatin, fluorouracil, and leucovorin for patients with unresectable liver-only metastases from colorectal cancer: a North Central Cancer Treatment Group phase II study. J Clin Oncol 2005;23:9243–9.
[46] Pozzo C, Basso M, Cassano A, et al. Neoadjuvant treatment of unresectable liver disease with irinotecan and 5-fluorouracil plus folinic acid in colorectal cancer patients. Ann Oncol 2004;15:933–9.
[47] Ellis LM, Curley SA, Grothey A. Surgical resection after downstaging colorectal liver metastasis in the era of bevacizumab. J Clin Oncol 2005;23:4853–5.
[48] Kraizer Y, Mawasi N, Seagal J, et al. Vascular endothelial growth factor and angiopoietin in liver regeneration. Biochem Biophys Res Commun 2001;287:209–15.
[49] Gordon Ms, Margolin K, Talpaz, et al. Phase I safety and pharmacokinetic data study of recombinant human anti-vascular endothelial growth factor in patients with advanced cancer. J Clin Oncol 2001;19:843–50.
[50] Scappaticci FA, Fehrenbacher L, Cartwright T, et al. Surgical wound healing complications in metastatic colorectal patients treated with bevacizumab. J Surg Oncol 2005;91: 173–80.
[51] Gruenberger T, Bruenberger B, Scheithauer W. Neoadjuvant therapy with bevacizumab. J Clin Oncol 2006;24:2592–3 [Letter to the editor].
[52] D'Angelica M, Kornprat P, Gonen M, et al. Lack of evidence for increased operative morbidity after hepatectomy with perioperative use of bevacizumab: a matched case-control study. Ann Surg Oncol 2007;14:759–65.
[53] Diaz Rubio E, Tabernero J, Van Cutsem E, et al. Cetuximab in combination with oxaliplatin 5-fluorouracil/folinic acid (FOLFOX4) in the first-line treatment of patients with epidermal growth factor receptor expressing metastatic colorectal cancer: an international phase II study. J Clin Oncol 2005;23:254.
[54] Leonard GD, Fong Y, Jarnagin W, et al. Liver resection after hepatic arterial infusion (HAI) plus systemic oxaliplatin (Oxal) combinations in pretreated patients with extensive unresectable colorectal liver metastases. Proc Am Soc Clin Ocnol 2004;23:256 [abstract 3535].
[55] Barnett K, Malafa M. Complications of hepatic arterial infusion: a review of 4580 reported cases. Int J Gastrointest Cancer 2001;30:147–60 [abstract 3542].
[56] Bilchik AJ, Poston G, Curley SA, et al. Neoadjuvant chemotherapy for metastatic colon cancer: a cautionary note. J Clin Oncol 2005;23:9073–8.
[57] Tisman G, MacDonald D, Shindell N, et al. Oxaliplatin toxicity masquerading as recurrent colon cancer. J Clin Oncol 2004;22:3202–4.
[58] Rubbia-Brandt L, Audard V, Sartoretti P, et al. Severe hepatic sinusoidal obstruction associated with oxaliplatin-based chemotherapy in patients with metastatic colorectal cancer. Ann Oncol 2004;15:460–6.
[59] Fernandez FG, Ritter J, Linehan DC, et al. Effect of steatohepatitis associated with irinotecan or oxaliplatin pre-treatment on resectability of hepatic colorectal metastases. J Am Coll Surg 2005;200:845–53.
[60] Peppercorn PD, Reznek RH, Wilson P, et al. Demonstration of hepatic steatosis by computerized tomography in patient receiving 5-fluorouracil-based therapy for advanced colorectal cancer. Br J Cancer 1998;77:2008–11.

[61] Vauthey JN, Pawlik TM, Ribero D, et al. Chemotherapy regimen predicts steatohepatitis and an increase in 90-day mortality after surgery for hepatic colorectal metastases. J Clin Oncol 2006;24:2065–72.

[62] Kooby DA, Fong Y, Suriawinata A, et al. Impact of steatosis on perioperative outcome following hepatic resection. J Gastrointest Surg 2003;7:1034–44.

[63] Elias D, Ouellet JF, Bellon N, et al. Extrahepatic disease does not contraindicate hepatectomy for colorectal liver metastases. Br J Surg 2003;90:567–74.

[64] Jaeck D, Oussoulzoglou E, Rosso E, et al. A two-stage hepatectomy procedure combined with portal vein embolization to achieve curative resection for initially unresectable multiple and bi-lobar colorectal liver metastases. Ann Surg 2004;240:1037–51.

[65] Benoist S, Brouquet A, Penna C, et al. Complete response of colorectal liver metastases after chemotherapy: does it mean cure? J Clin Oncol 2006;24:3939–45.

ELSEVIER
SAUNDERS

Surg Oncol Clin N Am
16 (2007) 557–577

SURGICAL
ONCOLOGY CLINICS
OF NORTH AMERICA

Patient Selection and Outcome of Hepatectomy for Noncolorectal Non-Neuroendocrine Liver Metastases

Eugene A. Choi, MD[a], Eddie K. Abdalla, MD[b,*]

[a]*The University of Texas M. D. Anderson Cancer Center, Department of Surgical Oncology, 1515 Holcombe Boulevard, Unit 444, Houston, TX 77030, USA*

[b]*Hepatobiliary Surgery and Surgical Oncology, The University of Texas M. D. Anderson Cancer Center, Department of Surgical Oncology, 1515 Holcombe Boulevard, Unit 444, Houston, TX 77030, USA*

The liver is a frequent site of metastasis from solid tumors. Treatment of colorectal liver metastases (LM) has been studied extensively; however, treatment of noncolorectal LM is less well defined. Patients with LM from primary neuroendocrine tumors (NET) represent the largest group of noncolorectal LM, and their treatment is addressed separately in the article by Wright and colleagues in this issue. The treatment of noncolorectal, non-neuroendocrine liver metastases (NCNNLM) is less well understood, particularly the role and utility of surgery as part of a multimodality approach. The development of newer, more effective treatment algorithms for colorectal LM, including safe, aggressive surgical approaches, have rekindled the interest in the treatment of NCNNLM.

In some cases, liver metastases from solid tumors may be regarded as evidence of systemic disseminated disease, wherein liver-directed surgical treatment should be considered only for palliation of symptoms related to liver involvement. In other cases, however, under the premise that the metastatic route via the portal vein confines metastatic disease to the liver, LM from solid tumors may also be considered as locoregional disease. Whether thought of as part of a systemic process or as part of a locoregional process, isolated LM from many sites of origin have been resected with acceptable outcomes. The potential utility of surgery in this setting likely relates to several factors: 1) advances in chemotherapy have led to effective control

* Corresponding author.
E-mail address: eabdalla@mdanderson.org (E.K. Abdalla).

1055-3207/07/$ - see front matter © 2007 Elsevier Inc. All rights reserved.
doi:10.1016/j.soc.2007.04.005 **surgonc.theclinics.com**

of extra hepatic disease for certain tumor types, supporting a rationale for surgical resection of LM in the presence of presumed or de facto systemic disease; 2) improvements in patient preparation for surgery, surgical technique and perioperative care have reduced the perioperative risk of hepatic resection, tipping the risk–benefit ratio in favor of surgical resection in selected cases; 3) the increased emphasis on and dissemination of multimodality treatment approaches has improved patient selection and strengthened the role of hepatic resection as a key component of integrated multidisciplinary care in selected patients with NCNNLM.

This chapter summarizes existing data regarding treatment of the most common of these uncommon diseases.

General overview of noncolorectal non-neuroendocrine liver metastases

Although it might appear that patients with isolated liver metastases can benefit from hepatic resection, the proper selection of patients that may potentially benefit from treatment remains the most critical issue. Patient selection criteria depend on the primary tumor type. After selection based on patient performance status and evaluation of comorbidities, staging studies are required not only to assess the overall disease status of the patient but also to characterize all liver lesions (benign and malignant) and their precise location relative to intrahepatic vascular structures. Assessment of the liver volume that will remain after resection is an equally important component of surgical planning for extensive hepatectomy.

Staging

Imaging modalities used to stage hepatic disease in patients include abdominal ultrasound scan, computed tomography (CT) scan, magnetic resonance imaging (MRI), and positron emission tomography (PET). Transabdominal ultrasound scan is used largely as a screening modality and to assist with biopsy procedures. Surgical planning requires cross-sectional imaging such as multiphase CT or MRI. Multiphase CT consists of preinfusion phase, arterial dominant phase, portal dominant phase, and, occasionally, late phase. CT is the preferred imaging test for most patients because 1) phase-specific enhancement patterns allow better characterization of lesions, ie, benign versus malignant; 2) it provides excellent rendering of intrahepatic anatomy; 3) it allows volumetric measurement of the liver remnant, greatly increasing safety of extended resection; and 4) it accurately stages lung, bowel, and peritoneum. MRI can be particularly useful for the characterization of very small hypervascular lesions and for the exclusion of benign processes such as cysts, hemangiomas, and nodular hyperplasia. It is less helpful for the diagnosis of extrahepatic disease (excluding the pancreas).

A frequently used whole-body imaging modality is the PET scan, a functional study most commonly using ^{18}F-2-fluoro-2-deoxy-D-glucose (FDG) [1]. Although whole-body PET does not provide the same anatomic detail as CT or MR imaging, it can be of significant value for staging. Additional advantages include high diagnostic sensitivity in some anatomic regions, multiplanar images, and the absence of CT contrast-related problems. PET does not detect nonhypermetabolic lesions; therefore, the results may be somewhat misleading after chemotherapy.

Principles of hepatic resection for metastatic disease

Patient selection and oncologic outcome of metastasectomy depends fundamentally on complete resection of all disease. In contrast, surgical outcome after major hepatic resection hinges on the postresection liver volume and function. Thus, preoperative studies are essential in defining both the extent and the limits of surgical resection. We have shown that hepatic volumetry to assess the planned future liver remnant (FLR) volume is a critical tool for the selection of patients who will undergo major hepatic resection [2]. To minimize the risk of liver failure and related complications, the FLR volume should be $\geq 20\%$ of the standardized total liver volume for nondiseased livers, $\geq 30\%$ in patients who have received extensive preoperative chemotherapy and $\geq 40\%$ in well-compensated cirrhotic patients [2]. If the future liver remnant is of inadequate volume, preoperative portal vein embolization can be used to induce hypertrophy of the future liver remnant to allow safe resection. Liver tumors are deemed resectable if preoperative evaluation shows that complete resection of the tumor-bearing liver leaves an adequate remnant volume with adequate vascular inflow, outflow, and biliary drainage [3]. Such a determination requires a multidisciplinary evaluation that includes evaluation by a surgeon with significant experience in hepatic surgery. This applies particularly to NCNNLM, because the treatment of each individual tumor type requires expertise in staging, systemic therapy, and hepatic surgery.

Nonresectional treatment

Surgical resection remains the gold standard for treatment of any liver tumor, primary or metastatic. However, percutaneous and intraoperative ablative techniques play a role in the treatment of many types of liver tumors because the therapy 1) can be performed percutaneously or with minimally invasive approaches, 2) is associated with low morbidity and mortality, and 3) can help preserve liver parenchyma in selected patients. The most common ablative method used today is radiofrequency ablation (RFA). Radiofrequency energy is delivered via a needle array to produce coagulation necrosis in the target tissue. Complications of RFA such as bleeding, hepatic fluid collections, and pleural effusions are relatively uncommon (< 10%) [4]. RFA is not effective for large tumors or tumors located near large branches of the portal veins, hepatic veins, and main bile ducts. Because of the relative paucity of data on the long-term outcome of RFA, indications for its use are even more difficult to define than for liver resection. RFA has been performed with curative intent alone or in combination with resection when all identifiable tumors can be resected or ablated. Long-term outcome data for RFA of liver lesions have consistently shown local failure rates of up to 30%, even for lesions <4 cm in diameter, suggesting caution when applying RFA with curative intent in lieu of resection [5–7]. In highly selected cases, RFA can be used to ablate large numbers of hepatic lesions (15 or more). This is usually done to palliate symptoms rather than with curative intent, for example, in patients with carcinoid LM suffering from carcinoid syndrome.

The role of nonresectional ablative approaches specifically for NCNNLM is not well defined. Data and experience are still accruing, and for now such treatment should be considered only in those centers that can provide the full spectrum of therapies for liver metastases.

Regional nonsurgical therapies

Hepatic artery infusion (HAI), transarterial embolization (TAE), and transarterial chemoembolization (TACE) are established liver-directed therapies for the treatment of CRC and neuroendocrine liver metastases [8]. Their utility in the treatment of NCNNLM is less well understood.

TACE is a combination of intraarterial chemotherapy and hepatic artery embolization, whereas TAE omits the chemotherapeutic agent. Hepatic arterial infusion therapy may be delivered as a single percutaneous transarterial injection or as bolus or continuous infusion via an implanted port or pump. All these treatments have been used in combination with ablation and hepatic resection. They rely on the fact that most malignant liver tumors derive their blood supply largely from the hepatic artery and that the liver rapidly clears chemotherapy agents before they can reach the systemic circulation.

In a small study, TAE was found to be effective for soft tissue sarcoma (STS) and gastrointestinal stromal tumor (GIST) liver metastases [9]. In an MD Anderson study of 110 patients with unresectable GIST LM treated with TACE, median overall survival was 17.2 months and the 3-year overall survival rate was 20% (75% had tumors >5 cm, 52% had >5 LM, and 36% had extrahepatic disease) [10]. Outcome was superior in patients with fewer than five tumors, after multiple TACE procedures and with the addition of imatinib therapy.

For ocular melanoma, TACE or HAI chemotherapy can be effective [11]. In one study, 18 of 24 patients treated with infusional 1,3-bis(2-chloroethyl)-1-nitrosourea (BCNU) derived a benefit including one complete response, four partial responses, and 13 cases of stable disease [12]. Despite good control of hepatic disease, 13 patients had extrahepatic progression.

TACE, TAE, and hepatic artery infusion are not considered standard therapy for NCNNLM. For certain tumor subtypes, including unresectable STS and GIST, these approaches hold promise.

Specific tumor types

Gastrointestinal tumors

NCNN gastrointestinal tumor patients with isolated LM are rare and represent a small proportion of the larger NCNNLM patient cohort. Collected series suggest poor survival rates after hepatic resection [13]. Overall reported survival rates for patients with LM from gastrointestinal tumors (esophageal, stomach, duodenum, pancreas, and small bowel) are worse than for those with nongastrointestinal LM.

Esophagus and stomach

Survival after treatment for esophageal carcinoma LM is dismal based on case reports using hepatic resection plus hepatic arterial infusion therapy and systemic therapy [14]. Currently, there are no accepted indications for resection of esophageal cancer LM, either for palliation or cure.

The justification for resection of gastric cancer liver metastases remains controversial [15]. A few published series from Japan and Korea, where the incidence of gastric cancer is high, specifically address gastric cancer LM. One of the first reported studies showed a median survival of 19 months with 4% of the patients surviving beyond 5 years [16]. Subsequent larger series suggest that better outcome may be achieved with careful patient selection. In a series of 90 patients with gastric adenocarcinoma and synchronous or metachronous hepatic metastases, 19 underwent curative resection with a 5-year survival rate of 34% and no operative mortality [17]. Eleven patients received additional systemic or locoregional chemotherapy. A subsequent series of 22 resected patients found overall 1-year, 3-year, and 5-year survival rates of 73%, 38%, and 38%, respectively. Only five patients survived recurrence-free for more than 3 years. The number of LM was the only significant prognostic factor [18]. Both studies suggest that most long-term survivors after hepatic resection for gastric LM had solitary liver lesions, well-differentiated tumors, and metachronous presentation. However, recurrences were common in both studies (up to 68% at 26 months of follow-up).

A larger series of 40 patients undergoing hepatic resection for gastric cancer metastases confirmed these findings [19]. Overall survival rate was 27% at 2 years but only 11% at 10 years with 6 patients surviving more than 5 years. Recurrences were seen in the majority of patients, mostly in the remaining liver. Disease-free interval and resection margin were significant prognostic factors by univariate analysis, but only disease-free interval was an independent prognostic factor for survival in multivariate analysis. Patients with solitary or few tumors, metachronous presentation, and a wide margin resection achieved a 37% 5-year overall survival [19], emphasizing the importance of patient selection.

Currently, hepatic resection for gastric adenocarcinoma cannot be recommended as standard of care. Data supporting hepatic resection in highly selected patients need confirmation by additional clinical studies.

Small bowel

Metastases from small bowel adenocarcinoma are most often widespread and associated with a dismal outcome regardless of treatment. Some larger mixed series contain a few patients with duodenal, jejunal, or ileal adenocarcinoma that underwent resection of LM with dismal reported survival [20]. There currently are no data to support resection of small bowel LM except in highly selected cases.

Anus

Liver metastases from anal adenocarcinoma are very uncommon, and a meaningful discussion of the indications for resection is difficult. In a large series, less than 1% of patients who underwent hepatic resection for NCNNLM had the primary diagnosis of anal cancer. The large European registry, which includes 1452 patients who had NCNNLM resected, reports on only 14 patients with resected anal carcinoma LM. Eight of the 14 patients had recurrence after hepatic resection at a median follow-up of 9 months [21].

Bile ducts and pancreas

In a collected series of patients with NCNNLM, fewer than ten patients had pancreatic, biliary, or periampullary primary tumors. Even in larger series of NCNNLM, only 1% to 5.5% of patients carry the diagnosis of primary ampullary, exocrine pancreatic, biliary, or gallbladder cancer [13,22–25]. Overall survival rarely exceeds 2 years and in many patients does not reach 6 months [23].

Gallbladder, hilar bile ducts, and ampulla. Fewer than 20 reports of patients with gallbladder, cholangiocarcinoma, and ampullary carcinoma treated for LM are available. Among 45 cases of hepatic metastases from gallbladder carcinoma, cholangiocarcinoma, and ampullary carcinoma, a total of two patients with gallbladder carcinoma and one with ampullary carcinoma survived 5 years. The European registry reported 15 patients who had liver metastases resected from ampullary carcinoma. Data suggest that highly selected patients who underwent hepatic resection for ampullary carcinoma metastases and to a lesser degree, gallbladder cancer metastases, derived a modest survival benefit. About half of the patients with primary ampullary carcinomas had recurrence at a median follow-up of 23 months; 29% of the patients had recurrence with extrahepatic disease [21].

There are small reports of hepatic resection for gallbladder liver metastasis after hepatic artery infusion (HAI) therapy. The largest is a retrospective analysis of 59 patients with stage IV primary gallbladder cancer treated either by surgery, chemotherapy (*cis*-diammine-dichloro-platinum-II and 5-fluorouracil), or best supportive therapy [26]. Twenty-nine patients underwent surgical resection for their primary gallbladder carcinoma, and 14 of the 29 had resected metastatic disease in lymph nodes (n = 8), liver (n = 5), and peritoneum (n = 1). Overall survival rate after resection of metastatic disease including the liver at 1 year was only 17%, and no patient was alive 2 years after resection. These results show no improvement of survival over systemic chemotherapy alone in patients who did not have resection [26]. Similarly, among five cases of resected hilar cholangiocarcinoma LM, there were no long-term survivors [21].

There currently are no generally accepted indications for hepatic resection in patients with gallbladder cancer, cholangiocarcinoma, or ampullary carcinoma. Judicious treatment recommendations should be made on a case-by-case basis.

Pancreas. Even for pancreatic carcinoma patients without LM, the overall survival is poor with few 5-year survivors and a median survival time of 18 to 24 months. In a total of 14 published series including 23 patients who underwent hepatic resection for metastatic pancreatic cancer, five patients (13%) were alive at 5 years. Takada and colleagues [27] reported one of the earliest series of patients with invasive ductal adenocarcinoma of the pancreatic head who underwent pancreatico-duodenectomy and simultaneous hepatic resection for metastatic disease. Of 33 patients found to have LM, only 11 underwent curative resection. The longest survival time was 10 months, and median survival time was 6 months. Significant operative mortality was observed.

Adam and colleagues [21] reported on 41 patients who underwent hepatic resection for metastatic pancreatic carcinoma (92% adenocarcinoma). The overall survival rate was 25% at 5 years (20% for adenocarcinoma) with three actual 5-year survivors. Yedibela and colleagues [28] reported a cohort of 161 patients with metastatic LM of, which 21 had primary pancreatic tumors. Although the exact survival of patients with pancreatic adenocarcinoma was not reported, the study suggests that patients with gastrointestinal tumors including the pancreas did poorly with a reported 5-year survival rate between 0 and 12% for surgical resection.

LM from pancreatic adenocarcinoma occurs nearly always in the setting of disseminated systemic disease. Five-year survival has been observed in anecdotal cases, but these patients uniformly succumb to recurrent disease. In the overwhelming majority of cases, benefit cannot be expected from hepatic resection for this disease.

Breast

A role for hepatic resection for breast LM in highly selected patients is gradually being clarified. Early series reported 9% to 22% 5-year overall survival rates, with a predominant pattern of recurrence in the liver (up to 67%) [29,30]. More recent studies suggest that with careful patient selection, resection of breast LM can produce long-term survival.

With aggressive staging using systematic intraoperative ultrasound scan and preoperative and intraoperative biopsy of all suspicious extrahepatic sites, we found a 61% 5-year overall survival rate with a median overall survival of 25 months in patients who had breast cancer LM resected [31]. Importantly, 80% of patients in our series received systemic chemotherapy. and 45% received hormonal therapy in conjunction with hepatic resection. A subsequent series of resected breast LM from Adam and colleagues [32] complemented these findings. In 85 patients, some of whom had known extrahepatic disease and clinical response to prehepatectomy chemotherapy, the 5-year overall survival rate was 37%, and median overall survival was 34 months; 83% of patients received chemotherapy, and 34% received hormonal therapy. Analysis of outcome predictors from these two studies show that a disease-free interval of less than 1 year from breast primary to liver metastasis diagnosis and a positive hepatic resection margins diminish the probability of long-term survival. Patients with relatively limited hepatic metastatic burden and long disease-free intervals are likely to benefit from hepatic resection. At our center, breast cancer patients who present with isolated synchronous LM are treated initially with systemic chemotherapy. In responders, hepatic resection is only contemplated if no other disease becomes evident during initial systemic treatment. Most candidates of hepatic resection, however, undergo treatment for metachronous disease and only undergo resection for metastatic disease confined to the liver.

Published studies on RFA for breast LM show disappointing results. Livraghi and colleagues [33] reported a series of 24 patients with breast cancer LM who were treated with RFA. All liver lesions had to be visible on transcutaneous ultrasound scan, and extrahepatic disease was ruled out by appropriate staging studies. Despite complete ablations in 59 of 64 lesions by postprocedure imaging, more than 50% of patients had recurrent disease at short follow-up intervals; 71% of all recurrences were seen in the liver. Outcome for RFA has not been comparable with liver resection.

Genitourinary

This category of tumors includes several histologic subtypes including bladder, kidney, prostate, testicles, cervix, uterus, and ovaries. Adrenal tumors, occasionally included in reviews of urologic tumors, are considered separately in this chapter. Prostate, bladder, and kidney tumors rarely metastasize to the liver [34,35]. Data on hepatic resection for prostate and bladder cancer essentially do not exist in the literature. Collected series suggest that among patients with NCNNLM, resection of genitourinary LM is generally associated with a better prognosis than for resection of gastrointestinal LM. More specific data are available for the following subgroups of genitourinary tumors.

Kidney

The number of studies evaluating renal tumors including Wilms' tumors, renal cell adenocarcinomas, and nephroblastomas are few, and the cohorts of patients are small. Data show that liver resection may improve overall survival in selected patients [36]. Beginning with reports in the mid 1990s, outcomes for resection of renal cell carcinoma and Wilms' tumors yielded encouraging results [37]. Alves and colleagues [38] reported a 3-year overall survival rate of 26% and median survival of 26 months in a cohort of 14 patients, ten with renal cell carcinoma and three with Wilms' tumor. Stratification of tumors by histologic subtypes showed better 2-year survival rates for patients with renal cell carcinoma versus other renal tumors (56% versus 38%, respectively). European Registry data confirmed the utility of hepatic resection for renal cell carcinoma [21]. Among 85 patients who underwent resection, the 5-year survival rate was 38% with a median survival time of 36 months. The majority of patients in that series had favorable clear cell carcinoma histology (95%), metachronous disease (84%), and solitary tumors (65%). The overall recurrence rate was 63%. Predictors of recurrence were tumors larger than 10 cm in diameter and a disease-free interval from nephrectomy to diagnosis of liver tumor of less than 2 years.

Testicle

Only 8% of patients with testicular cancer present with LM, but overall survival with chemotherapy is quite remarkable among patients with metastatic seminomatous and nonseminomatous testicular cancer. Five-year survival in the presence of visceral metastases is as high as 67%. Treatment with chemotherapy can lead to complete responses, either with or without residual teratomas. Surgical resection is considered a necessary salvage treatment in the absence of complete radiographic response to systemic therapy, because residual teratomas have been known to degenerate into invasive carcinoma.

In 1999, Hahn and colleagues [39] updated the initial series of patients reported by Goulet and colleagues [40] to include 57 patients who underwent a total of 60 resections. Histologic examinations of the resected liver specimens showed a complete pathologic response in nine, residual teratomas in 29, and viable malignant tumors in 19 patients. Patients with a complete response had the lowest recurrence rate at an average 47 months' follow-up. Patients with residual teratomas had eight recurrences and six deaths at an average follow-up of 57 months; 11 of 14 patients with residual active disease died of disease progression at an average follow-up of 20 months. The overall survival rate for the entire cohort of patients was 97% at 2 years. Similar data from Rivoire and colleagues [41] in 37 patients who underwent hepatic resection for germ cell tumors yielded a 5-year overall survival rate of 62% with 23 of 27 patients free of disease at a median follow-up of 66 months. Some investigators recommend close follow-up of small residual liver lesions after chemotherapy and reserve surgical resection for patients with lesions that increase in size during careful follow-up [42]. Based on existing data, including the European registry data (a 5-year overall survival rate of 51% in 78 patients who had resection), "salvage" hepatic resection should be considered because 1) resection is the only way to confirm a complete response in the residual liver masses, 2) teratomas may progress to malignant transformation in 30% of cases, 3) mortality and morbidity from hepatic resection is low, and 4) if feasible, concomitant resection of liver metastases and residual retroperitoneal disease is associated with favorable outcome.

Uterus and ovary

Published collected series of patients who underwent hepatic resection for uterine cancer metastases include 16 studies and a total of 38 patients with mixed tumor histologies. A combined 3-year survival rate of 31% was observed. Only four patients were alive after 5 years. Registry data [21] on 43 patients who underwent hepatic resection of primary uterine cancer include a majority of stromal tumors and squamous cancers (20 patients) with known better prognosis. In the entire cohort, 90% presented with metachronous disease and 75% with solitary metastasis, emphasizing a highly selected population. About half of the patients received some form of preoperative chemotherapy. The 5-year overall survival rate for the entire group was 35%. It is difficult to draw general recommendations from these limited data.

The concept of hepatic resection for LM from ovarian cancer has evolved from the fact that cytoreductive surgery can significantly alter the natural history of ovarian cancer metastatic to the peritoneum. Studies have found the value of hepatic metastasectomy during secondary cytoreductive surgery with a reported median survival of 43 months in patients with recurrent ovarian carcinomatosis. Yoon and colleagues [43] described 24 patients (21 with ovarian, three with fallopian tube carcinoma) with hepatic metastases resected as part of a secondary cytoreductive procedure. All patients had metachronous disease, with a median disease-free interval of 36.5 months and median time from first diagnosis of 69 months. Sixteen of 24 patients had solitary liver lesions, and 19 received preoperative chemotherapy. Median overall survival after LM resection and repeat peritoneal cytoreduction was 62 months. The Mayo Clinic reported a similar experience with resected ovarian cancer in 26 patients [44]. Most had stage III primary disease with a 30-month disease free interval. Two thirds of the patients had solitary liver lesions, and most underwent additional peritoneal cytoreduction at the time of liver resection. They reported a 27-month median survival in optimally cytoreduced patients. Both studies concluded that liver resection is beneficial for patients with limited hepatic involvement and a disease-free interval exceeding 1 year, provided that optimal cytoreduction of extrahepatic disease can be achieved. The European registry report [21] includes 65 patients with ovarian cancer LM. Hepatic metastasectomy led to a 50% 5-year overall survival rate.

Resection of ovarian LM may be considered in carefully selected patients that are candidates for complete cytoreduction after evaluation by a multidisciplinary team.

Melanoma

Isolated liver metastasis from cutaneous melanoma is uncommon. However, isolated LM from ocular melanoma occurs in 70% to 80% of those in whom metastatic disease develops. Hepatic resection has been performed in both populations, although outcomes differ based on the primary site of origin.

A large study from Rivoire and colleagues [45] screened 602 patients with uveal melanoma seen at their institution over a 14-year period using abdominal ultrasound scan every 6 months. Sixty-three (10%) patients were found to have LM after a median time of 29 months from primary diagnosis. Among those with LM, 28 were treated by hepatic resection followed by hepatic artery infusion chemotherapy, and 25 were treated by systemic therapy or supportive treatment. Half of the surgically resected patients (n = 14) underwent R0 resection; the other half underwent planned R2 debulking procedures (R2 resection). All patients who had resection received adjuvant hepatic artery infusion with fotemustine. The outcome analysis revealed little value for debulking R2 resections with a median survival of 16 months versus 11 months for nonsurgical therapy. R0 resections provided superior outcome with a 24-month median overall survival. The reported data suggested that those patients with nonciliary body tumors tended to fare better than those with ciliary-body uveal lesions.

A subsequent study by our group examined 16 patients with uveal melanoma and 24 with cutaneous melanoma hepatic metastases [46]. Most (65%) received adjuvant therapy, including hepatic artery embolization or infusion and bio-immunotherapy or vaccine therapy. Characteristics of patients who had resection were similar between ocular and cutaneous melanoma groups: the interval from primary diagnosis to LM diagnosis (62.9 versus 63.1 months), the proportion with solitary liver lesions (50% versus 67%), and the median tumor sizes (4.3 versus 4.2 cm). Outcomes, however, differed significantly. Five-year overall survival rate after resection was 20% in patients with ocular melanoma versus 0% in those with cutaneous melanoma. More than half (53%) of the resected ocular melanoma patients had recurrence in the liver compared with only 17% of those with cutaneous melanoma. Recurrences in cutaneous melanoma patients tended to be more disseminated and involved multiple extrahepatic sites. The disease-free interval after resection was twice as long for ocular (8.8 months) than cutaneous melanoma (4.7 months). Patients with smaller tumors (<5 cm) and response to systemic therapy tended to do better in both groups. Primary tumor factors such as tumor thickness, lymph node status, and tumor ulceration did not correlate with outcome after hepatic resection.

Hepatic resection for uveal or cutaneous melanoma should only be considered in a multidisciplinary setting and by experienced hepatic surgeons.

Adrenal

In the absence of exclusive reports on patients with adrenal carcinoma liver metastases, much of the information about their treatment is derived from studies on general reviews of NCNNLM.

Although a majority of adrenal tumors are nonsecretory, a small percentage of patients have subclinical Cushing's syndrome, pheochromocytomas, or aldosterone-producing adenomas. As shown in the largest series reported to date of 28 patients (17 pheochromocytomas, eight adrenocortical carcinoma, and two unknown type), hepatic metastasectomy is associated with a 66% 5-year overall survival rate and a 63-month median survival [21]. Most of the patients had fewer than three hepatic metastases, and 79% had metachronous disease. The median time from primary diagnosis to the development of liver metastasis was 31 months. The 5-year recurrence-free survival rate was 31%; 16 (57%) patients had recurrence, including nine with intrahepatic recurrences. Of those who had recurrence in the liver, five patients underwent successful repeat hepatic resections. With a reported 5-year overall survival rate of 10% and median survival of 8 months for unresected patients with stage IV adrenocortical carcinoma, these findings support the use of hepatic resection in these patients. Unfortunately, less than 10% of patients with adrenal LM are suitable candidates for hepatic surgery.

Overall, hepatic resection can provide acceptable results in selected patients with limited adrenal metastases, particularly for palliation of symptoms in patients with secreting hepatic tumors. For patients with symptomatic disease who are not candidates for surgery, ablative therapy such as RFA may be an effective alternative therapy for symptom control [47].

Soft tissue sarcoma and gastrointestinal stromal tumor

Hepatic resection for STS metastases is indicated for disease confined to the liver. Patients with retroperitoneal and intra-abdominal visceral STS and those with leiomyosarcomas are more likely to have liver-only metastatic disease than are patients with extra-abdominal STS [48]. GIST is a subset of leiomyosarcomas, distinguished by the presence of a mutation within the c-*Kit* gene, which codes for a 145 kilodalton transmembrane glycoprotein. A mutation, usually at codon 11, leads to the constitutive activation of receptor tyrosine kinase and is responsible for the particular sensitivity of this tumor to the molecular targeted agent imatinib mesylate, which blocks c-*Kit* activation, inhibits downstream signaling, and induces apoptosis. Therapy with imatinib has revolutionized the treatment of patients with GIST and has been used alone and in conjunction with hepatic resection for GIST LM. Non-GIST STSs generally do not respond to imatinib therapy. The evolving role for imatinib in the multidisciplinary treatment of patients with GIST LM is integrated in the discussion of hepatic resection for GIST below.

Although no prospective data are available regarding resection of STS LM, two retrospective studies [49,50] and two retrospective analyses of prospectively collected data [51,52] provide important information. Attention must be given to differences in the definition of "complete" resection among studies: R0 only (resection with grossly and microscopically negative surgical margins) versus R0 *or* R1 (inclusion of patients with grossly negative but microscopically positive surgical margins).

The first report [49] on 11 consecutive patients who underwent hepatic resection for leiomyosarcoma found a median overall survival of 39 months. Importantly, the median survival for the 6 patients who underwent R0 resections was not reached at 56 months' follow-up, whereas all five patients with R1 or R2 resection succumbed to disease by 39 months (median 25 months). In a subsequent report on leiomyosarcoma over a period of 15 years, 23 hepatic resections for metastases were reviewed [50]. For the 15 patients who underwent R0 resection, the median survival was 32 months and the 5-year survival rate was 33%. For the eight patients that underwent R1 or R2 resection, the median survival was 20.5 months. None of the 11 patients who underwent repeat resection for recurrences survived an additional 5 years, but the median overall survival after repeat resection was 31 months. Both studies emphasize the importance of R0 resection, the potential for long-term disease control with resection, and the value of repeat resection in selected patients.

A report from Memorial Sloan-Kettering Cancer Center [51] updated the institution's previously reported experience with resection of STS LM [53]. Among 331 patients with STS LM admitted from 1982 to 2000, 56 underwent grossly complete resection (R0 or R1). Patients were selected for resection based on performance status, estimated safety of procedure, control of primary tumor, resectability (distribution) of hepatic disease, and absence of extrahepatic disease. Of the 56 patients, 34 (61%) had GIST or gastrointestinal leiomyosarcomas. At 25 months' follow-up, the median survival for the entire R0/R1 group was 39 months, with a 5-year survival rate of 30% (with 10 actual 5-year survivors). The authors noted that patients who did not undergo complete resection (R2 resection, exploration without resection, or no exploration) had a median survival of only 12 months with a 5-year survival rate of 4%. Patterns of recurrence after resection of LM were predominantly in the liver (56%), at the primary site (41%), or in the lung (18%). A resection with a positive margin was the sole risk factor for recurrence and death after resection of STS liver metastases. Factors such as primary tumor site (retroperitoneal) and tumor grade (high grade) did not predict death or recurrence when liver resection margin was included in the analysis.

A recent report from the M. D. Anderson Cancer Center that included 66 patients with STS LM [52] showed a 5-year overall survival rate of 27% after liver resection. Recurrences were most common in the remnant liver (16 patients), at distant sites (11 patients), or both (17 patients) for an overall recurrence rate of 67%. Median overall survival with radiofrequency ablation alone or in combination with hepatic resection was worse (33 months) than for hepatic resection alone (54 months). Adjuvant chemotherapy provided a survival benefit when combined with hepatic resection. Patients with GIST tumors who underwent complete resection *and* were treated with imatinib had the longest median survival of all studied groups with metastatic STS (median survival not reached, 5-year survival approximately 50%). Patients with hepatic GIST metastases treated with resection but without imatinib showed a 5-year survival rate of 34% and a median survival of 36 months. Further data regarding the value of imatinib for resectable GIST tumors will come from an ongoing prospective trial sponsored by the American College of Surgeons Oncology Group (ACOSOG).

R0 resection of STS LM, especially for GIST, is associated with long-term survival when combined with systemic chemotherapy or molecular targeted therapy. Debulking surgery (R2 resection) is of questionable benefit. RFA shows results equivalent to an R2 resection and therefore should be discouraged if complete resection is safe and feasible. Finally, "complete" radiographic response assessed by CT or PET, including cystic changes after imatinib treatment of GIST, are not necessarily equivalent to complete pathologic response [54,55]. Because hepatic lesions contain viable tumor in >85% of cases after chemotherapy and biologic therapy, the goal of surgical treatment is complete removal of all residual disease including small residual cystic lesions and "scars."

Other tumors

For several other tumor types, anecdotal cases of hepatic resections have been reported. These include squamous cell carcinoma from many sites of origin and lung primary tumors of different histology.

Squamous cell carcinoma

For squamous cell carcinoma (SCCA), French registry data [21] report on 15 patients with head and neck primary tumors, a majority of who had SCCA. Hepatic resection for LM in this cohort led to a 3-year survival rate of 24% with a median survival of only 18 months. A multicenter US study analyzed 40 patients with SCCA LM from multiple sites of origin including anus (n = 23), head and neck (n = 6), lung (n = 3), gallbladder (n = 3), cervix (n = 2), and other (n = 3) [56]. Most patients presented with metachronous disease and received neoadjuvant chemotherapy. The majority of patients (n = 25) had solitary hepatic metastasis. The median diameter of the largest lesion was 3.5 cm. The median survival after hepatic resection was 34.9 months, and the 5-year overall survival rate was 32%. Despite a longer median time to recurrence, patients with anal cancer had shorter recurrence-free and 5-year survival times. Synchronous or bilobar disease and a positive surgical margin were associated with worse survival. At a median follow-up of 17 months, 23 patients (58%) had recurrence. The authors concluded that hepatic resection for metastatic SCCA can provide long-term survival, especially in patients with primary sites other than anus, in those with limited metachronous disease, and after obtaining a negative margin resection. Because the dataset is so heterogeneous, standard recommendations cannot be made, except that careful patient selection for hepatic resection is mandatory.

There are only 52 reported cases in the literature of hepatic resections for pulmonary LM. Five-year overall survival rates range from 8% to 10%, but data do not permit identification of a subset for which resection can be recommended.

Unknown primary cancer

The limited data on hepatic resection for highly selected patients with LM from unknown primary are encouraging. A large multi-institutional series [21] reported on 28 patients with unknown primary tumor LM and revealed a 5-year survival rate of 38% and median survival time of 30 months after resection, which was comparable to patients with primary tumors from adrenal, testicular, breast, and renal origin. Patients with stromal histology, adenocarcinoma, and sarcoma had 5-year survival rates >30%. Ultimately, hepatic resection can be considered in selected patients with localized metastases when all disease can be resected. Evidence regarding the value of preoperative chemotherapy is lacking. The treatment plan for these patients should be individualized and discussed in a multidisciplinary team.

Summary

The paradigm for the treatment of liver metastases is evolving rapidly because of improved patient selection, better staging, safe hepatic resection techniques, and significant advances in systemic therapies. Tumor biologies among NCNNLM vary widely, and their treatment requires dedicated multidisciplinary teams with expertise in diverse areas including hepatic surgery, surgical oncology, medical oncology, radiation oncology, diagnostic

Table 1
Overall survival in combined series for non-colorectal, non-neureoendocrine liver metastases

First author of study	Total No. of patients with LM	No. of patients[a] with NCNNLM	Gastrointestinal	Genitourinary	Breast	Melanoma	STS	HN/thyroid/ lung	NE	Other	5-year overall survival (%)	Median survival (mo)
Harrison [25]	96	96	7	34	—		41	HN 2	—	8	37	32
Lindell [23]	32	21	Stomach 3		—	3	2		11	—	36	32
Elias [13]	147	120	Stomach 11	Testis 20 Kidney 4 GYN 6	35	10	13	HN 5	27	10	36	NR
Hemming [24]	37	37	Esophagus 1 Small bowel 4 Pancreas 2	Renal 7 Adrenal 3	—	5	7	Thyroid 2	—	3	45	46
Yedibela [28]	162	150	50	11	24		15		12	20	26	23
Ercolani [57]	83	83	Esophagus 3 Stomach 10 Small bowel 2 Pancreas 3	15	29		10		—	19	34	NR

Weitz [22]	141	141	Stomach 3 Duodenal 1 Ampullary 2 Pancreas 5 Anal 1	50 Adrenal 15	29	17	—	Lung 4	—	14	30 (3 yr)	17
Adam [21]	1452	1452	GEJ 25 Esophagus 20 Stomach 64 Small bowel 28 Duodenal 12 Ampullary 15 Pancreas 40	Adrenal 28 Testis 78 Renal 85 Uterine 43	454	Cut 44 Oc 104	—	Lung 32 HN 15	—	28	36	35

Abbreviations: Cut, cutaneous; GEJ, gastroesophageal junction; GYN, gynecologic; HN, head and neck; LM, liver metastases; NE, neuroendocrine; NR, not reported; Oc, ocular; STS, soft tissue sarcoma.

[a] Some series did not report tumor origin when <2 patients per group; therefore, subgroups may not add up to total number of patients for each study.

Table 2
Outcome after treatment of subtypes of non-colorectal, non-neuroendocrine liver metastases: case series

Primary tumor	First author of study	No. of patients	5-year overall survival (%)	Median survival (mo)
Melanoma (ocular and cutaneous)	Pawlik [46]	40	11	28
Gastric adenocarcinoma	Ambiru [19]	40	18	Not reported
	Zacherl [15]	15	14	16
	Sakamoto [18]	22	38	21
	Okano [17]	90	34	Not reported
Pancreatic adenocarcinoma	Takada [27]	11	0	6
Breast	Selzner [30]	17	22	24
	Elias [29]	54	34	34
	Vlastos [31]	31	61	63
	Adam [21]	85	37	32
STS	DeMatteo [51]	56	51	39
	Pawlik [52]	35	27[a]	Not reached
Renal	Kierney [36]	41	31	41
Testicular	Hahn [39]	57	97 (2 yr)	Not reached
	Rivoire [41]	37	62	Not reached

[a] Includes patients who underwent radiofrequency ablation only.

imaging, and interventional radiology. Patient care must be individualized, especially in the absence of data to clearly guide therapy (Tables 1 and 2). When hepatic-directed therapy is deemed appropriate, complete resection of all hepatic disease using modern approaches to hepatic surgery are most likely to provide acceptable outcomes for palliation or potential cure. After review by an experienced multidisciplinary team, ablation techniques and arterial embolization can be effective adjuncts to therapy in selected patients who are not candidates for complete resection. Among liver-directed therapies for NCNNLM, hepatic resection remains the gold standard.

Improved patient selection, introduction of more effective systemic treatments including targeted biologic and combined therapies, and the low morbidity and mortality rates of hepatobiliary surgery in centers of excellence are likely to provide continued improvements in outcomes for patients with NCNNLM. Further advances in treatment may emerge from better understanding of the underlying tumor biology for each cancer type and application of individualized care to each patient.

References

[1] Choi J. Imaging of hepatic metastases. Cancer Control 2006;1:6–12.
[2] Abdalla EK, Adam R, Bilchik AJ, et al. Improving resectability of hepatic colorectal metastases: expert consensus statement. Ann Surg Oncol 2006;10:1271–80.

[3] Charnsangavej C, Clary B, Fong Y, et al. Selection of patients for resection of hepatic colorectal metastases: expert consensus statement. Ann Surg Oncol 2006;10:1261–8.
[4] Curley SA, Marra P, Beaty K, et al. Early and late complications after radiofrequency ablation of malignant liver tumors in 608 patients. Ann Surg 2004;4:450–8.
[5] Abdalla EK, Vauthey JN, Ellis LM, et al. Recurrence and outcomes following hepatic resection, radiofrequency ablation, and combined resection/ablation for colorectal liver metastases. Ann Surg 2004;6:818–25.
[6] Aloia TA, Vauthey JN, Loyer EM, et al. Solitary colorectal liver metastasis: resection determines outcome. Arch Surg 2006;141(5):460–6 [discussion: 466–7].
[7] Amersi FF, McElrath-Garza A, Ahmad A, et al. Long-term survival after radiofrequency ablation of complex unresectable liver tumors. Arch Surg 2006;6:581–7.
[8] Gupta S, Johnson MM, Murthy R, et al. Hepatic arterial embolization and chemoembolization for the treatment of patients with metastatic neuroendocrine tumors: variables affecting response rates and survival. Cancer 2005;8:1590–602.
[9] Maluccio MA, Covey AM, Schubert J, et al. Treatment of metastatic sarcoma to the liver with bland embolization. Cancer 2006;7:1617–23.
[10] Kobayashi K, Gupta S, Trent JC, et al. Hepatic artery chemoembolization for 110 gastrointestinal stromal tumors: response, survival, and prognostic factors. Cancer 2006;12: 2833–41.
[11] Vogl T, Eichler K, Zangos S, et al. Preliminary experience with transarterial chemoembolization (TACE) in liver metastases of uveal malignant melanoma: local tumor control and survival. J Cancer Res Clin Oncol 2007;3:177–84.
[12] Patel K, Sullivan K, Berd D, et al. Chemoembolization of the hepatic artery with BCNU for metastatic uveal melanoma: results of a phase II study. Melanoma Res 2005;4: 297–304.
[13] Elias D, Cavalcanti de Albuquerque A, Eggenspieler P, et al. Resection of liver metastases from a noncolorectal primary: indications and results based on 147 monocentric patients. J Am Coll Surg 1998;5:487–93.
[14] Yamamoto T, Tachibana M, Kinugasa S, et al. Esophagectomy and hepatic arterial chemotherapy following hepatic resection for esophageal cancer with liver metastasis. J Gastroenterol 2001;8:560–3.
[15] Zacherl J, Zacherl M, Scheuba C, et al. Analysis of hepatic resection of metastasis originating from gastric adenocarcinoma. J Gastrointest Surg 2002;5:682–9.
[16] Ochiai T, Sasako M, Mizuno S, et al. Hepatic resection for metastatic tumours from gastric cancer: analysis of prognostic factors. Br J Surg 1994;8:1175–8.
[17] Okano K, Maeba T, Ishimura K, et al. Hepatic resection for metastatic tumors from gastric cancer. Ann Surg 2002;1:86–91.
[18] Sakamoto Y, Ohyama S, Yamamoto J, et al. Surgical resection of liver metastases of gastric cancer: an analysis of a 17-year experience with 22 patients. Surgery 2003;5: 507–11.
[19] Ambiru S, Miyazaki M, Ito H, et al. Benefits and limits of hepatic resection for gastric metastases. Am J Surg 2001;3:279–83.
[20] Dabaja BS, Suki D, Pro B, et al. Adenocarcinoma of the small bowel: presentation, prognostic factors, and outcome of 217 patients. Cancer 2004;3:518–26.
[21] Adam R, Chiche L, Aloia T, et al. Hepatic resection for noncolorectal nonendocrine liver metastases: analysis of 1,452 patients and development of a prognostic model. Ann Surg 2006;4:524–35.
[22] Weitz J, Blumgart LH, Fong Y, et al. Partial hepatectomy for metastases from noncolorectal, nonneuroendocrine carcinoma. Ann Surg 2005;2:269–76.
[23] Lindell G, Ohlsson B, Saarela A, et al. Liver resection of noncolorectal secondaries. J Surg Oncol 1998;2:66–70.
[24] Hemming AW, Sielaff TD, Gallinger S, et al. Hepatic resection of noncolorectal nonneuroendocrine metastases. Liver Transpl 2000;1:97–101.

[25] Harrison LE, Brennan MF, Newman E, et al. Hepatic resection for noncolorectal, nonneuroendocrine metastases: a fifteen-year experience with ninety-six patients. Surgery 1997;6:625–32.
[26] Ishikawa T, Horimi T, Shima Y, et al. Evaluation of aggressive surgical treatment for advanced carcinoma of the gallbladder. J Hepatobiliary Pancreat Surg 2003;3:233–8.
[27] Takada T, Yasuda H, Amano H, et al. Simultaneous hepatic resection with pancreatoduodenectomy for metastatic pancreatic head carcinoma: does it improve survival? Hepatogastroenterology 1997;14:567–73.
[28] Yedibela S, Gohl J, Graz V, et al. Changes in indication and results after resection of hepatic metastases from noncolorectal primary tumors: a single-institutional review. Ann Surg Oncol 2005;10:778–85.
[29] Elias D, Maisonnette F, Druet-Cabanac M, et al. An attempt to clarify indications for hepatectomy for liver metastases from breast cancer. Am J Surg 2003;2:158–64.
[30] Selzner M, Morse MA, Vredenburgh JJ, et al. Liver metastases from breast cancer: long-term survival after curative resection. Surgery 2000;4:383–9.
[31] Vlastos G, Smith DL, Singletary SE, et al. Long-term survival after an aggressive surgical approach in patients with breast cancer hepatic metastases. Ann Surg Oncol 2004;9:869–74.
[32] Adam R, Aloia T, Krissat J, et al. Is liver resection justified for patients with hepatic metastases from breast cancer? Ann Surg 2006;6:897–907.
[33] Livraghi T, Goldberg SN, Solbiati L, et al. Percutaneous radio-frequency ablation of liver metastases from breast cancer: initial experience in 24 patients. Radiology 2001;1:145–9.
[34] Loberg RD, Fridman Y, Pienta BA, et al. Detection and isolation of circulating tumor cells in urologic cancers: a review. Neoplasia 2004;4:302–9.
[35] Alseidi A, Helton WS, Espat NJ. Does the literature support an indication for hepatic metastasectomy other than for colorectal primary? J Gastrointest Surg 2006;1:99–104.
[36] Kierney PC, van Heerden JA, Segura JW, et al. Surgeon's role in the management of solitary renal cell carcinoma metastases occurring subsequent to initial curative nephrectomy: an institutional review. Ann Surg Oncol 1994;4:345–52.
[37] Schwartz SI. Hepatic resection for noncolorectal nonneuroendocrine metastases. World J Surg 1995;1:72–5.
[38] Alves A, Adam R, Majno P, et al. Hepatic resection for metastatic renal tumors: is it worthwhile? Ann Surg Oncol 2003;6:705–10.
[39] Hahn TL, Jacobson L, Einhorn LH, et al. Hepatic resection of metastatic testicular carcinoma: a further update. Ann Surg Oncol 1999;7:640–4.
[40] Goulet RJ Jr, Hardacre JM, Einhorn LH, et al. Hepatic resection for disseminated germ cell carcinoma. Ann Surg 1990;3:290–3.
[41] Rivoire M, Elias D, De Cian F, et al. Multimodality treatment of patients with liver metastases from germ cell tumors: the role of surgery. Cancer 2001;3:578–87.
[42] Copson E, McKendrick J, Hennessey N, et al. Liver metastases in germ cell cancer: defining a role for surgery after chemotherapy. BJU Int 2004;4:552–8.
[43] Yoon SS, Jarnagin WR, Fong Y, et al. Resection of recurrent ovarian or fallopian tube carcinoma involving the liver. Gynecol Oncol 2003;2:383–8.
[44] Merideth MA, Cliby WA, Keeney GL, et al. Hepatic resection for metachronous metastases from ovarian carcinoma. Gynecol Oncol 2003;1:16–21.
[45] Rivoire M, Kodjikian L, Baldo S, et al. Treatment of liver metastases from uveal melanoma. Ann Surg Oncol 2005;6:422–8.
[46] Pawlik TM, Zorzi D, Abdalla EK, et al. Hepatic resection for metastatic melanoma: distinct patterns of recurrence and prognosis for ocular versus cutaneous disease. Ann Surg Oncol 2006;5:712–20.
[47] Wood BJ, Abraham J, Hvizda JL, et al. Radiofrequency ablation of adrenal tumors and adrenocortical carcinoma metastases. Cancer 2003;3:554–60.

[48] Abdalla EK, Pisters PW. Metastasectomy for limited metastases from soft tissue sarcoma. Curr Treat Options Oncol 2002;6:497–505.
[49] Chen H, Pruitt A, Nicol TL, et al. Complete hepatic resection of metastases from leiomyosarcoma prolongs survival. J Gastrointest Surg 1998;2:151–5.
[50] Lang H, Nussbaum KT, Kaudel P, et al. Hepatic metastases from leiomyosarcoma: A single-center experience with 34 liver resections during a 15-year period. Ann Surg 2000;4:500–5.
[51] DeMatteo RP, Shah A, Fong Y, et al. Results of hepatic resection for sarcoma metastatic to liver. Ann Surg 2001;4:540–7.
[52] Pawlik TM, Vauthey JN, Abdalla EK, et al. Results of a single-center experience with resection and ablation for sarcoma metastatic to the liver. Arch Surg 2006;6:537–43 [discussion: 543–4].
[53] Jaques DP, Coit DG, Casper ES, et al. Hepatic metastases from soft-tissue sarcoma. Ann Surg 1995;4:392–7.
[54] Bechtold RE, Chen MY, Stanton CA, et al. Cystic changes in hepatic and peritoneal metastases from gastrointestinal stromal tumors treated with Gleevec. Abdom Imaging 2003;6: 808–14.
[55] Goh BK, Chow PK, Chuah KL, et al. Pathologic, radiologic and PET scan response of gastrointestinal stromal tumors after neoadjuvant treatment with imatinib mesylate. Eur J Surg Oncol 2006;9:961–3.
[56] Pawlik TM, Bauer TW, Reddy SK, et al. Hepatic resection for metastatic squamous cell carcinoma to the liver: a multi-center analysis. Ann Surg Oncol 2007, in press.
[57] Ercolani G, Grazi GL, Ravaioli M, et al. The role of liver resections for noncolorectal, non-neuroendocrine metastases: experience with 142 observed cases. Ann Surg Oncol 2005;6: 459–66.

ELSEVIER
SAUNDERS

Surg Oncol Clin N Am
16 (2007) 579–605

SURGICAL
ONCOLOGY CLINICS
OF NORTH AMERICA

Surgical and Nonsurgical Therapy for Lung Metastasis: Indications and Outcomes

Todd L. Demmy, MD[a,c,*], Kelli Bullard Dunn, MD[b,c]

[a]*Department of Thoracic Surgery, Roswell Park Cancer Institute, Elm & Carlton Streets, Buffalo, NY 14231, USA*

[b]*Department of Surgical Oncology, Roswell Park Cancer Institute, Elm & Carlton Streets, Buffalo, NY 14231, USA*

[c]*Department of Surgery, State University of New York–Buffalo, Buffalo, NY, USA*

The management of pulmonary metastasis is a broad and multifaceted topic. Because of the filtration function and the favorable microenvironment of the lung, most malignancies cause pulmonary metastases. It is beyond the scope of this article to cite the numerous reports of pulmonary metastasectomy for all histologic subtypes. Comprehensive reviews can be found in several textbooks [1,2]. Rather, this article focuses on recent experience with secondary lung malignancies and their newer treatment options, indications, and technical aspects.

Pulmonary metastasectomy as an adjunct to chest wall resection was first reported in Germany in 1882 [3] and only much later developed into a stand-alone procedure in Europe (1926) and the United States (1930). Its survival benefit was demonstrated in 1947 by Alexander and Haight [4]. Accordingly these investigators are credited with increasing the global interest in metastasectomy. They were the first to require standards for patient selection, such as good primary tumor control and absence of extrathoracic disease.

The pathophysiology of pulmonary metastases is complex and still poorly understood. Tumor growth depends in large part on blood supply from the pulmonary circulation. In 10% to 20% of metastases that occur near the hilum, however, blood supply relies solely on bronchial circulation [5]. Only a small proportion of hematogenous tumor cells actually develop into a lung metastasis [6]. A complex cytokine and immune interaction,

* Corresponding author. Department of Thoracic Surgery, Roswell Park Cancer Institute, Elm & Carlton Streets, Buffalo, NY 14231.

E-mail address: todd.Demmy@roswellpark.org (T.L. Demmy).

1055-3207/07/$ - see front matter © 2007 Elsevier Inc. All rights reserved.
doi:10.1016/j.soc.2007.04.011 ***surgonc.theclinics.com***

successful angiogenesis, and cell trafficking between mediastinal and lymph nodes is necessary for this process [7,8]. Despite the histologic diversity of lung metastases and many different molecular profiles, there is a strikingly similar 5-year survival rate for patients subjected to surgical therapy. This is suggestive of a common fundamental proteomic or genomic profile for those patients who are long-term survivors after lung metastasectomy. Prognostication systems, such as the metagene profile recently shown for lung cancer, may someday improve patient selection for pulmonary metastasectomy [9].

Background and patient selection

Unlike primary lung tumors, it is unusual for pulmonary metastases to cause specific clinical symptoms. With reported diagnostic accuracy rates as low as 5% [10], history and physical examination are unlikely to uncover pulmonary metastatic disease. Documentation of the primary tumor-type and disease-free interval (DFI) is important. Also one has to be cognizant of diseases mimicking pulmonary metastases. On occasion sarcoidosis and Wegener' granulomatosis can be misdiagnosed as cancer metastases. For most histologic types of lung metastases tumor-specific markers are not available. Laboratory testing is therefore of limited value.

Imaging

Unfortunately with most imaging modalities lung metastases strongly resemble benign lesions. Chronic inflammatory conditions can easily be mistaken for malignant nodules [11] and calcified metastatic nodules can mimic calcified granulomas or hamartomas. The hallmarks of pulmonary metastases are multiple round nodules of variable size with possible diffuse thickening of the interstitium [12]. Several helpful imaging characteristics, such as indistinct edge, spiculation, pleural thickening, inhomogeneity, and ground-glass opacity of surrounding lung, determine nodule malignancy on chest CT. Cavitation is common with squamous cell metastases. Calcification is common in sarcomas (particularly osteogenic, chondro, and synovial cell) or giant cell tumor [13] and can often occur in epithelial tumors, such as papillary and mucinous adenocarcinomas. Cavitation and calcification can develop after antineoplastic therapy. Pneumothorax occurs occasionally, especially with osteosarcoma metastases. Endobronchial metastases cause atelectasis, and gastrointestinal malignancies induce air space consolidation. Because of their similar imaging characteristics on CT, colorectal carcinoma metastases can be mistaken for primary adenocarcinomas of the lung [14].

None of the imaging modalities provides reliable distinction between a metastasis sterilized by chemotherapy and residual viable tumor [12]. Position emission tomography (PET) imaging is helpful to separate a benign from a malignant solitary nodule. Its accuracy varies, however, particularly for osteosarcoma metastases [15–17]. PET imaging has limited sensitivity for nodules smaller than 11 mm [18].

New generations of CT scanners with improved resolution and speed of image acquisition have increased the ability to detect pulmonary nodules. With the routine acquisition of thin-sliced CT images, variations in pitch and detector conformation seem to have little effect on the number of malignant nodules found [19,20]. Whether or not the newest generation of scanners are able to detect all foci of metastatic disease, however, remains to be tested [21,22]. The surgeon's ability to remove small lung nodules is improved by CT-guided wire localizing. For intraoperative localization by fluoroscopy or hand-held gamma detectors, radio-opaque markers, visible dyes, and radioactive tracers can be used [23,24]. Operating rooms can be equipped with CT to localize deep-seated lung nodules [25]. Nuclear pharmaceuticals to localize tumors with specific biochemical function are available. Most notably, I^{131} whole body scanning improves detection of pulmonary nodules from thyroid malignancy [26]. Finally, CT scanning documents the response of pulmonary metastases to chemotherapy. Standard bidimensional measurement is used to assess response [27].

General treatment options

Control of primary tumor

Pulmonary metastasectomy should be considered only for patients in whom the primary tumor has been or can be completely resected. The ability to achieve a complete resection (microscopically negative margins; R0) is critical and has been shown to determine local recurrence rate and long-term survival in a wide variety of malignancies. Incomplete resection, either with microscopically positive (R1) or grossly positive (R2) margins, is associated with a high risk for local recurrence and decreased survival. In a clinical setting in which an R0 resection is not possible, pulmonary metastasectomy is contraindicated.

For patients in whom the primary tumor and pulmonary metastases are diagnosed simultaneously (synchronous lesions), the primary tumor is usually resected first and assessed pathologically for negative margins. Following primary tumor resection, adjuvant therapy (chemotherapy or radiation therapy) is sometimes given before lung resection. In this setting, clinical evaluation and imaging should be repeated after completion of adjuvant treatment to ensure that the pulmonary disease remains potentially resectable, additional systemic spread has not occurred, and the primary tumor has not recurred. Similarly in patients who develop metachronous pulmonary metastases, restaging and search for local and systemic recurrence is necessary. If the lung remains the sole site of metastasis in the absence of primary tumor recurrence, the patient is a candidate for pulmonary resection.

Significance of lymph node metastases

Pulmonary metastases often represent only a fraction of the residual tumor burden. In two large series of pulmonary metastasectomy for various histologic subtypes, approximately 30% of patients had positive mediastinal lymph nodes [28,29]. Depending on the histology positive lymph nodes decreased 3-year survival rates by approximately 30%. Nevertheless there were long-term survivors in both groups, and some investigators recommend performing lymph node dissections to improve staging and outcome.

Patient- and physician-controlled factors

Several patient- and physician-controlled factors affect the development or treatment of pulmonary metastases. For instance, smokers increase their risk for developing lung metastases proportionate to the number of cigarettes consumed during their lifetime [30]. Although smoking cessation improves survival even in patients who have advanced lung cancer, it is unclear whether it changes the outcome in metastasectomy patients.

The complex interplay of physician-driven therapeutics on the outcomes of patients is difficult to analyze. Many clinical studies and most experimental research show that stress response adversely affects survival for certain neoplasms. An important review of the adverse effects of surgical trauma on ablative therapy has been published [6]. Some of these findings fuel the debate over the optimal surgical approach for patients who have lung metastases. Surgeons favoring a less invasive approach emphasize the role of the immune system to fight residual disease [31]. Perioperative factors, including the use of blood transfusions, perioperative hypothermia, metabolic control (in particular diabetes), length of ventilatory support, and degree of tissue trauma, are causes for concern. Many of these factors are emerging as important outcome criteria after surgical treatment for metastatic disease.

Surgical approaches to thoracic metastasectomy

The optimal approach for lung metastases resection depends on surgeon experience (or preference) and the anatomic characteristics of the lesion. Rather than relying on one technique, a versatile surgeon can apply any method to fit the unique clinical scenario.

General considerations

Most commonly a surgical stapling system is used to divide the lung parenchyma. A 3.5-mm staple length is most common, but a thicker, 4.8-mm load may be needed in the presence of fibrosis, edema, or cellular infiltration. Endoscopic staplers are reliable but more expensive. Because they are practical in tight spaces, endostaplers are sometimes used in open thoracotomies.

The linear cutter stapler is applied so as to minimize parenchymal loss without compromising margin. Characteristically this creates a specimen with a pie-shaped wedge appearance. When the nodule is deep-seated, a tongue-shaped resection can be created by stapling parallel to the nodule and dividing the base (deep margin) with a transverse stapler or a laser. Generally it is easier to excise nodules in the middle or lower lobes, because thinner edges and fissures allow for easier stapler application.

The difficulty in excising a nodule is directly related to its size and depth of location [32]. Formal lobectomy or pneumonectomy becomes necessary if the lesion is deep, large, or intimately associated with central lobar vessels or bronchi. A large number of metastases within one portion of the lung may also dictate a formal resection with lobectomy or even pneumonectomy.

Median sternotomy

Median sternotomy offers the advantage of simultaneous access to both thoracic cavities. If stable approximation of the sternum is achieved, the patient generally has less pain and respiratory compromise than after unilateral thoracotomy. A disadvantage of median sternotomy is the high morbidity of sternal wound complications. In addition, access to posterior lung lesions can be difficult, particularly on the left side, because of the presence of the heart.

Thoracotomy and trans-sternal thoracotomy

A traditional posterolateral thoracotomy performed through the fifth or sixth interspace provides excellent exposure for ipsilateral pulmonary resections. Comparing median sternotomy with thoracotomy, the National Cancer Institute reported a higher yield for occult pulmonary nodules with sternotomy. Despite finding more nodules overall survival was not improved, questioning the need to discover all pulmonary metastases at the first surgical intervention [33]. The argument for unilateral explorations has been strengthened by findings that delaying contralateral thoracotomy until disease becomes clinically detectable did not affect outcome [34].

For surgeons who prefer to maximize the number of occult nodules discovered at the first operation, a trans-sternal approach or clamshell incision made by extending an anterolateral thoracotomy through the lower half of the sternum offers optimal exposure [35,36]. It provides excellent access to both pleural spaces. The patient is supine, and because of the sternal release, less force is applied to fewer rib interspaces. Consequently postoperative pain may be less than that after bilateral traditional thoracotomies. Pain can be further diminished by additional stabilization of the sternal cut with K-wires or stents placed within the sternal cortex (Fig. 1). The disadvantage of this approach lies in the need to sacrifice both internal thoracic arteries, reducing the options of subsequent flap reconstruction, particularly after chest wall resections.

In highly selected patients, bilateral posterolateral thoracotomies can be performed at the same operation. In most cases a staged procedure is preferable. Axillary thoracotomy is considered less invasive and painful than

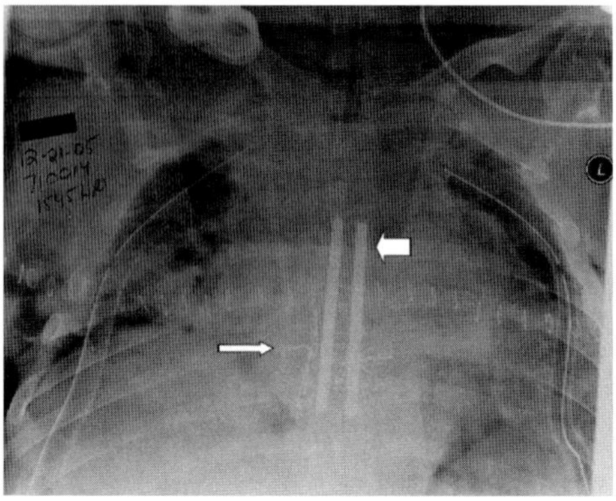

Fig. 1. Chest roentgenogram showing pins (*thick arrow*) placed between sternal tables to prevent override that would occur if only wires (*thin arrow*) held transverse sternotomy.

traditional thoracotomy because fewer shoulder girdle muscles are divided, but access to the thoracic cavity is limited [37]. Because rib spreading is required, this is not considered a thoracoscopic approach.

Laser resection for pulmonary metastases

The neodymium-yttrium aluminum garnet (Nd-YAG) laser has shown promise in the management of patients who have multiple pulmonary metastases. A randomized study showed better tissue sparing, air leak control, and postsurgical recovery [38]. Several large centers have shown that laser technology facilitates resection of multiple nodules (up to 20) deep within lobes with low mortality and good survival rates. The lobectomy rate was only 7% in two large series [39]. Although lasers can excise the nodule with a rim of ablated tissue, they can also be used to create heat within the tumor to ablate metastases. Although the experience with this technology is new, it seems to have similar tissue effects as other ablative technologies such as radio frequency ablation [40,41].

Extended resection

As long as the patient can be rendered disease-free, more extended resections such as pneumonectomy with en bloc resections of chest wall or diaphragm may be indicated [42]. Completion pneumonectomy or initial pneumonectomy for metastatic disease can have acceptable outcomes in selected patients with reported 5-year survival rates of 30% [43,44]. These operations require careful planning because of the increased morbidity and uncertain oncologic benefit, particularly if a completion pneumonectomy after repeat thoracotomy for metastatic disease is contemplated [45].

Minimally invasive resection methods

Following a general trend in medicine to use less invasive therapies with better preservation of the host function, thoracoscopic lung surgery has gained more acceptance in the treatment of pulmonary metastases. Broad interest in such techniques has fostered rapid innovations in the technical aspects of this operative approach over the last decade. In certain centers thoracoscopic lobectomy is now the preferred method for resection of lung metastases [46]. Compared with open procedures, thoracoscopy has been shown to have better postoperative pulmonary function, survival, and immunologic function [47–49]. Adjuvant chemotherapy may be started sooner or may be given with better tolerance after thoracoscopic resection. Although the arguments for less invasive operations are compelling, the oncologic equivalency is still a matter of debate, and surgeons have achieved excellent results with extended open exposures and maximal complete resection for pulmonary metastatic disease.

A large prospective trial comparing open thoracotomy to video-assisted thoracic surgery (VATS) showed open thoracotomy to be superior to VATS in finding pulmonary lesions [50]. By performing an open thoracotomy immediately following VATS the study found that 56% of lung lesions were missed by the VATS procedure. The investigators concluded that VATS is inadequate for pulmonary metastasectomy with curative intent. Newer CT scanning technologies have improved the rate of preoperative identification for metastatic lung nodules. It is uncertain, however, when imaging will equal the discriminative power of manual palpation at open thoracotomy. Thoracoscopic procedures most often only allow palpation in the lung areas immediately subjacent to the access ports using a single digit. Because of the growing popularity of thoracoscopic lung resections there has been renewed interest in refining the indications for VATS in pulmonary metastatic disease [51].

Accordingly investigators have applied thoracoscopic metastasectomy selectively to achieve acceptable oncologic results [52]. The selection criteria restrict this approach to patients who have peripheral lesions less than 3 cm in diameter. In a cooperative trial, resection of colorectal pulmonary metastases achieved a 31% 5-year survival rate using VATS [53]. Conversion to thoracotomy was recommended when the lesions could not be found or when an acceptable surgical margin could not be achieved.

Nonsurgical methods for treatment of pulmonary metastases

In general interventional techniques are used when the patient has prohibitive comorbidities for surgical resection. One of the most common interventional methods for ablating pulmonary metastasis is radio frequency ablation (RFA). RFA is performed by an imaged-guided probe that delivers high-frequency current by thin electrodes placed into the tumor tissue. A targeted lesion is thereby heated to 60° C for approximately 12 minutes. This creates an area of tissue injury emanating around the probe and resulting in a "light bulb" appearance on subsequent CT scan (Fig. 2) [54]. Pneumothorax formation and a persistent cavity or scar at the ablation site is

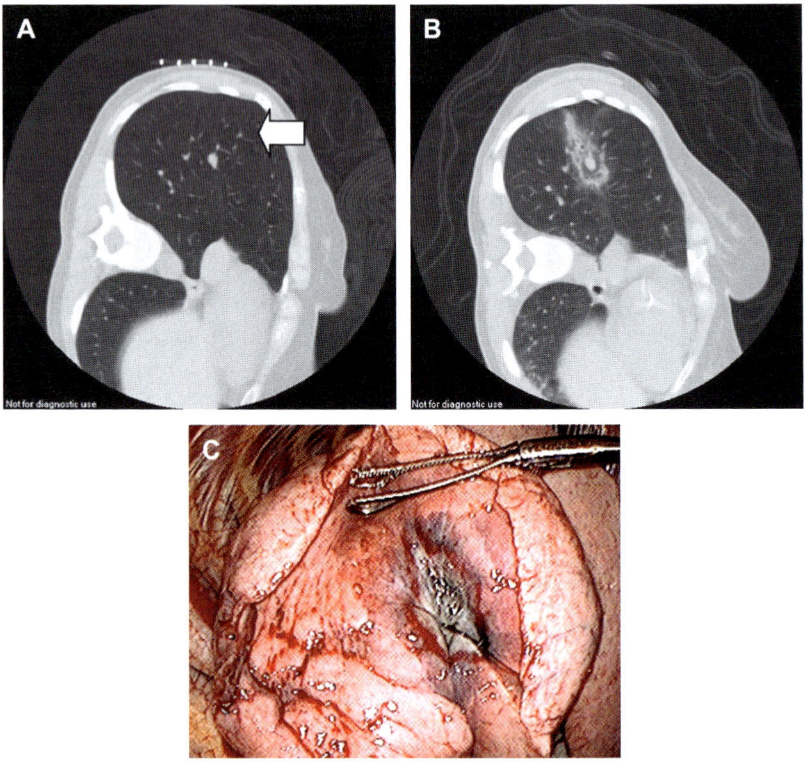

Fig. 2. Chest CT scan showing (*A*) pre-RFA ablation of small metastatic sarcoma nodule in right lower lobe (*arrow*) and (*B*) post-ablation appearance with light bulb-shaped area of injury. Intraoperative photo (*C*) of same patient shows concentric zones of injury (target appearance) of ablation.

common [55]. In a large series reported by Yan, 3-year survival reached 46% in patients not suitable for surgical resection [56]. Metastases greater than 3 cm were associated with poor survival. Because of local recurrence rates as high as 50%, RFA for lung metastases is still considered investigational and should only be used in selected patients otherwise unable to undergo open surgical resection [57].

Endobronchial metastases

Endobronchial metastases are rare. The most common types of tumors that metastasize to the airway are breast, colorectal, and renal [58]. Other malignancies presenting with endobronchial metastases include melanoma, sarcoma, pheochromocytoma, upper gastrointestinal malignancy, Hodgkin disease, and thyroid cancer. Most patients present with symptoms of dyspnea, cough, and hemoptysis in increasing order of frequency. The mean time to diagnosis is 3 years and average survival time is 15 to 18 months [59]. Ablation of these unusual tumors can be done with photodynamic therapy, which relieves hemoptysis and dyspnea in 85% of patients [60] or with intraluminal radiotherapy and Nd-YAG laser ablation [61,62].

Stereotactic radiosurgery

The advances in diagnostic imaging and respiratory gating have increased the popularity of radiation therapy for pulmonary metastases. Tumors are treated with tight radiation fields confined around the lesion and total dose rates of 50 Gy using multiple fractions or 30 Gy in a single treatment [63,64]. With single-dose treatment, 5-year survival rates of 42% have been reported, which is comparable to other methods of ablation [64].

Investigational regional chemotherapy

Many metastases have isolated blood supply from the pulmonary circulation. Accordingly there has been a steady interest in delivering chemotherapeutic or other agents to the pulmonary circulation for regional treatment either by perfusion or static infusion. Isolated lung infusion with platinum or tumor necrosis factor has been used for soft-tissue sarcoma [65,66]. Burt and colleagues [67] reported a phase I trial of doxorubicin for sarcoma metastases. High doses were achieved with acceptable toxicity, but treatment responses were disappointing without any partial or complete responses. Others have successfully used melphalan for resectable lung metastasis in a phase I clinical trial [68]. Transpulmonary chemoembolization can achieve tumor volume regression using mitomycin-C and microspheres [69]. Despite its theoretic appeal, regional lung chemotherapy for pulmonary metastases has not shown a potential for broader clinical application and remains investigational.

Other experimental options

Whole lung radiation for pulmonary metastases has been used in investigational trials for the treatment of radiosensitive cancers such as Wilms tumor and as an adjunct treatment for unusual tumors such as alveolar soft part sarcoma [70–73]. Cryotherapy has been applied in some centers with limited results [74]. Whole body hyperthermia achieves an augmented immune response and microvascular inhibition [75,76]. In addition, focal hyperthermia delivered by microwave technology can achieve thermal ablation of metastases. Radiofrequency or laser-induced interstitial thermal ablation has been shown to have additional effectiveness in selected tumors, such as colorectal carcinoma [77].

The evidence

Prognostic factors

Given favorable tumor biology, surgical resectability, and low comorbidity, pulmonary metastasectomy can yield acceptable oncologic results [78].

Over the past quarter century, specialized centers compiled and reported the outcomes of patients who had various tumor histologies. Over the same period, staging systems for most tumors evolved so that only patients who have reasonable expectations of systemic disease control are referred for thoracic metastasectomy.

Table 1 shows prognostic factors uncovered in these studies in decreasing order of frequency. Table 2 [79] lists the major studies of pulmonary metastasectomy. Despite the wide range of tumor histologies, diverse patient populations, and differing geographic regions, 5-year survival rates are remarkably similar.

The operative mortality rates for metastasectomy range from 2% to 4% (see Table 2) and morbidity rates range from 7% to 14% [80,81]. In their landmark study, Pastorino and others published the most relevant prognostic factors for pulmonary metastasectomy [82]. Multifactorial analysis of 5206 cases revealed three pre-eminent risk factors (Fig. 3): (1) complete resection, (2) disease-free interval, and (3) number of metastases. These factors were used to establish a simple scoring system (Table 3) [83].

Complete resection

Complete resection with negative microscopic margin is paramount to a curative result of pulmonary metastasectomy. The chance to fail in achieving this goal should be minimized. Historically palliative operations for metastasectomy resulted in survival rates of less than 10% [84,85]. The survival for incomplete resections noted in Fig. 3 is somewhat better, because some of these may represent R1 resections. Palliative debulking (R2) operations are not recommended.

Disease-free interval

Short DFI usually implies the presence of numerous occult metastatic deposits. Because tumor volume has to reach 1 billion cells before it becomes

Table 1
Commonly cited predictors of pulmonary metastasectomy failure (decreasing order of frequency)

Predictor	Abbreviation
Disease-free interval (brief)	DFI
Histologic cell type	Histo
Multiple nodules	Mult
Incomplete resection	Inc
Volume of tumor	Vol
Metastatic route (eg, portal versus caval vein)	Route
Nodal metastases present	Nodes
Tumor doubling time (brief)	TDT
Chemotherapy not given	Chemo
Extension past visceral pleura	Ext
Recurrence after previous metastasectomy	Recur
Symptom presence	Sx

Table 2
Series of pulmonary metastasectomy (mixed histology, chronologic order)

Author/reference	Year	N	Survival[a]	Predictors and comments
Morrow	1980	167	29%	Ext, Mult
Takita	1981	243	21.4 m	(median survival) Mult, Nodes
Blondet	1981	50	30%	Chemo, DFI ± 4 years, Histo
Wright	1982	142	24%–29%	—
Roeslin	1983	55	21%	—
Rendina	1984	93	32%	DFI, Histo
van de Wal	1986	80	53%	DFI, Histo, Node, TDT, Vol
Swoboda	1986	157	43%	—
Vogt-Moykopf	1986	261	38%	DFI, Inc, Route
van Dongen	1986	107	46%	Mult, TDT, Vol
Eckersberger	1988	122	38%	(28% for sarcoma) Mult, PFI, Vol
Vogt-Moykopf	1988	368	33%	DFI, Histo
Roberts	1989	132	20%	DFI, Histo, Mult, Sx
McCormack	1990	415	—	DFI, Histo, Multi, TDT
Metzger	1990	110	37%	Chemo, Ext, Route
Silber	1990	215	31%	Inc, Nodes, Route, Sx
Ris	1991	83	38%	Inc, Histo
Vogt-Moykopf	1992	655	31%	DFI, Histo, Mult
Girard	1994	186	35%	Inc, Mult
van Geel	1996	255	38%	DFI, Histo, Inc
Girard	1997	575	37%	DFI, Multi
Abecasis	1999	85	29%	Inc, Vol
Koodziejski	1999	93	35%	DFI, Histo
Maniwa et al. [92]	2000	120	37%	Recur
Hendriks et al. [90]	2001	56	46%	Histo
Monteiro et al. [79]	2004	78	47%	DFI
Rena et al. [80]	2006	202	43%	DFI, Inc, Mult
Rolle et al. [39]	2006	328	41%	Inc

[a] Five-year actuarial except as noted in comments. Reference information on listed studies (those before 2000) can be found in comprehensive reviews [1,2].

apparent on plain film imaging, many tumor doublings occur before disease can be detected. Accordingly tumor doubling time can be seen as a surrogate for DFI and can be used as a prognostic factor. This has been a consistent finding and there is consensus for the intervals cited in the International Registry (<1, 1–3, and >3 years) [82]. The belief that a long DFI is always equal to a better prognosis and a reduced need for intense follow-up is questionable. Despite long DFIs (including those greater than 10 years) early death from disease can occur [86].

Number of metastases

In numerous studies the number of lesions is directly correlated to survival rate, with one single lesion providing the best results. Beyond that the number of lesions does not seem to matter as much as the ability to achieve complete resection. Clearly the number of lesions is inversely related

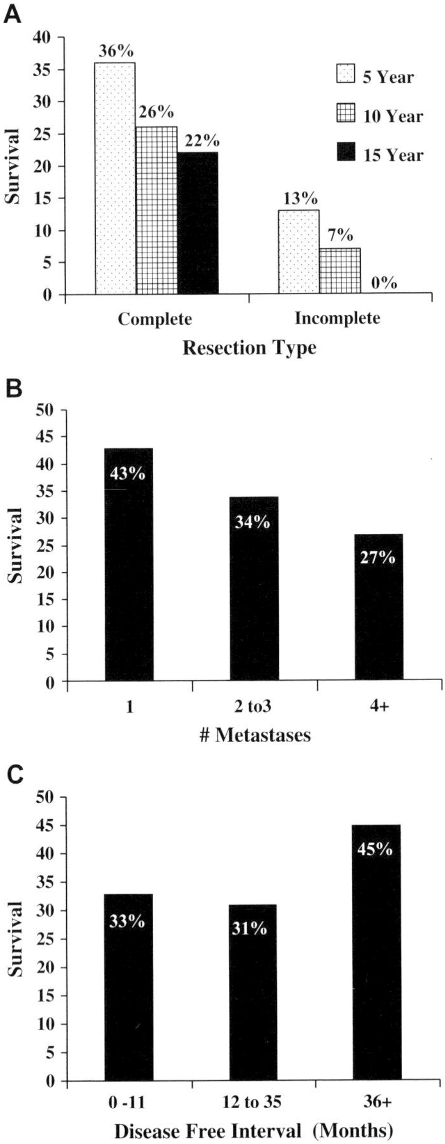

Fig. 3. Bar graphs showing the three major predictors of success for pulmonary metastasectomy from the International Registry series: (*A*) complete resection, (*B*) number of metastases, and (*C*) disease-free interval. (*Data from* The International Registry of Lung Metastases. Long-term results of lung metastasectomy: prognostic analyses based on 5206 cases. J Thorac Cardiovasc Surg 1997;113(1):37–49.)

Table 3
Median survival based on survival groupings

Risk grouping	Median survival (months)
No risk factors[a]	61
One risk factor	34
Both risk factors	24
Unresectable	14

[a] Risk factors for resectable patients (see Fig. 3) are: DFI $\leq$36 m, more than one metastasis.
Data from The International Registry of Lung Metastases. Long-term results of lung metastasectomy: prognostic analyses based on 5206 cases. J Thorac Cardiovasc Surg 1997;113(1):37–49.

to achieving a complete resection. Recurrence with a large number of lesions and a short DFI predicts the presence of microscopic residual disease [87].

Histology

It remains unclear how tumor histology affects the results of metastasectomy. Interpretations of reported survival statistics are rendered difficult because of improved patient selection, changes in the staging systems, and an improved understanding of tumor biology. Because of the increased ability to detect and predict incurable systemic disease, patients are now less likely to be considered for futile pulmonary metastasectomy. At the same time, much improved chemotherapy regimens for certain tumor types have increased the ability to control systemic disease after pulmonary metastasectomy. In earlier series, long-term survival for sarcomas was superior to that of carcinomas [88,89]. Also risk factors for osteogenic sarcomas were found to be different from those of soft-tissue sarcomas [88]. Head and neck cancers and testicular and germ cell tumors tend to have better prognoses [78,83,90]. Tumor types with consistently lower survival rates after pulmonary metastasectomy are breast cancer and melanoma [90,91].

Repeat resections

The benefit of repeated resections for recurrent pulmonary metastases remains controversial. In general multiple resections are adequate as long as the selection criteria are kept the same. In a large series of repeat surgical resections for pulmonary metastases, short DFI was found to be a poor prognostic indicator [88]. Maniwa and colleagues [92] found poor prognoses after extended resections and pneumonectomies when disease-free interval was less than 6 months. Oncologic acceptable results have been reported with up to four re-resections for pulmonary metastases [88].

Pulmonary metastasectomy for specific tumor types

Colorectal cancer

Colorectal cancer is one of the most common adult malignancies in the United States [93]. Nearly a third of those patients who undergo resection of metastases develop recurrent disease [94]. The most common metastatic site is the liver, followed by the lung. Approximately 20% of patients who have colorectal cancer develop pulmonary metastases [95]. Most present with multiple bilateral nodules or extrapulmonary disease and therefore are not candidates for metastasectomy. The subset of patients who have potentially resectable pulmonary metastases is small and represents only 1% to 2% of all patients who have colorectal cancer. The mainstay of therapy for metastatic colorectal cancer is systemic chemotherapy, but cure with chemotherapy alone remains elusive. For this reason surgery plays an important part in the multimodality treatment of stage IV colorectal cancer. This is evident in the increased use of resection for liver and pulmonary metastases. Although some studies have reported 5-year survival after resection of lung metastases as high as 55%, most studies show 5-year survival closer to 30% to 40% [96–103]. The calculated probability of 10-year survival is estimated at 20%, with one series reporting actual 10-year survival of 37% [99,104]. Expected operative mortality is as low as 2%, suggesting that in well-selected patients, pulmonary metastasectomy for colorectal cancer is appropriate and beneficial [96,105].

Combined surgical resection of isolated hepatic and lung metastases has met with relative success. Several small studies report 5-year survival after combined resections ranging from 11% to 43% [104,106–109]. This is almost within the range of survival rates reported for hepatic resections alone (21%–43%) [103,110–114]. These results suggest that in selected patients who have both liver and lung metastases, metastasectomy may yield long-term benefit.

Relapse after pulmonary resection is high, and more than 70% of patients have recurrent disease in the chest. A minority of these patients fulfill criteria for re-resection (isolated pulmonary recurrence, anatomic resectability, and medically fit for repeat pulmonary resection). In these highly selected patients, oncologic results can reach those seen after the first resection. Several investigators report 5-year survival rates of more than 30% in these patients, suggesting that some recurrences of pulmonary metastases are confined to the lung and are not a sign of recurrent systemic disease [96,99,105].

The presence of a single metastasis, long DFI of greater than 36 months, and normal preoperative carcinoembryonic antigen (CEA) are generally regarded as predictors of good outcome [96,104,107]. Other studies, however, have suggested that preoperative CEA does not predict outcome, and that hilar or mediastinal lymph node status may be more important [102]. At present the role of these factors in predicting long-term outcome and in guiding clinical decision-making requires further refinement.

New chemotherapeutic combination regimens, including biologic agents, show improved tumor response in advanced disease and hold promise for further improving treatment of patients who have metastatic colorectal cancer. The impact of these emerging technologies on treatment of patients who have metastatic colorectal cancer to the lung remains to be seen.

Other gastrointestinal malignancy

Hepatocellular carcinoma (HCC) is the only other gastrointestinal cancer for which successful pulmonary metastasectomy has been reported. In highly selected patients (small case series with fewer than 10 patients) greater than 5-year survival rates after pulmonary metastasectomy for HCC has been demonstrated [115–118]. Despite these reports, the prognosis for most patients who have metastatic HCC remains extremely poor. Pulmonary resection should only be considered in patients who have low-volume disease, isolated pulmonary metastases, low alpha feta protein levels, and DFIs greater than 12 months [119].

The paucity of metastasectomy reports for other gastrointestinal malignancies (esophageal, gastric, small bowel, appendiceal, pancreatic carcinoma, and cholangiocarcinoma) likely reflects the more aggressive natural history and poorer prognosis of these tumors. On occasion resection of a solitary pulmonary lesion is performed, mainly to exclude primary malignant lung disease [120].

Sarcoma

The discussion of pulmonary metastasectomy for sarcoma can be divided into that of osteogenic sarcoma (particularly of the extremities) and soft-tissue sarcoma. In general pulmonary metastasectomy for soft-tissue sarcomas confers a better survival chance than for osteogenic sarcoma. With the introduction of more effective chemotherapy, survival rates after pulmonary resections of osteogenic sarcoma metastases have improved.

Osteogenic sarcoma

Osteogenic sarcoma (OS) metastasizes to the lung in up to 80% of cases. Before the availability of effective chemotherapy, pulmonary metastasectomy for OS was only entertained for metachronous disease. Today effective chemotherapy makes pulmonary resection for some patients who have synchronous disease appropriate. Presentation of pulmonary metastases for OS can be divided into four categories: those identified at initial presentation, those apparent during preoperative chemotherapy, those found during adjuvant chemotherapy following primary resection, and those diagnosed after completing treatment for the primary tumor. The last group of patients has by far the best 5-year survival rates, with 31% compared with 0% for those who developed pulmonary metastases during induction chemotherapy [121]. Another way of analyzing the outcomes of metastasectomy for patients who have OS is to evaluate the results from the time of relapse. Patients who can undergo surgery for recurrent disease have a 39% 5-year survival rate versus 0% for those who are not surgical candidates [122,123]. An isolated lung relapse confers a better prognosis than other sites. Survival chances are higher for relapses occurring beyond 2 years and for less than three lung metastases [122]. The Cooperative Osteosarcoma Study Group found similar results in their multivariate analysis [124]. They reported pleural disruption by the tumor to confer a higher rate of recurrence. High levels of necrosis after neoadjuvant therapy were associated with improved survival. Combination chemotherapy provided only limited improvement in outcomes [124]. In another study recurrence was predicted by the degree of tumor necrosis at the time of the original lung metastasectomy [125]. Patients can benefit from multiple resections (up to four), provided a complete resection is obtained each time. With a complete resection, anticipated survival curves are similar after each iteration [126]. The number of pulmonary metastases resected for OS seems to interfere less with results. Resection of large numbers of metastases can be entertained with a reasonable expectation for cure as shown by Saltzman and colleagues [127]. On average 10.2 pulmonary metastases per patient were resected during each of a mean of three open thoracotomies. A 24% 5-year survival rate was observed [127].

Soft-tissue sarcomas

In the same Saltzman study the survival rate at 5 years was 71% for nonosteogenic sarcomas. In a large registry trial the following predictors of failure for pulmonary metastasectomy in soft-tissue sarcoma (STS) were identified: greater than two metastases, DFI less than 16 months, size greater than 2 cm, malignant fibrous histiocytoma histology, and age greater than 50 years [128]. In another large multivariate analysis, age greater than 50 years and liposarcoma or malignant peripheral nerve sheath histology predicted recurrence [129]. More than three pulmonary nodules, size greater than 2 cm, and high-grade histology were independent poor prognostic factors [130].

Because of its questionable efficacy, chemotherapy after pulmonary metastasectomy for STS is still controversial [128,131]. A recent meta-analysis showed some overall recurrence-free survival improvement with the use of adjuvant doxorubicin-based chemotherapy [132].

Two unusual types of sarcoma deserve separate mention. Ewing sarcoma and alveolar soft part sarcoma are treated by multiple lung resections and multiagent chemotherapy. Whole lung radiation therapy or aggressive resections (exceeding 130 nodulectomies) have been performed with variable success [73,133].

Melanoma

Overall survival for metastatic melanoma is poor. Not surprisingly any clinical scenario with more than one or two metastatic foci is unlikely to benefit from any surgical intervention. In one of the largest studies on pulmonary metastases for melanoma, Duke University reported more than 7500 patients, of whom 945 went on to develop pulmonary metastatic disease (12%) [134]. The risk for developing metastases by 10 years is 19%

in the affected population; once metastatic disease is present, 3- and 5-year survival rates decrease to 9% and 4%, respectively. Independent factors were complete resection, long DFI, one or two pulmonary nodules, and absence of lymph node metastases. The International Melanoma Registry reported 328 patients having pulmonary metastasectomies [135]. Patients who did best had a complete resection, single lesions, and a DFI exceeding 36 months. Survival rate was 29% if all good prognostic factors were present but decreased to 0% with incomplete resection [135]. A high percentage of benign pulmonary nodules were found in patients explored for suspected metastatic melanoma [136].

Breast cancer

Isolated lung metastases occur in 10% to 20% of women who have breast cancer, excluding unresectable lymphangitic pulmonary infiltration [137]. Similar to melanoma it is imperative to rule out primary lung cancer. In a series of 30 breast cancer patients biopsied for pulmonary nodules, only 9 patients had metastatic breast cancer. The remaining 21 patients were diagnosed with primary lung cancer [138]. Because of the rapid evolution of systemic chemotherapy, only recent series looking at pulmonary breast cancer metastases should be considered for review. The importance of chemotherapy in the setting of metastatic breast cancer is highlighted by the fact that incomplete resection of metastatic disease is not necessarily a poor prognostic factor, as shown in a recent series by Planchard and colleagues [137]. In two larger series 5-year survival rate for isolated pulmonary metastasectomy was approximately 45% [137,139]. In Planchard's study, metastases greater than 2 cm and DFI less than 3 years predicted poor outcome. In the International Registry series [139], more than one metastases and DFI less than 3 years were poor prognostic factors. Breast cancer tends to have a very long average DFI of 43 months [140]. Lymph node involvement did not predict risk for pulmonary metastases. In summary, patients who have isolated pulmonary breast metastases and long DFIs are best suited for metastasectomy.

Germ cell tumors

The introduction of cisplatin-based chemotherapy caused a dramatic change in the management of patients who have germ cell tumors. Approximately 30% of patients who have testicular primaries develop intrathoracic lesions [141]. Follow-up studies after successful chemotherapy reveal metastatic disease in up to 50% of patients [142]. Most are surgically resectable. Well-selected patients can undergo simultaneous resection of retroperitoneal, cervical, and thoracic metastases [143]. Five-year survival in these patients can reach 82% as reported by Liu and others and confirmed in a more recent review of 103 patients [141,144]. In approximately 44% of resected specimens, residual viable tumor is found on pathologic examination, translating into reduced long-term survival. Unfortunately normalized serum tumor markers, such as beta HCG and AFP, cannot serve as a surrogate for complete pathologic response and resection is always indicated, even after apparent successful chemotherapy. A residual mass after a complete pathologic response can display one of three histologic patterns: mature teratoma, diffuse necrosis, or fibrous tissue [141]. In summary pulmonary metastasectomy and thoracic lymph node dissections still play an important role in the treatment of germ cell tumors despite effective chemotherapy.

Genitourinary

Twenty-one percent of patients who have renal cancer develop metastatic disease, of which 10% is evident at the time of diagnosis [145]. The lungs represent the second most frequent site of metastases and are often the only disease location [3]. Five-year survival rates for pulmonary metastasectomy are approximately 40% [3,146,147]. Renal cell metastases of the lung or adrenal glands confer superior survival compared with other sites [145]. Important poor prognostic factors are large nodule size, incomplete resection, and positive lymph node status [146]. In the International Registry study, the number of metastases and disease-free survival were shown to be significant risk factors. The adjuvant treatment of renal cancer is immune-based, and spontaneous resolution of pulmonary metastases has been reported. Prostate cancer patients generally have lymphangitic spread treated by androgen deprivation and are not candidates for metastasectomy [148].

Head and neck malignancy

Pulmonary metastases occur in approximately 6% of all head and neck cancer patients [149]. After metastasectomy the overall 5-year survival rate is 50% [149,150]. Patients who have squamous cell carcinomas have a poorer prognosis with 5-year survival rates reaching 35% compared with a survival rate of 70% for glandular tumor patients. For glandular tumors, survival after surgical metastasectomy is equivalent to that after chemotherapy alone, whereas patients who have squamous cell cancer metastases treated nonsurgically can expect only 4% 5-year survival rates [149].

The patient who has prior head and neck cancer and a new pulmonary lesion is more likely to have primary lung cancer; however, confirming the diagnosis remains a difficult problem. Genomic classification systems are being developed to identify the origin of a malignant pulmonary lesion in this setting. For example, micro satellite instability has been associated with head and neck origin of solitary squamous cell cancer lesions in the lung [151].

Gynecologic malignancy

Most commonly pulmonary metastases originate from ovarian, uterine body, and cervical malignancies. Choriocarcinoma metastases have good prognosis because of effective chemotherapy. An isolated ovarian carcinoma metastasis to the lung without associated systemic disease is unusual. In one of the few large series of ovarian pulmonary metastases, only three patients had no other evidence of metastases elsewhere [152]. Endometrial cancer metastasizes to the lung in approximately 5% of cases and is associated with poor prognosis. The few patients who are candidates for metastasectomy can reach 50% 5-year survival [153,154]. Short DFI, more than four metastases, and large size predict failure. In one study, a DFI of less than 12 months was associated with low survival rates [153].

In patients who have early cervical cancer, pulmonary metastases are uncommon (0.37%) [155]. Primary tumor histology is of special importance: patients who have squamous cell carcinoma do much better (47% 5-year disease-free survival) than those who have adenocarcinomas (0%) [155].

Miscellaneous adult tumors

"Benign" giant cell tumor of the bone has been known to cause pulmonary metastases that can be resected with good prognosis [156,157]. The mortality rate directly related to metastasis of this giant cell tumor is approximately 23%. Occasionally meningioma can cause pulmonary metastases [158]. Carefully selected patients who have endocrine tumor (carcinoid, thyroid, pheochromocytoma, and parathyroid) metastases can be considered for surgical resection [159]. Although metastasectomy is generally not considered appropriate for primary lung cancer, isolated ipsilateral lesions without mediastinal lymph node spread may warrant resection in highly selected patients.

Pediatric tumors

Treatment of pulmonary metastases in children is generally considered an adjunct to systemic chemotherapy. It does seem to prolong survival after careful selection, but cure is less likely compared with adults [160]. Patients who have hepatoblastoma may undergo thoracotomies as an adjunct to chemotherapy and patients who have osteosarcoma may benefit from salvage surgery also [161,162]. The benefit for patients who have Ewing tumors, Wilms tumors, and soft-tissue sarcoma is uncertain [163]. Like in adults, incomplete resection, short DFI, and multiple metastases are unfavorable [164].

Summary

The defining principles of acceptable pulmonary metastasectomy, ie, control of the primary lesion, no extrathoracic disease, and sufficient cardiopulmonary reserve, although intuitive and simple, require detailed knowledge of tumor biology and clinical behavior. To fulfill these selection criteria, physicians must understand the basic behavior of the primary lesion, must use sophisticated staging tests, and must perform sufficient physiologic testing. Given some histologic variability, following this approach uniformly leads to an anticipated 5-year survival of approximately 40%. The emergence of more accurate (eg, molecular-based) staging systems should eliminate unnecessary metastasectomy cases and increase the enthusiasm for others. Better chemotherapy, regionally delivered compounds, and minimally invasive technologies to control pulmonary metastasis deserve ongoing attention.

Acknowledgments

The authors express our appreciation to Nancy Sikora, Elicia Schmitt, and Dr. Donald Klippenstein for their assistance in the preparation of this manuscript.

References

[1] Temeck BK, Pass HI, et al. Intrathoracic metastases. In: Aisner J, Arriagada R, Green MR, editors. Comprehensive textbook of thoracic oncology. Baltimore (MD): Williams & Wilkins; 1996. p. 906–20.
[2] Rodriguez E, Cohn HE, Friedberg JS. Secondary lung tumors. In: Selke F, Swanson S, del Nido PJ, editors. Sabiston & Spencer surgery of the chest. Philadelphia: Elsevier Saunders; 2005. p. 337–54.
[3] Pfannschmidt J, Hoffmann H, Muley T, et al. Prognostic factors for survival after pulmonary resection of metastatic renal cell carcinoma. Ann Thorac Surg 2002;74(5):1653–7.
[4] Alexander J, Haight C. Pulmonary resection for solitary metastatic sarcomas and carcinomas. Surg Gynecol Obstet 1947;85:129–46.
[5] Milne EN, Zerhouni EA. Blood supply of pulmonary metastases. J Thorac Imaging 1987; 2(4):15–23.
[6] Coffey JC, Wang JH, Smith MJ, et al. Excisional surgery for cancer cure: therapy at a cost. Lancet Oncol 2003;4(12):760–8.
[7] Strieter RM, Belperio JA, Phillips RJ, et al. Chemokines: angiogenesis and metastases in lung cancer. Novartis Found Symp 2004;256:173–84.
[8] Skitzki J, Craig RA, Okuyama R, et al. Donor cell cycling, trafficking, and accumulation during adoptive immunotherapy for murine lung metastases. Cancer Res 2004;64(6): 2183–91.
[9] Potti A, Mukherjee S, Petersen R, et al. A genomic strategy to refine prognosis in early-stage non-small-cell lung cancer. N Engl J Med 2006;355(6):570–80.
[10] Johnston MR. Median sternotomy for resection of pulmonary metastases. J Thorac Cardiovasc Surg 1983;85(4):516–22.
[11] Seemann MD, Seemann O, Luboldt W, et al. Differentiation of malignant from benign solitary pulmonary lesions using chest radiography, spiral CT and HRCT. Lung Cancer 2000; 29(2):105–24.
[12] Seo JB, Im JG, Goo JM, et al. Atypical pulmonary metastases: spectrum of radiologic findings. Radiographics 2001;21(2):403–17.
[13] Maile CW, Rodan BA, Godwin JD, et al. Calcification in pulmonary metastases. Br J Radiol 1982;55(650):108–13.

[14] Kawaguchi T, Kusumoto M, Maeshima A, et al. High-resolution computed tomography appearances of surgically resected pulmonary metastases from colorectal cancer, with histopathologic correlation. Radiat Med 2005;23(6):418–26.

[15] Hsu WH, Hsu NY, Shen YY, et al. Differentiating solitary pulmonary metastases in patients with extrapulmonary neoplasms using FDG-PET. Cancer Invest 2003;21(1):47–52.

[16] Franzius C, drup-Link HE, Sciuk J, et al. FDG-PET for detection of pulmonary metastases from malignant primary bone tumors: comparison with spiral CT. Ann Oncol 2001;12(4): 479–86.

[17] Iagaru A, Chawla S, Menendez L, et al. 18F-FDG PET and PET/CT for detection of pulmonary metastases from musculoskeletal sarcomas. Nucl Med Commun 2006;27(10): 795–802.

[18] Reinhardt MJ, Wiethoelter N, Matthies A, et al. PET recognition of pulmonary metastases on PET/CT imaging: impact of attenuation-corrected and non-attenuation-corrected PET images. Eur J Nucl Med Mol Imaging 2006;33(2):134–9.

[19] Kozuka T, Johkoh T, Hamada S, et al. Detection of pulmonary metastases with multidetector row CT scans of 5-mm nominal section thickness: autopsy lung study. Radiology 2003;226(1):231–4.

[20] Zhao B, Schwartz LH, Moskowitz CS, et al. Pulmonary metastases: effect of CT section thickness on measurement—initial experience. Radiology 2005;234(3):934–9.

[21] Margaritora S, Porziella V, D'Andrilli A, et al. Pulmonary metastases: can accurate radiological evaluation avoid thoracotomic approach? Eur J Cardiothorac Surg 2002;21(6): 1111–4.

[22] Parsons AM, Detterbeck FC, Parker LA. Accuracy of helical CT in the detection of pulmonary metastases: is intraoperative palpation still necessary? Ann Thorac Surg 2004;78(6): 1910–6.

[23] Watanabe K, Nomori H, Ohtsuka T, et al. Usefulness and complications of computed tomography-guided lipiodol marking for fluoroscopy-assisted thoracoscopic resection of small pulmonary nodules: experience with 174 nodules. J Thorac Cardiovasc Surg 2006; 132(2):320–4.

[24] Daniel TM. A proposed diagnostic approach to the patient with the subcentimeter pulmonary nodule: techniques that facilitate video-assisted thoracic surgery excision. Semin Thorac Cardiovasc Surg 2005;17(2):115–22.

[25] Gaffke G, Stroszczynski C, Rau B, et al. [CT-guided resection of pulmonary metastases]. Rofo 2005;177(6):877–83 [in German].

[26] Kucuk ON, Gultekin SS, Aras G, et al. Radioiodine whole-body scans, thyroglobulin levels, 99mTc-MIBI scans and computed tomography: results in patients with lung metastases from differentiated thyroid cancer. Nucl Med Commun 2006;27(3):261–6.

[27] Prasad SR, Saini S, Sumner JE, et al. Radiological measurement of breast cancer metastases to lung and liver: comparison between WHO (bidimensional) and RECIST (unidimensional) guidelines. J Comput Assist Tomogr 2003;27(3):380–4.

[28] Ercan S, Nichols FC III, Trastek VF, et al. Prognostic significance of lymph node metastasis found during pulmonary metastasectomy for extrapulmonary carcinoma. Ann Thorac Surg 2004;77(5):1786–91.

[29] Pfannschmidt J, Klode J, Muley T, et al. Nodal involvement at the time of pulmonary metastasectomy: experiences in 245 patients. Ann Thorac Surg 2006;81(2):448–54.

[30] Scanlon EF, Suh O, Murthy SM, et al. Influence of smoking on the development of lung metastases from breast cancer. Cancer 1995;75(11):2693–9.

[31] Carter JJ, Feingold DL, Kirman I, et al. Laparoscopic-assisted cecectomy is associated with decreased formation of postoperative pulmonary metastases compared with open cecectomy in a murine model. Surgery 2003;134(3):432–6.

[32] Demmy TL, Wagner-Mann CC, James MA, et al. Feasibility of mathematical models to predict success in video-assisted thoracic surgery lung nodule excision. Am J Surg 1997; 174(1):20–3.

[33] Roth JA, Pass HI, Wesley MN, et al. Comparison of median sternotomy and thoracotomy for resection of pulmonary metastases in patients with adult soft-tissue sarcomas. Ann Thorac Surg 1986;42(2):134–8.

[34] Younes RN, Gross JL, Deheinzelin D. Surgical resection of unilateral lung metastases: is bilateral thoracotomy necessary? World J Surg 2002;26(9):1112–6.

[35] Bains MS, Ginsberg RJ, Jones WG, et al. The clamshell incision: an improved approach to bilateral pulmonary and mediastinal tumor. Ann Thorac Surg 1994;58(1):30–2.

[36] Shimizu N, Ando A, Matsutani T, et al. Transsternal thoracotomy for bilateral pulmonary metastasis. J Surg Oncol 1992;50(2):105–9.

[37] Margaritora S, Cesario A, Galetta D, et al. Staged axillary thoracotomy for bilateral lung metastases: an effective and minimally invasive approach. Eur J Cardiothorac Surg 1999; 16(Suppl 1):S37–9.

[38] Mineo TC, Ambrogi V, Pompeo E, et al. The value of the Nd:YAG laser for the surgery of lung metastases in a randomized trial. Chest 1998;113(5):1402–7.

[39] Rolle A, Pereszlenyi A, Koch R, et al. Is surgery for multiple lung metastases reasonable? A total of 328 consecutive patients with multiple-laser metastasectomies with a new 1318-nm Nd:YAG laser. J Thorac Cardiovasc Surg 2006;131(6):1236–42.

[40] Vogelsang H, Haas S, Hierholzer C, et al. Factors influencing survival after resection of pulmonary metastases from colorectal cancer. Br J Surg 2004;91(8):1066–71.

[41] Weigel C, Rosenberg C, Langner S, et al. Laser ablation of lung metastases: results according to diameter and location. Eur Radiol 2006;16(8):1769–78.

[42] Putnam JB Jr, Suell DM, Natarajan G, et al. Extended resection of pulmonary metastases: is the risk justified? Ann Thorac Surg 1993;55(6):1440–6.

[43] Jungraithmayr W, Hasse J, Stoelben E. Completion pneumonectomy for lung metastases. Eur J Surg Oncol 2004;30(10):1113–7.

[44] Koong HN, Pastorino U, Ginsberg RJ. Is there a role for pneumonectomy in pulmonary metastases? International registry of lung metastases. Ann Thorac Surg 1999;68(6): 2039–43.

[45] Grunenwald D, Spaggiari L, Girard P, et al. Completion pneumonectomy for lung metastases: is it justified? Eur J Cardiothorac Surg 1997;12(5):694–7.

[46] McKenna RJ Jr, Houck W, Fuller CB. Video-assisted thoracic surgery lobectomy: experience with 1,100 cases. Ann Thorac Surg 2006;81(2):421–5.

[47] Kaseda S, Aoki T, Hangai N, et al. Better pulmonary function and prognosis with video-assisted thoracic surgery than with thoracotomy. Ann Thorac Surg 2000;70(5):1644–6.

[48] Leaver HA, Craig SR, Yap PL, et al. Lymphocyte responses following open and minimally invasive thoracic surgery. Eur J Clin Invest 2000;30(3):230–8.

[49] Sugiura H, Morikawa T, Kaji M, et al. Long-term benefits for the quality of life after video-assisted thoracoscopic lobectomy in patients with lung cancer. Surg Laparosc Endosc Percutan Tech 1999;9(6):403–8.

[50] McCormack PM, Bains MS, Begg CB, et al. Role of video-assisted thoracic surgery in the treatment of pulmonary metastases: results of a prospective trial. Ann Thorac Surg 1996; 62(1):213–6.

[51] Sonett JR. Pulmonary metastases: biologic and historical justification for VATS. Video assisted thoracic surgery. Eur J Cardiothorac Surg 1999;16(Suppl 1):S13–5.

[52] Mutsaerts EL, Zoetmulder FA, Meijer S, et al. Long term survival of thoracoscopic metastasectomy vs metastasectomy by thoracotomy in patients with a solitary pulmonary lesion. Eur J Surg Oncol 2002;28(8):864–8.

[53] Landreneau RJ, De GT, Mack MJ, et al. Therapeutic video-assisted thoracoscopic surgical resection of colorectal pulmonary metastases. Eur J Cardiothorac Surg 2000;18(6): 671–6.

[54] Dupuy DE, DiPetrillo T, Gandhi S, et al. Radiofrequency ablation followed by conventional radiotherapy for medically inoperable stage I non-small cell lung cancer. Chest 2006;129(3):738–45.

[55] Steinke K, King J, Glenn D, et al. Radiologic appearance and complications of percutaneous computed tomography-guided radiofrequency-ablated pulmonary metastases from colorectal carcinoma. J Comput Assist Tomogr 2003;27(5):750–7.
[56] Yan TD, King J, Sjarif A, et al. Percutaneous radiofrequency ablation of pulmonary metastases from colorectal carcinoma: prognostic determinants for survival. Ann Surg Oncol 2006;13(11):1529–37.
[57] Ketchedjian A, Daly B, Luketich J, et al. Minimally invasive techniques for managing pulmonary metastases: video-assisted thoracic surgery and radiofrequency ablation. Thorac Surg Clin 2006;16(2):157–65.
[58] Akoglu S, Ucan ES, Celik G, et al. Endobronchial metastases from extrathoracic malignancies. Clin Exp Metastasis 2005;22(7):587–91.
[59] Sorensen JB. Endobronchial metastases from extrapulmonary solid tumors. Acta Oncol 2004;43(1):73–9.
[60] Litle VR, Christie NA, Fernando HC, et al. Photodynamic therapy for endobronchial metastases from nonbronchogenic primaries. Ann Thorac Surg 2003;76(2):370–5.
[61] Quantrill SJ, Burt PA, Barber PV, et al. Treatment of endobronchial metastases with intraluminal radiotherapy. Respir Med 2000;94(4):369–72.
[62] Quin JA, Letsou GV, Tanoue LT, et al. Use of neodymium yttrium aluminum garnet laser in long-term palliation of airway obstruction. Conn Med 1995;59(7):407–12.
[63] Okunieff P, Petersen AL, Philip A, et al. Stereotactic Body Radiation Therapy (SBRT) for lung metastases. Acta Oncol 2006;45(7):808–17.
[64] Fritz P, Kraus HJ, Muhlnickel W, et al. Stereotactic, single-dose irradiation of stage I non-small cell lung cancer and lung metastases. Radiat Oncol 2006;1:30.
[65] Ratto GB, Toma S, Civalleri D, et al. Isolated lung perfusion with platinum in the treatment of pulmonary metastases from soft tissue sarcomas. J Thorac Cardiovasc Surg 1996;112(3): 614–22.
[66] Pass HI, Mew DJ, Kranda KC, et al. Isolated lung perfusion with tumor necrosis factor for pulmonary metastases. Ann Thorac Surg 1996;61(6):1609–17.
[67] Burt ME, Liu D, Abolhoda A, et al. Isolated lung perfusion for patients with unresectable metastases from sarcoma: a phase I trial. Ann Thorac Surg 2000;69(5):1542–9.
[68] Hendriks JM, Grootenboers MJ, Schramel FM, et al. Isolated lung perfusion with melphalan for resectable lung metastases: a phase I clinical trial. Ann Thorac Surg 2004;78(6): 1919–26.
[69] Vogl TJ, Wetter A, Lindemayr S, et al. Treatment of unresectable lung metastases with transpulmonary chemoembolization: preliminary experience. Radiology 2005;234(3):917–22.
[70] Baeza MR, Barkley HT Jr, Fernandez CH. Total-lung irradiation in the treatment of pulmonary metastases. Radiology 1975;116(1):151–4.
[71] Kayton ML, Meyers P, Wexler LH, et al. Clinical presentation, treatment, and outcome of alveolar soft part sarcoma in children, adolescents, and young adults. J Pediatr Surg 2006; 41(1):187–93.
[72] Sherman N, Vavilala M, Pollock R, et al. Radiation therapy for alveolar soft-part sarcoma. Med Pediatr Oncol 1994;22(6):380–3.
[73] Spunt SL, McCarville MB, Kun LE, et al. Selective use of whole-lung irradiation for patients with Ewing sarcoma family tumors and pulmonary metastases at the time of diagnosis. J Pediatr Hematol Oncol 2001;23(2):93–8.
[74] Xiang J, Xie D, Qiu J. [Cryosurgical resection of pulmonary metastases (experience of twenty years)]. Zhonghua Wai Ke Za Zhi 1995;33(10):639–40 [in Chinese].
[75] Richel O, Zum Vorde Sive Vording PJ, Rietbroek R, et al. Phase II study of carboplatin and whole body hyperthermia (WBH) in recurrent and metastatic cervical cancer. Gynecol Oncol 2004;95(3):680–5.
[76] Shen RN, Hornback NB, Shidnia H, et al. Whole-body hyperthermia decreases lung metastases in lung tumor-bearing mice, possibly via a mechanism involving natural killer cells. J Clin Immunol 1987;7(3):246–53.

[77] Weigel C, Schuchmann S, Kirsch M, et al. [Percutaneous thermoablation of lung metastases. Indication, performance, initial results, and imaging findings]. Radiologe 2004;44(5): 491–9 [in German].
[78] McCormack P. Surgical resection of pulmonary metastases. Semin Surg Oncol 1990;6(5): 297–302.
[79] Monteiro A, Arce N, Bernardo J, et al. Surgical resection of lung metastases from epithelial tumors. Ann Thorac Surg 2004;77(2):431–7.
[80] Rena O, Papalia E, Oliaro A, et al. Pulmonary metastases from epithelial tumours: late results of surgical treatment. Eur J Cardiothorac Surg 2006;30(2):217–22.
[81] Kick J, Schelzig H, Heinecke A, et al. [Resection of lung metastases—risk or chance?]. Zentralbl Chir 2005;130(6):534–8 [in German].
[82] Long-term results of lung metastasectomy: prognostic analyses based on 5206 cases. The international registry of lung metastases. J Thorac Cardiovasc Surg 1997;113(1):37–49.
[83] Pastorino U. Lung metastasectomy: why, when, how. Crit Rev Oncol Hematol 1997;26(3): 137–45.
[84] van de Wal HJ, Verhagen A, Lecluyse A, et al. Surgery of pulmonary metastases. Thorac Cardiovasc Surg 1986;34(Spec No 2):153–6.
[85] Silber R, Elert O, Englmaier S. [Surgical treatment and prognosis of lung metastases]. Langenbecks Arch Chir Suppl II Verh Dtsch Ges Chir 1990;795–9 [in German].
[86] Kamiyoshihara M, Hirai T, Kawashima O, et al. Resection of pulmonary metastases in six patients with disease-free interval greater than 10 years. Ann Thorac Surg 1998;66(1): 231–3.
[87] Girard P, Spaggiari L, Baldeyrou P, et al. Should the number of pulmonary metastases influence the surgical decision? Eur J Cardiothorac Surg 1997;12(3):385–91.
[88] Kandioler D, Kromer E, Tuchler H, et al. Long-term results after repeated surgical removal of pulmonary metastases. Ann Thorac Surg 1998;65(4):909–12.
[89] Vogt-Moykopf I, Bulzebruck H, Kryza S, et al. Results in surgery of pulmonary metastases. Chirurg 1992;118(5):263–71.
[90] Hendriks JM, Romijn S, van PB, et al. Long-term results of surgical resection of lung metastases. Acta Chir Belg 2001;101(6):267–72.
[91] Koodziejski L, Goralczyk J, Dyczek S, et al. The role of surgery in lung metastases. Eur J Surg Oncol 1999;25(4):410–7.
[92] Maniwa Y, Kanki M, Okita Y. Importance of the control of lung recurrence soon after surgery of pulmonary metastases. Am J Surg 2000;179(2):122–5.
[93] Cancer Facts and Figures 2006. American Cancer Society page. Available at: http://www.cancer.org/docroot/STT/stt_0.asp. Accessed December 12, 2006.
[94] Bullard K, Rothenberger D, et al. Colon, rectum, and anus. In: Brunicardi FC, Andersen DK, Billiar TR, editors. Schwartz's principles of surgery. New York: McGraw Hill; 2004. p. 1055–177.
[95] Galandiuk S, Wieand HS, Moertel CG, et al. Patterns of recurrence after curative resection of carcinoma of the colon and rectum. Surg Gynecol Obstet 1992;174(1):27–32.
[96] Rena O, Casadio C, Viano F, et al. Pulmonary resection for metastases from colorectal cancer: factors influencing prognosis. Twenty-year experience. Eur J Cardiothorac Surg 2002; 21(5):906–12.
[97] Pfannschmidt J, Muley T, Hoffmann H, et al. Prognostic factors and survival after complete resection of pulmonary metastases from colorectal carcinoma: experiences in 167 patients. J Thorac Cardiovasc Surg 2003;126(3):732–9.
[98] Sakamoto T, Tsubota N, Iwanaga K, et al. Pulmonary resection for metastases from colorectal cancer. Chest 2001;119(4):1069–72.
[99] Saito Y, Omiya H, Kohno K, et al. Pulmonary metastasectomy for 165 patients with colorectal carcinoma: a prognostic assessment. J Thorac Cardiovasc Surg 2002;124(5):1007–13.
[100] Inoue M, Ohta M, Iuchi K, et al. Benefits of surgery for patients with pulmonary metastases from colorectal carcinoma. Ann Thorac Surg 2004;78(1):238–44.

[101] Zink S, Kayser G, Gabius HJ, et al. Survival, disease-free interval, and associated tumor features in patients with colon/rectal carcinomas and their resected intra-pulmonary metastases. Eur J Cardiothorac Surg 2001;19(6):908–13.
[102] Yedibela S, Klein P, Feuchter K, et al. Surgical management of pulmonary metastases from colorectal cancer in 153 patients. Ann Surg Oncol 2006;13(11):1538–44.
[103] Iwasaki A, Shirakusa T, Yamashita Y, et al. Characteristic differences between patients who have undergone surgical treatment for lung metastasis or hepatic metastasis from colorectal cancer. Thorac Cardiovasc Surg 2005;53(6):358–64.
[104] Girard P, Ducreux M, Baldeyrou P, et al. Surgery for lung metastases from colorectal cancer: analysis of prognostic factors. J Clin Oncol 1996;14(7):2047–53.
[105] McAfee MK, Allen MS, Trastek VF, et al. Colorectal lung metastases: results of surgical excision. Ann Thorac Surg 1992;53(5):780–5.
[106] Headrick JR, Miller DL, Nagorney DM, et al. Surgical treatment of hepatic and pulmonary metastases from colon cancer. Ann Thorac Surg 2001;71(3):975–9.
[107] Iizasa T, Suzuki M, Yoshida S, et al. Prediction of prognosis and surgical indications for pulmonary metastasectomy from colorectal cancer. Ann Thorac Surg 2006;82(1):254–60.
[108] Smith JW, Fortner JG, Burt M. Resection of hepatic and pulmonary metastases from colorectal cancer. Surg Oncol 1992;1(6):399–404.
[109] Gough DB, Donohue JH, Trastek VA, et al. Resection of hepatic and pulmonary metastases in patients with colorectal cancer. Br J Surg 1994;81(1):94–6.
[110] Steele G Jr, Ravikumar TS. Resection of hepatic metastases from colorectal cancer. Biologic perspective. Ann Surg 1989;210(2):127–38.
[111] Hughes KS, Rosenstein RB, Songhorabodi S, et al. Resection of the liver for colorectal carcinoma metastases. A multi-institutional study of long-term survivors. Dis Colon Rectum 1988;31(1):1–4.
[112] Ohlsson B, Stenram U, Tranberg KG. Resection of colorectal liver metastases: 25-year experience. World J Surg 1998;22(3):268–76.
[113] Minagawa M, Makuuchi M, Torzilli G, et al. Extension of the frontiers of surgical indications in the treatment of liver metastases from colorectal cancer: long-term results. Ann Surg 2000;231(4):487–99.
[114] Simmonds PC, Primrose JN, Colquitt JL, et al. Surgical resection of hepatic metastases from colorectal cancer: a systematic review of published studies. Br J Cancer 2006;94(7): 982–99.
[115] Tomimaru Y, Sasaki Y, Yamada T, et al. The significance of surgical resection for pulmonary metastasis from hepatocellular carcinoma. Am J Surg 2006;192(1):46–51.
[116] Gwak GY, Jung JO, Sung SW, et al. Long-term survival after pulmonary metastasectomy of hepatocellular carcinoma; treatment outcome or natural history? Hepatogastroenterology 2004;51(59):1428–33.
[117] Lam CM, Lo CM, Yuen WK, et al. Prolonged survival in selected patients following surgical resection for pulmonary metastasis from hepatocellular carcinoma. Br J Surg 1998; 85(9):1198–200.
[118] Nakajima J, Tanaka M, Matsumoto J, et al. Appraisal of surgical treatment for pulmonary metastasis from hepatocellular carcinoma. World J Surg 2005;29(6):715–8.
[119] Nakagawa T, Kamiyama T, Nakanishi K, et al. Pulmonary resection for metastases from hepatocellular carcinoma: factors influencing prognosis. J Thorac Cardiovasc Surg 2006; 131(6):1248–54.
[120] Kanemitsu Y, Kondo H, Katai H, et al. Surgical resection of pulmonary metastases from gastric cancer. J Surg Oncol 1998;69(3):147–50.
[121] Tsuchiya H, Kanazawa Y, bdel-Wanis ME, et al. Effect of timing of pulmonary metastases identification on prognosis of patients with osteosarcoma: the Japanese Musculoskeletal Oncology Group study. J Clin Oncol 2002;20(16):3470–7.
[122] Ferrari S, Briccoli A, Mercuri M, et al. Postrelapse survival in osteosarcoma of the extremities: prognostic factors for long-term survival. J Clin Oncol 2003;21(4):710–5.

[123] Kempf-Bielack B, Bielack SS, Jurgens H, et al. Osteosarcoma relapse after combined modality therapy: an analysis of unselected patients in the Cooperative Osteosarcoma Study Group (COSS). J Clin Oncol 2005;23(3):559–68.
[124] Harting MT, Blakely ML. Management of osteosarcoma pulmonary metastases. Semin Pediatr Surg 2006;15(1):25–9.
[125] Antunes M, Bernardo J, Salete M, et al. Excision of pulmonary metastases of osteogenic sarcoma of the limbs. Eur J Cardiothorac Surg 1999;15(5):592–6.
[126] Briccoli A, Rocca M, Salone M, et al. Resection of recurrent pulmonary metastases in patients with osteosarcoma. Cancer 2005;104(8):1721–5.
[127] Saltzman DA, Snyder CL, Ferrell KL, et al. Aggressive metastasectomy for pulmonic sarcomatous metastases: a follow-up study. Am J Surg 1993;166(5):543–7.
[128] Choong PF, Pritchard DJ, Rock MG, et al. Survival after pulmonary metastasectomy in soft tissue sarcoma. Prognostic factors in 214 patients. Acta Orthop Scand 1995;66(6): 561–8.
[129] Billingsley KG, Burt ME, Jara E, et al. Pulmonary metastases from soft tissue sarcoma: analysis of patterns of diseases and postmetastasis survival. Ann Surg 1999;229(5):602–10.
[130] Weiser MR, Downey RJ, Leung DH, et al. Repeat resection of pulmonary metastases in patients with soft-tissue sarcoma. J Am Coll Surg 2000;191(2):184–90.
[131] Lanza LA, Putnam JB Jr, Benjamin RS, et al. Response to chemotherapy does not predict survival after resection of sarcomatous pulmonary metastases. Ann Thorac Surg 1991; 51(2):219–24.
[132] Adjuvant chemotherapy for localised resectable soft-tissue sarcoma of adults: meta-analysis of individual data. Sarcoma Meta-Analysis Collaboration. Lancet 1997;350(9092): 1647–54.
[133] Kodama K, Doi O, Higashiyama M, et al. Surgery for multiple lung metastases from alveolar soft-part sarcoma. Surg Today 1997;27(9):806–11.
[134] Harpole DH Jr, Johnson CM, Wolfe WG, et al. Analysis of 945 cases of pulmonary metastatic melanoma. J Thorac Cardiovasc Surg 1992;103(4):743–8.
[135] Leo F, Cagini L, Rocmans P, et al. Lung metastases from melanoma: when is surgical treatment warranted? Br J Cancer 2000;83(5):569–72.
[136] Pogrebniak HW, Stovroff M, Roth JA, et al. Resection of pulmonary metastases from malignant melanoma: results of a 16-year experience. Ann Thorac Surg 1988;46(1):20–3.
[137] Planchard D, Soria JC, Michiels S, et al. Uncertain benefit from surgery in patients with lung metastases from breast carcinoma. Cancer 2004;100(1):28–35.
[138] Chang EY, Johnson W, Karamlou K, et al. The evaluation and treatment implications of isolated pulmonary nodules in patients with a recent history of breast cancer. Am J Surg 2006;191(5):641–5.
[139] Friedel G, Pastorino U, Ginsberg RJ, et al. Results of lung metastasectomy from breast cancer: prognostic criteria on the basis of 467 cases of the international registry of lung metastases. Eur J Cardiothorac Surg 2002;22(3):335–44.
[140] Kayser K, Biechele U, Kayser G, et al. Pulmonary metastases of breast carcinomas: ligandohistochemical, nuclear, and structural analysis of primary and metastatic tumors with emphasis on period of occurrence of metastases and survival. J Surg Oncol 1998;69(3): 137–46.
[141] Liu D, Abolhoda A, Burt ME, et al. Pulmonary metastasectomy for testicular germ cell tumors: a 28-year experience. Ann Thorac Surg 1998;66(5):1709–14.
[142] Hartmann JT, Candelaria M, Kuczyk MA, et al. Comparison of histological results from the resection of residual masses at different sites after chemotherapy for metastatic nonseminomatous germ cell tumours. Eur J Cancer 1997;33(6):843–7.
[143] Brenner PC, Herr HW, Morse MJ, et al. Simultaneous retroperitoneal, thoracic, and cervical resection of postchemotherapy residual masses in patients with metastatic nonseminomatous germ cell tumors of the testis. J Clin Oncol 1996;14(6):1765–9.

[144] Eskicorapci SY, Ekici S, Atsu MN, et al. Resection of pulmonary metastases following chemotherapy for high stage testicular tumors. Int J Urol 2004;11(8):634–9.
[145] Antonelli A, Zani D, Cozzoli A, et al. Surgical treatment of metastases from renal cell carcinoma. Arch Ital Urol Androl 2005;77(2):125–8.
[146] Piltz S, Meimarakis G, Wichmann MW, et al. Long-term results after pulmonary resection of renal cell carcinoma metastases. Ann Thorac Surg 2002;73(4):1082–7.
[147] Kavolius JP, Mastorakos DP, Pavlovich C, et al. Resection of metastatic renal cell carcinoma. J Clin Oncol 1998;16(6):2261–6.
[148] Fabozzi SJ, Schellhammer PF, el-Mahdi AM. Pulmonary metastases from prostate cancer. Cancer 1995;75(11):2706–9.
[149] Wedman J, Balm AJ, Hart AA, et al. Value of resection of pulmonary metastases in head and neck cancer patients. Head Neck 1996;18(4):311–6.
[150] Liu D, Labow DM, Dang N, et al. Pulmonary metastasectomy for head and neck cancers. Ann Surg Oncol 1999;6(6):572–8.
[151] Leong PP, Rezai B, Koch WM, et al. Distinguishing second primary tumors from lung metastases in patients with head and neck squamous cell carcinoma. J Natl Cancer Inst 1998; 90(13):972–7.
[152] Kerr VE, Cadman E. Pulmonary metastases in ovarian cancer. Analysis of 357 patients. Cancer 1985;56(5):1209–13.
[153] Anraku M, Yokoi K, Nakagawa K, et al. Pulmonary metastases from uterine malignancies: results of surgical resection in 133 patients. J Thorac Cardiovasc Surg 2004;127(4):1107–12.
[154] Tangjitgamol S, Levenback CF, Beller U, et al. Role of surgical resection for lung, liver, and central nervous system metastases in patients with gynecological cancer: a literature review. Int J Gynecol Cancer 2004;14(3):399–422.
[155] Yamamoto K, Yoshikawa H, Shiromizu K, et al. Pulmonary metastasectomy for uterine cervical cancer: a multivariate analysis. Ann Thorac Surg 2004;77(4):1179–82.
[156] Dominkus M, Ruggieri P, Bertoni F, et al. Histologically verified lung metastases in benign giant cell tumours—14 cases from a single institution. Int Orthop 2006.
[157] Tubbs WS, Brown LR, Beabout JW, et al. Benign giant-cell tumor of bone with pulmonary metastases: clinical findings and radiologic appearance of metastases in 13 cases. AJR Am J Roentgenol 1992;158(2):331–4.
[158] Murrah CP, Ferguson ER, Jennelle RL, et al. Resection of multiple pulmonary metastases from a recurrent intracranial meningioma. Ann Thorac Surg 1996;61(6):1823–4.
[159] Khan JH, McElhinney DB, Rahman SB, et al. Pulmonary metastases of endocrine origin: the role of surgery. Chest 1998;114(2):526–34.
[160] Karnak I, Emin SM, Kutluk T, et al. Pulmonary metastases in children: an analysis of surgical spectrum. Eur J Pediatr Surg 2002;12(3):151–8.
[161] Pastorino U, Gasparini M, Tavecchio L, et al. The contribution of salvage surgery to the management of childhood osteosarcoma. J Clin Oncol 1991;9(8):1357–62.
[162] Perilongo G, Brown J, Shafford E, et al. Hepatoblastoma presenting with lung metastases: treatment results of the first cooperative, prospective study of the International Society Of Paediatric Oncology on childhood liver tumors. Cancer 2000;89(8):1845–53.
[163] Heij HA, Vos A, de KJ, et al. Prognostic factors in surgery for pulmonary metastases in children. Surgery 1994;115(6):687–93.
[164] Temeck BK, Wexler LH, Steinberg SM, et al. Reoperative pulmonary metastasectomy for sarcomatous pediatric histologies. Ann Thorac Surg 1998;66(3):908–12.

ELSEVIER
SAUNDERS

Surg Oncol Clin N Am
16 (2007) 607–625

SURGICAL
ONCOLOGY CLINICS
OF NORTH AMERICA

The Role of Minimal Access Surgery for Metastasectomy and Cytoreduction

Horacio J. Asbun, MD[a,b,*], Michaela Straznicka, MD[c], Vivian E. Strong, MD[d]

[a]*John Muir Health, 401 Gregory Lane, # 204, Walnut Creek, CA 94523, USA*
[b]*Hepatobiliary and Pancreas Cancer Program, John Muir Cancer Institute, 1601 Ygnacio Valley Road, Walnut Creek, CA 94598, USA*
[c]*Thoracic Oncology Program, John Muir Cancer Institute, 1601 Ygnacio Valley Road, Walnut Creek, CA 94598, USA*
[d]*Memorial Sloan-Kettering Cancer Center, Weill Medical College of Cornell University, 1275 York Ave. # 1217, New York, NY 10021, USA*

The role of minimal-access surgery for resection of malignant neoplasms has been widely debated and remains an area of controversy for surgical oncologists. Since the early years of advanced laparoscopic procedures, concerns about port-site metastases [1–3] and dissemination of tumor cells via carbon dioxide insufflation [4] prevented laparoscopic surgeons from further developing innovative approaches for oncologic resections. Controversy developed even for the most common gastrointestinal cancers, such as colon cancer. More recent prospective, randomized trials have put these controversies to rest and have demonstrated the safety of the laparoscopic approach [5]. The key goals are to ensure safe, complete oncologic resections and, at the same time, provide the benefits of decreased pain, shorter hospital stay, fewer incisional hernias, and earlier return to work. Decreased blood loss and immunosuppression after minimally invasive surgery may specifically benefit cancer patients [6].

The slow progress and acceptance of minimal-access cancer surgery may also be related to limited training and experience within the field of surgical oncology. While this factor is difficult to measure, most advanced laparoscopic surgery training programs, with the exception of those for colon cancer, have limited access to major oncologic pathologic processes, such as those involving liver, pancreas, or esophageal cancers. It is therefore less

* Corresponding author.
E-mail address: asbun@bayareasurgical.net (H.J. Asbun).

1055-3207/07/$ - see front matter © 2007 Elsevier Inc. All rights reserved.
doi:10.1016/j.soc.2007.04.008 **surgonc.theclinics.com**

likely for a highly skilled advanced laparoscopic surgeon to be as experienced and well trained in surgical oncology as in other areas of laparoscopic surgery. Meanwhile, the large majority of surgical oncology training programs have not widely embraced advanced laparoscopic techniques. This gap should narrow as more general surgeons are trained and become proficient in advanced laparoscopic techniques and as more specific and appropriate minimal-access approaches are developed for oncologic surgery.

By design, minimally invasive procedures are ideally suited for clinical scenarios where palliation is the main goal. Because of important recent advances in systemic, regional cytotoxic and biologic therapy as well as in nonresectional ablation techniques, the strict separation of curative and palliative surgical interventions has been somewhat obscured. In patients selected for cytoreductive surgery and metastasectomy, the intent is less likely cancer cure and more likely improved quality of life and prolonged survival with cancer. In this setting, surgery is just one more modality within a therapeutic framework rather than the traditional single modality for cure.

In this context, minimal-access surgery may have a significant role beyond palliative procedures alone. Because of its implicit advantages, the development of innovative minimal-access procedures may find increased acceptance with surgeons and affected patients by way of providing less traumatic and debilitating surgery when life span is limited and surgery likely noncurative.

In this article, we summarize findings on the applicability of minimal-access techniques for thoracic and upper gastrointestinal cancers, including those affecting the lung, liver, stomach, and adrenal gland. If metastasectomy and cytoreductive surgery are rapidly evolving, minimal-access surgery in this setting is in its introductory stages. Even though minimal-access metastasectomy and cytoreductive surgery may harbor great potential for selected cancer patients, its benefits are not well understood and need further elucidation in clinical studies.

Liver cancer

The advantages of metastasectomy are best illustrated in the treatment of colorectal cancer liver metastases. The expected outcomes of colorectal cancer liver metastasectomy are well established and indications for such a metastasectomy are traditionally restricted to assure resection in curable patients only [7]. The recent development of vastly more efficient cytotoxic and biologic therapies for metastatic colorectal cancer have led to the inclusion of patients for metastasectomy who traditionally would have been judged unresectable for cure [8]. Furthermore, the introduction of safe nonresectional ablative techniques has further challenged the classic resection indications, such as number of metastases and/or presence of bilobar disease. Along with newer systemic agents, combined ablation and resection as well as staged and repeat hepatectomies are now practiced with low mortality and promising results in patients previously deemed unresectable [9]. Patient selection, indications, and outcomes for open surgical resection are extensively discussed in other articles in this issue. We will focus our discussion on the minimal-access approach to liver metastases.

Laparoscopy and laparoscopic ultrasound was first used in liver surgery for malignant disease as a diagnostic and staging tool. Several studies have shown the significant impact of laparoscopic ultrasonography on staging based on its ability to detect small lesions missed by preoperative CT and MRI (Table 1) [10,11]. With the emergence of high-resolution CT scanners and the routine use of multiphase scanning, the accuracy of preoperative staging has improved and the impact of laparoscopic ultrasound staging may not be as significant in the future. Nevertheless, as in its open counterpart, laparoscopic ultrasound plays a critical role in minimal-access surgery for liver metastases. Adequate exposure of the liver is mandatory and division of the ligamentus teres, falciform ligament, right and left triangular ligaments, and possibly the coronary ligament are required to fully mobilize the liver, depending on the location of the lesion.

Laparoscopic radiofrequency ablation plays an important role in minimal-access surgery for liver metastases. It allows tumor destruction when resection is not possible because of concerns regarding the preservation of residual hepatic function. It is associated with very low morbidity and mortality. Its main disadvantage resides in relatively high rates of local recurrence. For a variety of reasons, ablation is the method of choice for nonresectional approaches to liver metastases and, in many cases, the laparoscopic approach is preferable to percutaneous ablation. The procedure can be applied safely for superficial lesions and lesions on the dome of the liver that may otherwise require transdiaphragmatic access. Neighboring viscera and other structures can be retracted to avoid injury, and direct visualization of the hepatic puncture site facilitates hemostasis. The laparoscopic approach can also be used for staging extrahepatic and peritoneal disease, performing biopsy procedures, and assessing other suspicious lesions.

Table 1
Influence of intraoperative laparoscopic ultrasound in staging for patients with liver malignancies

Author/reference	Number of patients	Stage changed by intraoperative laparoscopic ultrasound
Awad et al, [10] 2002	14	28%
Terrosu et al, 2000	76	28%
Velasco et al, 2000	33	18%
Rahusen et al, [11] 1999	47	38%
Marchesa et al, 1996	22	12%
Hunnerbein et al, 1995	20	15%
John et al, 1994	43	33%

Even though laparoscopic resection of benign disease has become relatively commonplace, laparoscopic resection for malignant disease has remained controversial and limited to those surgeons with extensive experience in both hepatic and laparoscopic surgery. After the first use of laparoscopic liver resection in 1993 [12], several articles about the procedure have been published [12–20] (Table 2). Many of these articles report a significant number of major hepatectomies with acceptable morbidity and mortality rates [13,17]. Dissemination of cancer cells has not been an issue in experienced hands [15,16,21,22]. It is evident from these investigations that blood loss as well as operative time significantly improve as more experience is gained. The surgeon embarking in laparoscopic liver resections should be facile with the surgical principles of open hepatic surgery.

Patients are positioned supine, with the right side elevated if a right hepatectomy is planned. The number and location of ports vary with the procedure and the surgeon's preference. One should plan for the possibility of performing a hand-assisted laparoscopic surgery (HALS) when placing the ports. HALS is particularly helpful when performing formal right hepatic lobectomies, when dealing with a large specimen, and when manual palpation is required for evaluating extent of disease. HALS can facilitate retraction of a bulky lobe during right hepatectomy, shorten operative time, and decrease blood loss. Mobilization of the liver is readily obtained by dividing the ligamentus teres, falciform, triangular, and coronary ligaments. Some surgeons prefer to delay division of the triangular ligament and coronary ligaments so that the ligaments can be used for traction and support during the parenchymal resection [23]. The technical aspects of hilar dissection and ligation of the hilar vessels and bile ducts are similar to those for open surgery using suture or appropriate staple devices. The ligation of the hepatic veins is usually performed during parenchymal transection. It is advisable to identify and expose the suprahepatic vena cava and its tributaries before parenchymal dissection. Laparoscopic identification of the left or right hepatic veins as they join the vena cava is feasible and provides for additional control of hepatic blood flow.

In recent years, laparoscopic ultrasonic energy devices, improved electrothermal and bipolar devices, water jet dissectors, and cavitational ultrasonic surgical applicators have facilitated the minimal-access approach to parenchymal dissection. The surgeon experienced with open liver surgery can seamlessly apply these technologies to laparoscopic hepatic resections. Metallic clips are helpful for medium-sized vessels and bile ducts. Major vascular structures are either suture-ligated or transected with laparoscopic staplers. Because three-dimensional visualization during laparoscopy can be suboptimal, the direction of the dissection is constantly reassessed to assure parenchymal transsection in the desired plane. Early identification and localization of the suprahepatic vein branches significantly aids in delineating the direction of dissection. The general principles of adequate suction, irrigation, and retraction are as crucial in laparoscopic surgery as they are

Table 2
Outcomes of laparoscopic liver resection for malignant disease

Author/ reference	Number of patients	Malignancies (%)	Morbidity	Mortality	Conversion to open	Operating room time (minutes)	Length of hospital stay (days)
Dagher et al [13], 2007	70	38 (54%)	16%	2.6%	10%	227 ± 109	5.9
Vibert et al [14], 2006	89	65 (73%)	21%	1.1%	13.5%	NA	NA
Cherqui et al [15], 2006	27	27 (100%)	33%	0%	26%	240 ± 75	15.2
Kaneko et al [12], 2005	30	30 (100%)	10%	0%	3.3%	182 ± 38	14.9
Mala et al [16], 2005	53	53 (100%)	16%	0%	NA	NA	3.5
Buell et al [17], 2005	100	35 (35%)	23%	1%	0%	132	3
Gigot et al [18], 2002	37	37 (100%)	22%	0%	13.5%	NA	6
Descottes et al [19], 2002	87	81 (93%)	5%	0%	10%	NA	5
Huscher et al [20], 1998	38	32 (84%)	43%	2.5%	5.3%	189 ± 80	10

Abbreviation: NA, information not available.

in the open procedure. Having an experienced laparoscopic surgeon as an assistant is a significant benefit during the parenchymal dissection, particularly when performing a major hepatic resection. Once a major hepatic vein branch is identified, it is usually divided with an endo-stapler under direct visualization. If HALS is being performed, the vein is circumferentially exposed with careful finger-dissection and the stapler is guided accordingly. Newer laparoscopic hydro-dissection and coagulation devices allow safe circumferential exposure of major vascular structures without injury to the vessel itself and greatly facilitate laparoscopic parenchymal dissection.

Gas embolism in laparoscopic hepatic surgery, a potentially serious complication, is rare [24]. The main steps of prevention include (1) maintaining the lowest possible intraabdominal pressure that still allows for adequate exposure during parenchymal dissection and (2) avoiding exposed open venous branches by clamping or ligating them before division.

Once the specimen is completely freed, it should be placed in an endoscopic retrieval bag and removed from the abdomen. Except for cirrhotic livers, specimens usually can be removed through a relatively small incision by gentle traction maneuvers. Placement of a wound protector and expander greatly facilitates this step and avoids direct contact of the specimen with the wound. It is important to remove the specimen en bloc for correct pathologic margin assessment.

The residual raw surface of the liver is inspected for complete hemostasis and for any bile leaks, which are dealt with in a manner similar to that used in open surgery. Drains are used at the surgeon's discretion.

Gastric cancer

Gastric adenocarcinoma is the fourth leading cause of cancer deaths in the United States and affects roughly 25,000 patients per year [25]. Despite these alarming statistics, little progress has been made for this disease, perhaps largely due to the late stage at which the diagnosis is made. In countries such as Japan, South Korea, Costa Rica, and those of the former Soviet Union the death rates from gastric cancer range between 38 to 55 patients per 100,000 population. In the United States, the incidence of gastric cancer is lower but remains at 1:100,000 per year [26–28]. Japanese investigators have been leaders in developing both screening techniques and minimal-access approaches to treatment of early gastric cancers. Unfortunately, in the United States, few patients present with early stage disease amenable to minimally invasive surgery.

Despite these issues, the role of minimal-access surgery for gastric cancer is expanding. Laparoscopic wedge resection for gastrointestinal stromal tumors and carcinoids is now well established and has enabled patients to have earlier intervention for diagnostic and therapeutic purposes, without the morbidity of a laparotomy. The indications for laparoscopic approaches to treat gastric adenocarcinoma are growing as we improve our understanding of the disease process. Japanese cancer centers have heralded this effort and continue to evaluate the utility and technique of minimal-access surgery for gastric cancer. Studies in other countries have resulted in similar experiences and recommendations. For instance, Huscher and colleagues [29] reported on 5-year clinical outcomes of laparoscopic-assisted subtotal gastrectomy compared with open subtotal gastrectomy for stage-matched adenocarcinomas, and demonstrated both safety and feasibility of the laparoscopic approach. Five-year survival numbers showed no significant difference between the two groups. Other studies have demonstrated similar outcomes [30,31].

Meanwhile, interest has grown in the use of cytoreduction in the management of advanced gastric cancer. Currently, clinical trials are being performed using multimodality treatments comparing intraperitoneal and systemic chemotherapy, cryoablation, radiofrequency ablation, and surgical debulking. A prospective study by Jeung and colleagues [32] reported on the feasibility of using intraperitoneal chemotherapy to treat advanced gastric cancer in 49 patients after palliative gastrectomy. Aggressive cytoreduction yielded a progression-free interval of 7 months and an overall survival of 12 months. Farma and colleagues [33] evaluated the response of 18 patients, including 9 with gastric cancer, who presented with peritoneal carcinomatosis. After optimal cytoreduction, intraperitoneal chemotherapy with 5-fluorouracil and paclitaxel achieved a median overall survival of only 8 months [33]. These investigators concluded that other novel approaches should be evaluated. A number of other reports, including those on peritonectomy as treatment for peritoneal dissemination of gastric cancer, yielded varying results [34–36]. Clearly, additional studies to validate the benefits of cytoreduction for gastric cancer are needed. Table 3 summarizes some of the current studies examining cytoreduction therapies combined with intraperitoneal chemotherapy for advanced gastric cancer. The main difficulty in advanced gastric cancer remains the high rate of peritoneal recurrence. After curative resection of T3/T4 tumors, about 60% recur in the peritoneal cavity.

Minimal access surgery has greatly contributed to more accurate staging of patients to avoid unnecessary open procedures. In 2001, Conlon [37] described staging laparoscopy for gastric cancer and noted that peritoneal washings obtained from 103 consecutive patients demonstrated metastatic disease in 37% of patients judged to have only localized disease before laparoscopy. A study by Bentrem and colleagues [38] has shown that positive peritoneal cytology is associated with a particularly poor prognosis and median survival of only 15 months. In such a setting, metastatic peritoneal disease portends such a poor prognosis that many groups believe surgical resection should not be offered with therapeutic intent [39]. Virally directed fluorescent imaging compounds may one day provide better localization of peritoneal metastases [40].

For patients with unresectable gastric adenocarcinoma, minimal-access options exist as well. Sarela and colleagues [41] found that 50% of 165

Table 3
Cytoreduction therapies combined with intraperitoneal chemotherapy for advanced gastric cancer

Author/ reference	Year	Number of patients with gastric cancer	Total number of patients	Survival
Jeung et al [32]	2002	49	49	12-month median
Farma et al [33]	2005	9	18	8-month median (all patients)
Yonemura et al [35]	2002	32	57	18% of gastric cancer patients survived 5 years
Roviello et al [43]	2006	12	59	51% of gastric cancer patients survived 5 years
Glehen et al [44]	2006	125	376	3-month median
Kusamura et al [34]	2005	12	205	Not reported

patients with metastatic gastric adenocarcinoma required invasive procedures at a median time of 4 months, mostly percutaneous endoscopic procedures for nutrition or obstruction. Only 12% of the patients in this series required surgical intervention. Laparoscopic gastrojejunostomy for palliation in such patients is an ideal option. Choi [42] described 78 patients with unresectable gastric cancer who underwent laparoscopic gastrojejunostomy resulting in lower perioperative morbidity and earlier recovery of gastrointestinal function compared with patients who underwent open gastrojejunostomy. A laparoscopic wedge resection or laparoscopic distal gastrectomy is ideally suited to palliate selected patients with minimal morbidity and mortality.

In summary, although debulking and cytoreduction remain controversial and require further systematic investigation, improvements in early diagnosis, refinements in instrumentation, and demand for more effective palliative and cytoreductive procedures will likely increase the role of laparoscopy as part of a multimodality strategy for gastric cancer patients [43,44].

Adrenal neoplasms

Neoplasms of the adrenal gland are rare and paucity of data makes treatment recommendations difficult. Laparoscopic adrenalectomy is accepted by most surgeons as the gold standard for benign disease, but recommendations of laparoscopic techniques for malignant tumors remain controversial because of possible dissemination of tumor cells.

Approximately 5% to 6% of pheochromocytomas are malignant, with an annual prevalence of 0.3 to 0.7 cases per million in the United States for malignant pheochromocytomas [45]. Differentiating a benign pheochromocytoma from a malignant pheochromocytoma is often difficult, relying on the presence of tumor deposits in sites that do not usually have chromaffin cells or on imaging or histologic proof of local invasion [46]. Malignant tumors may only reveal themselves through a clinical course of recurrence, a process that may take 5 or more years after initial resection [47,48]. Because nonsurgical treatment is unavailable and determination of malignancy often impossible before resection [45], laparoscopic resection of a biochemically proven pheochromocytoma remains a valuable option. If local invasion is encountered intraoperatively, conversion to an open procedure should be considered to ensure that the capsule is not violated and to make certain the tumorectomy is complete. A preoperative CT is critical to assess tumor size and to help guide the surgical approach [49].

Adrenal cortical carcinoma (ACC) is an aggressive malignancy with an overall 5-year survival of $<30\%$ and with two of three patients developing recurrence within 2 years [50]. Given the poor prognosis of this disease and the lack of effective adjuvant therapies, resection is the only possible cure. Some investigators have advocated a more aggressive approach to incidentalomas in an attempt to detect early adrenal cortical carcinomas [51]. Although some groups advocate open resections for any suspected ACC, no large-scale study has evaluated the efficacy of laparoscopic adrenalectomy for ACC. The three largest series to date include six patients each. Each patient underwent laparoscopic adrenalectomy for ACC. The investigation reported local recurrence in two of six, three of six, and two of six patients, respectively [52,53]. The group from MD Anderson additionally reported 100% recurrence in patients who underwent a laparoscopic resection versus 35% recurrence in open adrenalectomy [54]. Five of the patients developed carcinomatosis, consistent with the natural history of this aggressive neoplasm. Complete resection is a critical component of treatment, as demonstrated by a series from Memorial Sloan-Kettering Cancer Center, where complete primary resection was associated with a 55% 5-year survival, as opposed to a 5-year survival of 5% with incomplete resection [55]. Because this is a rare cancer, the suitability of laparoscopy in this application remains uncertain. As with any cancer operation, a minimal-access approach is feasible for well-circumscribed, smaller lesions that are within the safe technical abilities of the operating surgeon. For large and obviously invasive lesions, the open approach is usually advocated.

The role of minimal-access techniques for metastatic lesions to the adrenal is becoming clearer [53,56]. Studies have established that resection of isolated metastases to the adrenal gland is associated with improved survival when compared with chemotherapy alone [57]. A retrospective study from Memorial Sloan-Kettering Cancer Center reported 11 patients undergoing laparoscopic resection for adrenal metastases, compared with a group of open resections. The overall 5-year actuarial survival was 29% and there was no difference in overall survival in either group [56]. Another series from the Cleveland Clinic reported on 26 patients having laparoscopic adrenalectomy for isolated adrenal metastases and demonstrated safety and efficacy. There were no port-site metastases, no operative mortalities, and no differences in survival [53]. Other series similarly have shown safe and efficacious results [52,58]. Part of the difficulty in assessing minimal-access techniques for metastatic lesions is the small number of cases and the inherent bias of studying a highly selected group of patients who have favorable tumor biology and are candidates for surgical resection. The guiding principle for such resections includes a technically safe, complete excision without violation of the lesion capsule. Emerging evidence suggests that patients who respond to treatment of their primary malignancy benefit significantly from adrenal metastasectomy.

Pulmonary metastases

Retrospective studies have documented a survival benefit for well-selected patients who develop pulmonary metastases. Patients who are most likely to obtain clinical benefit should ideally have certain characteristics: control of the primary tumor, no evidence of extra thoracic metastases, complete removal of thoracic tumor burden possible, and acceptable decrease in pulmonary function [59]. A longer disease-free interval from initial diagnosis to metastatic presentation is associated with improved survival. These criteria were confirmed in the largest series of pulmonary metastectomy trial reports by the International Registry of Lung Metastasis [60].

The standard approach for pulmonary metastasectomy has been thoracotomy or median sternotomy with bimanual palpation of the lung parenchyma. Bimanual palpation allows for careful examination of the entire lung tissue and identification of all but micrometastatic disease. Although the open approach is considered the standard of care, it can be associated with significant morbidity. This has led to an increased application of minimally invasive approaches to pulmonary metastectomy, specifically thoracoscopy or video-assisted thoracic surgery (VATS). Minimally invasive treatments offer decreased pain, decreased morbidity, and the potential to preserve pulmonary and physical function, especially in patients who are considered high risk for open procedures or are candidates for palliation only [61]. The major disadvantage of a thoracoscopic approach is the loss of tactile tumor localization. Several novel approaches have been proposed to replace tactile localization. The relative risks and benefits of these approaches are discussed in this section.

VATS for pulmonary metastasis was first documented at the University of Pittsburgh in 1992. Dowling and colleagues [62] successfully resected a solitary renal cell carcinoma metastasis using the Nd:YAG garnet laser and a thoracoscopic approach. The same institution subsequently reported a series of 72 patients treated with thoracoscopic metastectomy. The investigators concluded that thoracoscopy was a feasible technique for the treatment of pulmonary metastasis.

The use of thoracoscopy for pulmonary metastasis has technical limitations. The inherent characteristics of the technique make bimanual palpation of the lung not possible. There is argument that macroscopic disease may be missed without manual examination. This could compromise oncologic outcome since complete resection of all disease is associated with significantly improved survival [63,64]. The International Registry of Lung Metastases study documented 36% 5-year survival in completely resected patients as compared with 13% when resection was incomplete [61].

The use of VATS for metastectomy has also been challenged. McCormack and colleagues [65] from Memorial Sloan-Kettering Cancer Center conducted a prospective trial comparing VATS to thoracotomy for metastectomy. The trial was suspended after accrual of 18 patients because of a statistically significant benefit for thoracotomy patients. In 83% of the patients, all nodules seen on CT scan were resected by VATS approach. These same patients were then explored via thoracotomy. Additional nodules not seen on CT or by thoracoscopy were identified at thoracotomy in 10 of 18 patients (56%). The investigators conclude that VATS was inadequate as a therapeutic modality and should be reserved for diagnosis only. This study used older-generation CT scans with thick cuts (1 cm), decreasing the ability to detect smaller nodules. Modern helical scans have significantly increased the sensitivity of finding small (< 10 mm) nodules preoperatively.

A Dutch study used a similar design for 28 patients, explored first by thoracoscopy and then thoracotomy [66]. VATS resection was not possible in 10 patients secondary to central location of the tumor nodules. One patient with carcinoid tumor was excluded. In the remaining 17 patients, 12 had a single lesion. Of these, 11 were successfully resected (92%) via thoracoscopy. Only 1 of the 5 patients with multiple lesions was completely resected (20%). The investigators concluded that VATS resection should be reserved for patients with solitary nodules located in the lung periphery.

Multiple studies were conducted to measure the physiologic impact of thoracoscopy versus thoracotomy with the expectation that thoracoscopy patients would demonstrate decreased morbidity and faster recovery. Ninomiya and colleagues [67] compared pulmonary function tests before and after thoracoscopy or thoracotomy. They compared changes in vital capacity in the early and late postoperative phase. The VATS group demonstrated significantly better outcomes with a decrease in early and late vital capacity of 16% and 2% respectively, compared with 33% and 18% in the thoracotomy group. The decrease in early vital capacity was greater in patients requiring repeat thoracotomy (61%) compared with repeat thoracoscopy (21%). Landreneau and colleagues [61] compared postoperative pain and shoulder function after thoracoscopy or thoracotomy. Patients were divided into two groups: less than 1 year (n = 239) and more than 1 year postoperative (n = 104). Patients less than 1 year after surgery had less pain and shoulder dysfunction after thoracoscopy compared with thoracotomy. These differences disappeared after more than 1 year postsurgery. In a separate study, the same investigators reviewed changes after thoracoscopy and thoracotomy in $FEV_1\%$, which is forced expiratory volume in 1 second (FEV_1) as a percentage of forced vital capacity (FVC) times 100 [68]. Patients underwent comparable pulmonary resections. The decrease in $FEV_1\%$ was significantly worse 1 week after thoracotomy compared with thoracoscopy. No differences between the two procedures were seen after postoperative week three.

Another critical aspect of pulmonary metastasectomy is completeness of resection. The International Registry of Lung Metastases demonstrated that patients with incomplete resections after thoracotomy had significantly worse prognosis than those with complete resections [59]. The identification of radiologically occult nodules at the time of surgery using bimanual palpation is one argument for open thoracotomy, although a statistical survival benefit is difficult to prove. Roth and colleagues [69] examined this issue in patients with pulmonary sarcoma metastases, matching two groups for number of nodules, tumor-doubling time, and disease-free interval. Patients with apparent unilateral disease were subjected to either sternotomy with bimanual palpation and metastasectomy of both lungs or unilateral thoracotomy of the affected side with manual palpation and metastasectomy. Forty-five percent of the sternotomy patients were found to have occult disease in the contralateral lung. However, survival was not improved when compared with the unilateral thoracotomy group.

Recurrence in either the ipsilateral or contralateral lung after metastasectomy is common, even after complete resection [70,71]. Re-resection has been shown to provide a benefit in patients with recurrent pulmonary metastases. Repeat thoracotomy is difficult because of significant adhesions from previous thoracotomy. It can be argued that using a VATS approach for the first operation may minimize adhesions, allowing for a VATS approach for subsequent operations as well.

Colorectal cancer is one of the most common malignancies to metastasize to the lung. Isolated pulmonary metastases occur in 2% to 4% of patients [59]. A large multicenter trial studied the use of VATS resection in 80 patients with metastatic colon cancer [59]. A solitary lesion was resected in 60 (75%) patients, and multiple lesions were resected in 20 (25%) patients. Four patients required conversion to thoracotomy, either because the lesions could not be identified or margins would have been compromised. Mean survival was 30.4 months for patients with single tumors compared with 26.5 months for patients with multiple lesions. In 69% of patients, disease recurred, predominantly with distant metastases. The mean disease-free interval in recurrence-free patients was 38.7 months. The investigators advocate the use of VATS for colorectal cancer metastases if all lesions can be identified and if clear margins can be obtained [59].

Clearly, the greatest challenge for the thoracic surgeon performing VATS for metastatic disease is the identification of the lesions without reliance on tactile sensation. Some investigators report up to 11% of cases complicated by the inability to identify the nodule at the time of surgery [72]. The classic "puckering" or retraction that occurs for lesions invading the visceral pleura after the lung is deflated can help identification by VATS. Lesions located immediately subpleural can be identified by a "mound" that develops as the surrounding lung becomes atelectatic. If the mass is deeper, a blunt probe passed over the surface or a finger palpation through a port site can be helpful. However, in many cases, the metastatic nodule is too small or too deep to be identified by these methods. Several additional techniques to assist with localization and minimize the need for conversion to thoracotomy have been described.

The two most common techniques are percutaneous hook-wire placement under CT guidance and methylene blue injection, sometimes used in combination. Similar to mammographic needle localization, a CT-guided hook wire can be placed into pulmonary lesions immediately before surgical resection. Small quantities of methylene blue can be injected at the same time as the hook wire is placed, which can be helpful in case the hook wire is dislodged during transport from the CT room to the operating room. In a report by Thaete and colleagues [73] on 101 lesions localized in 94 patients, 20% had dislodgement of the wire, but the methylene blue allowed for localization without extra ports or conversion. The success rate for metastasectomy was 98% in this series. The failure rate for methylene blue injection alone is around 13% [74]. The amount of injected dye is critical for success, since too much dye may obscure the localization of metastases. Several investigators advise thoracoscopy within 3 hours of dye injection [75]. Wire localization carries the risk of pneumothorax, pulmonary hemorrhage, poor localization, and dislodgement between placement and time of surgery. Dislodgement has been documented in 6% to 10% of cases [76].

These drawbacks have led to the development of methods with decreased risks of dislodgement or localization errors. Powell and colleagues [77] recently described a technique using platinum microcoils for small pulmonary nodules. Under CT guidance, coils are placed adjacent to the nodule and the pleural surface. These coils are localized in the operating room using fluoroscopy. In a pilot study involving 12 patients, the success rate was 100%. Potential risks include pneumothorax and pulmonary hemorrhage.

A similar technique has been developed in Japan for localization of small and deep pulmonary nodules during thoracoscopy. The technique is called fluoroscopy-assisted thoracoscopic surgery after CT-guided bronchoscopic metallic coil marking (FATS-CM) [78]. Lesions should preferentially be approximately 10 mm in size and located not more than 30 mm from a pleural edge. After mapping the lesion using virtual bronchoscopy and thin-cut CT, metal coils are placed proximal and distal to the target lesion in the closest bronchus with an ultrathin bronchoscope. After confirming correct placement with CT, the patient is taken to the operating room for resection within 30 days of coil placement. After coil localization with fluoroscopic guidance, the target area is resected with endostaplers and the specimen immediately analyzed to determine completeness of resection. In a report of this technique on 9 patients with 11 pulmonary lesions, all but one nodule were removed without complications using three port sites [78]. One nodule required a mini-thoracotomy for resection. This pilot study suggests that despite its complexity, FATS-CM is a feasible option for identifying small lesions within the lung parenchyma at thoracoscopy. It does require a team that includes a skilled bronchoscopist, a thoracic surgeon, and a fluoroscopist.

Ultrasonographic localization of pulmonary nodules at the time of thoracoscopy has been described by Yamamoto and colleagues [79] in 26 patients who underwent VATS for solitary pulmonary nodules between 8 and 40 mm in size. Localization with a 7.5-MHz flexible endosonographic probe identified 21 of 26 nodules (81%). Five patients had to be converted to open palpation because of failure to visualize the lesion secondary to either retained air within severely emphysematous lung or excessive depth of the mass. These results suggest that thoracoscopic sonography is safe and effective for lesions close to the lung surface. It is mandatory to completely collapse the lung before ultrasound examination. The addition of Doppler examination can help determine benign versus malignant lesions [79].

Davini and colleagues [80] describe their experience with radioguided localization in 30 patients with solitary pulmonary nodules. They randomized patients with nodules <3 cm in maximum diameter and at a maximum depth of 3 cm from the visceral pleura to either hooked-needle localization or the Scinti-probe technique before thoracoscopy. The Scinti-probe technique requires CT-guided needle localization of the lesion followed by injection of 0.2 to 0.5 mL of technetium Tc 99m (5–10 megabecquerel) labeled albumin microspheres containing 0.2 mL of nonionic contrast medium. After CT confirmation of correct localization, standard thoracoscopy for resection was performed in both groups. The area of highest signal was resected using endo-staplers. The remaining lung parenchyma was evaluated for appropriately low background counts to assure complete resection. All specimens were evaluated by frozen section. For the diagnosis of primary lung cancer, patients were converted to thoracotomy and lobectomy. There were no complications related to Scinti-probe technique. In the group localized by hook wire, 1 patient suffered a pneumothorax (6.5%) and 1 patient had dislodgement of the wire (6.5%) requiring a mini-thoracotomy. In this study, the radioguided technique successfully localized 100% of the nodules and was less expensive than the hook-wire technique (not including the initial cost of the reusable gamma probe).

Finally, HATS has been described for nodule localization. HATS uses a 7- to 8-cm incision 2 cm below the costal margin and extending through the rectus muscle. The surgeon's hand passes through the extraperitoneal space behind the costal margin. The diaphragm is split near the periphery to avoid injury to the phrenic nerve. The "hand port" allows for tactile examination of the lung for excellent localization of pulmonary nodules without rib spreading. Wright and colleagues [81] described the use of HATS in 46 patients with conversion to open procedure in only 2 patients. Detterbeck [82] and his group used a similar hand-assisted procedure in 24 patients. Their approach involved resection of the xyphoid and dissection of the diaphragm attachments in an extrapleural plane. Their success was 67% with 23% conversion to an open procedure.

In conclusion, thoracoscopy is an appropriate treatment option for many patients with pulmonary metastases. Suggested selection criteria are similar to those for open metastectomy, and include:

- A primary neoplasm that can be controlled
- A thin-cut helical scan that identifies all but microscopic disease
- No more than two lesions within the same hemithorax
- Cardiac and pulmonary tolerance for the proposed pulmonary resection
- Tumor nodules within the outer one third of the lung or within 30 mm of the closest pleural surface
- Conditions that permit all nodules to be resected [83].

Patients with more than two lesions or patients with lesions in both hemithoraces should be strongly considered for open resection, possibly via median sternotomy. VATS is an excellent tool for diagnosis of indeterminate nodules. Alternately, VATS may be an acceptable option in patients at high risk for complications after thoracotomy. The principles of oncologic surgery, such as complete resection and negative margins, need to be adhered to.

Summary

Major recent advances in medical and radiation oncology as well as in ablative therapy have had a significant impact in patients with advanced metastatic disease. These advances have forced the surgical oncology community to reassess the indications for surgery for these patients. Patients with noncurable disease where surgery would traditionally not have been considered may now benefit from metastasectomy and/or cytoreductive surgery. In these patients, where surgical intent is centered on prolonging and improving quality of life, minimal-access surgery holds great potential because of decreased trauma, decreased imunosuppression, and faster recovery.

Despite major accomplishments in advanced minimal-access surgery over the past 15 years, its role in the treatment of malignant neoplasms continues to be widely debated and in many aspects remains controversial. When curative-intent surgery is performed, minimal-access approaches should not compromise the oncologic outcome. The procedures are technically demanding and experience in both advanced laparoscopic surgery and open surgical oncology is required. For example, a laparoscopic surgeon with limited training in open hepatectomy should not perform laparoscopic liver resections alone. Similarly, an experienced hepato-biliary surgeon should not venture into the minimal-access approach before mastering the necessary advanced laparoscopic skills. Unfavorable initial results significantly delay the development of these operations. These lessons were learned during the development of laparoscopic colon surgery for cancer, where early reports of an increased number of port-sites metastases and substandard oncologic resections appear now secondary to limitations in technical experience and skills.

References

[1] Dhobada S, Patankar S, Gorde V. Case report: port-site metastasis after laparoscopic radical nephrectomy for renal-cell carcinoma. J Endourol 2006;20:119–22.
[2] Giuliante F, Ardito F, Vellone M, et al. Port-sites excision for gallbladder cancer incidentally found after laparoscopic cholecystectomy. Am J Surg 2006;191:114–6.
[3] Wexner SD, Cohen S. Port site metastases after laparoscopic colorectal surgery for cure of malignancy. Br J Surgery 1995;33:295–8.
[4] Knolmayer TJ, Asbun HJ, Shibata G, et al. An experimental model of cellular aerosolization during laparoscopic surgery. Surg Laparosc Endosc 1997;7(5):399–402.
[5] Nelson H, Sargent DJ, Weiand S. Clinical outcomes of surgical therapy study group: a comparison of laparoscopically assisted and open colectomy for colon cancer. N Engl J Med 2004;350(20):2050–9.
[6] Burpee SE, Kurian M, Murakame Y, et al. The metabolic and immune response to laparoscopic versus open liver resection. Surg Endosc 2002;16(6):899–904.
[7] Asbun HJ, Hughes K. Management of recurrent and metastatic colorectal carcinoma. Surg Clin North Am; 73(1):145–65.
[8] Elias D, Sideris L, Marc Pocard M, et al. Results of R0 resection for colorectal liver metastases associated with extrahepatic disease. Ann Surg Oncol 2004;11:274–80.
[9] Adam R, Delvart V, Pascal G, et al. Rescue surgery for unresectable colorectal liver metastases downstaged by chemotherapy: a model to predict long-term survival. Ann Surg 240(4):644–58.
[10] Awad SS, Fagan S, Abudayyeh S, et al. Preoperative evaluation of hepatic lesions for the staging of hepatocellular and metastatic liver carcinoma using endoscopic ultrasonography. Am J Surg 2002;184(6):601–4.
[11] Rahusen F, Cuesta M, Borgstein P, et al. Selection of patients for resection of colorectal metastases to the liver using diagnostic laparoscopy and laparoscopic ultrasonography [abstract]. Ann Surg 1999;230:31–7.
[12] Kaneko H, Takagi S, Oksuka Y, et al. Laparoscopic liver resection of hepatocellular carcinoma. Am J Surg 2005;189(2):190–4.
[13] Dagher I, Proske JM, Carloni A, et al. Laparoscopic liver resection: results for 70 patients. Surg Endosc 2007 [Epub ahead of print].
[14] Vibert E, Perniceni T, Levard H, et al. Laparoscopic liver resection. Br J Surg 2006;93(1): 67–72.
[15] Cherqui D, Laurent A, Tayar C, et al. Laparoscopic liver resection for peripheral hepatocellular carcinoma in patients with chronic liver disease: midterm results and perspectives. Ann Surg 2006;243(4):499–506.
[16] Mala T, Edwin B, Rosseland AR, et al. Laparoscopic liver resection of hepatocellular carcinoma. J Hepatobiliary Pancreat Surg 2005;12(4):298–303.
[17] Buell JF, Koffron AJ, Thomas MJ, et al. Laparoscopic liver resection. J Am Coll Surg 2005; 200(3):472–80.

[18] Gigot JF, Glineur D, Santiago Azagra J, et al. Laparoscopic liver resection for malignant liver tumors: preliminary results of a multicenter European study. Ann Surg 2002;236:90–7.
[19] Descottes B, Glineur D, Lachachi F, et al. Laparoscopic liver resection of benign liver tumors. Surg Endosc 2002;17(1):23–30.
[20] Huscher CG, Lirici MM, Chiodini S. Laparoscopic liver resections. Semin Laparosc Surg 1998;5(3):204–10.
[21] Champault A, Dagher I, Vons C, et al. Laparoscopic hepatic resection for hepatocellular carcinoma: retrospective study of 12 patients. Gastroenterol Clin Biol 2005;29(10):969–73.
[22] Lang BH, Poon RT, Fan ST, et al. Influence of laparoscopy on postoperative recurrence and survival in patients with ruptured hepatocellular carcinoma undergoing hepatic resection. Br J Surg 2004;91(4):444–9.
[23] Palanivelu C. Laparoscopic hepatic surgery. In: Palanivelu C, editor. Art of laparoscopic surgery. 1st edition. Coimbatore (India): Jaya Publications; 2005. p. 785–806.
[24] O'Rourke N, Fielding G. Laparoscopic right hepatectomy: surgical technique. J Gastrointest Surg 2004;8:213–6.
[25] Brennan MF. Current status of surgery for gastric cancer: a review. Gastric Cancer 2005;8: 64–70.
[26] Wanebo HJ, Kennedy BJ, Chmiel J, et al. Cancer of the stomach: a patient care study by the American college of surgeons. Ann Surg 1993;218:583–92.
[27] Fuchs CS, Mayer RJ. Gastric carcinoma. N Engl J Med 1995;333:32–41.
[28] Salvon-Harman JC, Cady B, Nikulasson S, et al. Shifting proportions of gastric adenocarcinomas. Arch Surg 1994;129:381–8.
[29] Huscher CG, Mingoli A, Sgarzini G, et al. Laparoscopic versus open subtotal gastrectomy for distal gastric cancer: five-year results of a randomized prospective trial. Ann Surg 2005; 241:232–7.
[30] Dulucq JL, Wintringer P, Stabilini C, et al. Laparoscopic and open gastric resections for malignant lesions; a prospective comparative study. Surg Endosc 2005;19:933–8.
[31] Mochiki E, Kamiyama Y, Aihara R, et al. Laparoscopic assisted distal gastrectomy for early gastric cancer: five years' experience. Surgery 2005;137:317–22.
[32] Jeung HC, Rha SY, Jang WI, et al. Treatment of advanced gastric cancer by palliative gastrectomy, cytoreductive therapy and postoperative intraperitoneal chemotherapy. Br J Surg 2002;89:460–6.
[33] Farma JM, Pingpank JF, Libutti SK, et al. Limited survival in patients with carcinomatosis from foregut malignancies after cytoreduction and continuous hyperthermic peritoneal perfusion. Gastrointest Surg 2005;9:1346–53.
[34] Kusamura S, Younan R, Baratti D, et al. Cytoreductive surgery followed by intraperitoneal hyperthermic perfusion: analysis of morbidity and mortality in 209 peritoneal surface malignancies treated with closed abdomen technique. Cancer 2006;106:1144–53.
[35] Yonemura Y, Fujimura T, Fushida S, et al. Peritonectomy as a treatment modality for patients with peritoneal dissemination from gastric cancer. In: Nakashima T, Yonemura Y, editors. Multimodality therapy for gastric cancer: appendix: database of the cancer institute hospital. Tokyo: Springer-Verlag; 1999. p. 71–80.
[36] Gretschel S, Siegel R, Estevez-Schwarz L, et al. Surgical strategies for gastric cancer with synchronous peritoneal carcinomatosis. Br J Surg 2006;93:1530–5.
[37] Conlon KC. Staging laparoscopy for gastric cancer. Ann Ital Chir 2001;72:33–7.
[38] Bentrem DJ, Wilton A, Mazumdar M, et al. The value of peritoneal cytology as a preoperative predictor in patients with gastric carcinoma undergoing a curative resection. Ann Surg Oncol 2005;12:347–53.
[39] Gold JS, Jaques DP, Bentrem DJ, et al. Outcome of patients with known metastatic gastric cancer undergoing resection with therapeutic intent. Ann Surg Oncol 2007;14(2):365–72.
[40] Adusumilli PS, Eisenberg DP, Chun YS, et al. Virally directed fluorescent imaging improves diagnostic sensitivity in the detection of minimal residual disease after potentially curative cytoreductive surgery. J Gastrointest Surg 2005;9:1138–47.

[41] Sarela AI, Miner TJ, Karpeh MS, et al. Clinical outcomes with laparoscopic stage M1, unresected gastric adenocarcinoma. Ann Surg 2006;243:189–95.
[42] Choi YB. Laparoscopic gastrojejunostomy for palliation of gastric outlet obstruction in unresectable gastric cancer. Surg Endosc 2002;16:1620–6.
[43] Roviello F, Marrelli D, Neri A, et al. Treatment of peritoneal carcinomatosis by cytoreductive surgery and intraperitoneal hyperthermic chemoperfusion (IHCP): postoperative outcome and risk factors for morbidity. World J Surg 2006;30:2033–40.
[44] Glehen O, Mohamed F, Gilly FN. Peritoneal carcinomatosis from digestive tract cancer: new management by cytoreductive surgery and intraperitoneal chemohyperthermia. Lancet Oncol 2004;5:219–28.
[45] Zarnegar R, Kebebew E, Duh QY, et al. Malignant pheochromocytoma. Surg Oncol Clin N Am 2006;115:555–71.
[46] Thompson LD. Pheochromocytoma of the adrenal gland scaled score (PASS) to separate benign from malignant neoplasms: a clinicopathologic and immunophenotypic study of 100 cases. Am J Surg Pathol 2002;26:551–66.
[47] Baba T, Machid K, Ozaki I, et al. A malignant pheochromocytoma with ileus, polyuria and hypercalcemia: a case of recurrence 17 years after the initial operation. Endocr J 1985;32: 337–45.
[48] Tanaka S, Ito T, Tomoda J, et al. Malignant pheochromocytoma with hepatic metastasis diagnosed 20 years after resection of the primary adrenal lesion. Intern Med 1993;32:789–94.
[49] Shen WT, Sturgeon C, Clark OH, et al. Should pheochromocytoma size influence surgical approach? A comparison of 90 malignant and 60 benign pheochromocytomas. Surgery 2004;136:1129–37.
[50] Vassilopoulou-Sellin R, Schultz PN. Adrenocortical carcinoma. Clinical outcome at the end of the 20th century. Cancer 2001;92:1113–21.
[51] Paton BL, Novitsky YW, Zerey M, et al. Outcomes of adrenal cortical carcinoma in the United States. Surgery 2006;140(6):914–20.
[52] Kebebew E, Siperstein AE, Clark OH, et al. Results of laparoscopic adrenalectomy for suspected and unsuspected malignant adrenal neoplasms. Arch Surg 2002;137:948–51.
[53] Moinzadeh A, Gill IS. Laparoscopic radical adrenalectomy for malignancy in 31 patients. J Urol 2005;173:519–25.
[54] Gonzalez RJ, Shapiro S, Sarlis N, et al. Laparoscopic resection of adrenal cortical carcinoma: a cautionary note. Surgery 2005;138:1078–85.
[55] Pommier RF, Brennan MF. An eleven-year experience with adrenocortical carcinoma. Surgery 1992;112:963–70.
[56] Sarela AI, Murphy I, Coit DG, et al. Metastasis to the adrenal gland: the emerging role of laparoscopic surgery. Ann Surg Oncol 2003;10:1191–6.
[57] Luketich JD, Burt ME. Does resection of adrenal metastases from non-small cell lung cancer improve survival? Ann Thorac Surg 1996;6:1614–6.
[58] Heniford BT, Arca MJ, Walsh RM, et al. Laparoscopic adrenalectomy for cancer. Semin Surg Oncol 1999;16:293–306.
[59] Landreneau RJ, De Giacomo T, Mack MJ, et al. Therapeutic video-assisted thoracoscopic surgical resection of colorectal pulmonary metastases. Eur J Cardiothorac Surg 2000;18: 671–6.
[60] Long-term results of lung metastasectomy: prognostic analyses based on 5206 cases. The international registry of lung metastases. J Thorac Cardiovasc Surg 1997;113:37–49.
[61] Landreneau RJ, Mack MJ, Hazelrigg SR, et al. Prevalence of chronic pain after pulmonary resection by thoracotomy or video-assisted thoracic surgery. J Thorac Cardiovasc Surg 1994; 107:1079–85.
[62] Dowling RD, Wach ME, Ferson PF, et al. Thoracoscopic neodymium: yttrium aluminum garnet laser resection of a pulmonary metastasis. Cancer 1992;70:1873–5.
[63] Girard P, Baldeyrou MS, Begg CB, et al. Surgery for pulmonary metastases. Who are the 10-year survivors? Cancer 1994;74:2791–7.

[64] Gadd MA, Casper ES, Woodruff JM, et al. Development and treatment of pulmonary metastases in adult patients with extremity soft tissue sarcoma. Ann Surg 1993;218:715–12.
[65] McCormack PM, Bains MS, Begg CB, et al. Role of video-assisted thoracic surgery in the treatment of pulmonary metastases: results of a prospective trial. Ann Thorac Surg 1996; 62:213–6.
[66] Mutsaerts EL, Zoetmulder FA, Meijer S, et al. Outcome of thoracoscopic pulmonary metastasectomy evaluated by confirmatory thoracotomy. Ann Thorac Surg 2001;72:230–3.
[67] Ninomiya M, Nakajima J, Tanaka M, et al. Effects of lung metastastectomy on respiratory function. Jpn J Thorac Cardiovasc Surg 2001;49:17–20.
[68] Landreneau RJ, Mack MJ, Keenan RJ, et al. Strategic planning for video-assisted thoracic surgery. Ann Thorac Surg 1993;56:615–9.
[69] Roth JA, Pass HI, Wesley MN, et al. Comparison of median sternotomy and thoracotomy for resection of pulmonary metastases in patients with adult soft-tissue sarcomas. Ann Thorac Surg 1986;42:134–8.
[70] Martini N, McCormack PM, Bains MS, et al. Surgery for solitary and multiple pulmonary metastases. N.Y. State J Med 1978;78:1711–4.
[71] Weiser MR, Downey RJ, Leung DH, et al. Repeat resection of pulmonary metastases in patients with soft tissue sarcoma. J Am Coll Surg 2000;191:184–90.
[72] Hazelrigg SR, Nunchack SK, Landreneau RJ, et al. Cost analysis for thoracoscopy: thoracoscopic wedge resection. Ann Thorac Surg 1993;56:633–5.
[73] Thaete FL, Peterson MS, Plunkett MB, et al. Computed tomography-guided wire localization of pulmonary lesions before thoracoscopic resection: results in 101 cases. J Thorac Imaging 1999;14:90–8.
[74] Kerrigan DC, Spence PA, Crittenden MD, et al. Methylene blue guidance for simplified resection of a lung lesion. Ann Thorac Surg 1992;53:163–4.
[75] Vandori RE, Cuttat JF, Wicky S, et al. CT-guided methylene blue labeling before thoracoscopic resection of pulmonary nodules. Eur J Cardiothorac Surg 1998;14:265–70.
[76] Plunkett MB, Peterson MS, Landreneau RJ. Peripheral pulmonary nodules: preoperative percutaneous needle localization with CT guidance. Radiology 1992;185:274–6.
[77] Powell TI, Jangra D, Clifton JC, et al. Peripheral lung nodules: fluoroscopically guided video-assisted thoracoscopic resection after computer tomography-guided localization using platinum micro-coils. Ann Surg 2004;240:481–8.
[78] Takanori T, Kazuya K, Hiromitsu T, et al. Fluoroscopy-assisted thoracoscopic resection of pulmonary nodules after computed tomography-guided bronchoscopic metallic coil marking. J Thor and Cardiovasc Surg 2006;131:704–10.
[79] Yamamoto M, Takeo M, Meguro F, et al. Sonographic evaluation for peripheral pulmonary nodules during video-assisted thoracoscopic surgery. Surg Endosc 2003;17:825–7.
[80] Davini F, Gonfiotti A, Vaggell L, et al. Thoracoscopic localization techniques for patients with solitary pulmonary nodule: radioguided surgery versus hook-wire localization. J Card Surg 2006;47:355–9.
[81] Wright GM, Clarke CP, Paica JM. Hand assisted thoracoscopic surgery. Ann Thorac Surg 2003;75:1665–7.
[82] Detterbeck FC, Egan TM. Thoracoscopy using a substernal hand port for palpation. Ann Thorac Surg 2004;78:1031–6.
[83] Ketchedjian A, Daly B, Luketich J, et al. Minimally invasive techniques for managing pulmonary metastases: video-assisted thoracic surgery and radiofrequency ablation. Thor Surg Clin 2006;16:157–65.

ELSEVIER
SAUNDERS

Surg Oncol Clin N Am
16 (2007) 627–637

SURGICAL
ONCOLOGY CLINICS
OF NORTH AMERICA

Hepatic Cytoreductive Surgery for Neuroendocrine Cancer

Byron E. Wright, MD, FACS, Chris C. Lee, MD, Anton J. Bilchik, MD, PhD, FACS*

Department of Surgical Oncology, John Wayne Cancer Institute at Saint John's Health Center, 2200 Santa Monica Boulevard, Santa Monica, CA 90404, USA

Neuroendocrine tumors (NET) of the gastrointestinal tract are uncommon neoplasms that display unique features and characteristics in comparison to other malignancies. These tumors are typically slow-growing, low-grade malignancies that can remain clinically silent for long periods. Gut NET often disseminate during this period of asymptomatic growth. The characteristic feature of these tumors is the secretion of biologically active compounds that, when produced in large amounts from disseminated disease, can overwhelm the physiologic control systems and produce a constellation of clinical symptoms. This coincides typically with the time of definitive diagnosis.

Like most gastrointestinal-based malignancies, the pattern and route of hematogenous metastatic spread for NET are through the liver. A large hepatic burden of disease often is the dominant focus throughout the patient's illness. Although patients with advanced metastatic NET are not considered surgically curable, they may have a lengthy survival time. However, their quality of life can be significantly impaired by the often uncontrollable symptoms associated with the tumor burden and hormone production. These patients are often referred to a surgeon with expertise in the treatment of metastatic hepatic malignancy in hopes that surgical cytoreduction might help reduce or resolve hormonal symptoms and improve quality of life.

This research was supported by funding from the Rod Fasone Memorial Cancer Fund (Indianapolis, IN), the William Randolph Hearst Foundations (San Francisco, CA), and the Davidow Charitable Fund (Los Angeles, CA).

* Corresponding author.
E-mail address: bilchika@jwci.org (A.J. Bilchik).

1055-3207/07/$ - see front matter © 2007 Published by Elsevier Inc.
doi:10.1016/j.soc.2007.04.009

surgonc.theclinics.com

Overview of neuroendocrine tumors

As mentioned earlier, the term NET refers to a rather diverse spectrum of relatively uncommon neoplasms. Their common embryologic or stem cell origin enables them to take up and secrete bioactive amines, hence the term APUDomas for tumors arising from amine precursor uptake and decarboxylation (APUD) cells [1]. A common protodifferentiated adult stem cell may give rise to a number of different NET [2].

Gastroenteropancreatic NET arise from the stomach, the pancreas, and the small or large bowel, including the rectum, and are uncommon and slow growing [3]. The primary tumor is often small (<1 cm in diameter) and clinically indolent until metastases occur. Their presenting symptoms may be unrecognized and/or misdiagnosed for years and diagnosis requires careful laboratory and radiographic screening. Table 1 summarizes the types and symptoms of NET [4].

Patients typically present with either metastatic carcinoid or metastatic pancreatic islet cell neoplasm (noncarcinoid NET). Carcinoid tumors are the most common NET of the gut [5]. They are classically divided into foregut, midgut, and hindgut neoplasms, with the midgut location being the most common [5,6]. The carcinoid syndrome typically occurs with midgut tumors and is only seen in roughly 5% to 10% of all carcinoid patients. Serotonin is the major biologically active peptide produced by these lesions. Other peptides include prostaglandins and kinins. Cutaneous flushing, persistent diarrhea, and bronchial constriction with wheezing comprise the classic triad of symptoms. Other symptoms include those related to progressive valvular heart disease secondary to prolonged and direct hormone exposure.

Table 1
Common gastrointestinal neuroendocrine tumors with their dominant hormone symptoms

Tumor type	Percentage of cases	Dominant hormone	Classic symptoms
Carcinoid	56	Serotonin	Flushing, diarrhea, wheezing
Insulinoma	17	Insulin	Symptomatic hypoglycemia
Pancreatic polypeptidoma (PPoma)	15	Pancreatic polypeptide	Clinically silent
Gastrinoma	9	Gastrin	Peptic ulcer disease, diarrhea
Vasoactive intestinal peptide-producing tumor (VIPoma)	2	Vasoactive intestinal polypeptide	Secretory diarrhea
Glucagonoma	1	Glucagon	Characteristic rash, glucose intolerance
Somatostatinoma	1	Somatostatin	Gallstones, diabetes, diarrhea

With carcinoid tumors, the latency period between symptom onset and diagnosis may be as long as 10 years. Occasionally the patient will exhibit carcinoid syndrome at the time of definitive diagnosis.

Pancreatic islet cell tumors are a diverse group of neoplasms that can each give rise to their own characteristic spectrum of symptoms (see Table 1). Insulinomas, the most common noncarcinoid NET, classically present with the so-called "Whipple's triad" of symptomatic hypoglycemia with low documented blood glucose levels and resolution of symptoms with oral ingestion of glucose. A 72-hour monitored fast along with establishment of insulin-to-glucose ratios >0.3 can generally confirm the diagnosis [7]. Only 10% of these tumors demonstrate malignant behavior with evidence of invasion or metastatic disease. Glucagonomas secrete large amounts of glucagon with the resultant distinct symptoms of anemia, weight loss, glucose intolerance, and characteristic rash. These tumors can be quite large by the time they are diagnosed and 40% to 80% of patients have hepatic-based metastatic disease at the time of diagnosis. Gastrinomas are gastrin-secreting islet cell neoplasms typically found in and around the pancreas. These tumors have a high propensity to metastasize and over 50% of patients with gastrinoma of pancreatic origin present with hepatic metastases. Other well-described islet cell neoplasms include somatostatinomas, vasoactive intestinal peptide-producing tumors (VIPomas), and pancreatic polypeptidomas (PPomas). The overall 5-year survival rate for patients with untreated metastatic NET is 25% to 30%.

The cornerstone of medical management for symptomatic metastatic NET is antisecretory therapy. Hepatic metastases of NET produce and secrete large amounts of bioactive amines that eventually overwhelm physiologic mechanisms of control and produce characteristic and debilitating symptoms. Treatment with the somatostatin analog octreotide can dramatically reduce tumor hormonal production and often leads to early and complete symptom control. Multiple daily injections have been replaced by once or twice monthly injections of long-acting formulas (eg, Octreotide-LAR) [8]. With progression of disease, symptoms often become increasingly resistant to antisecretory therapy [9] as tumor burden and hormonal secretion increase. Hence, the concept of surgical cytoreduction, which decreases the tumor burden and prolongs or restores the effectiveness of targeted antisecretory therapies.

A multitude of chemotherapeutic drugs and biologic agents have been used, either alone or in combination, in this patient population with disappointing results. Streptozotocin, doxorubicin, and dacarbazine have all typically shown poor response rates of 30% or less with short-lived benefit. Interferon has shown slightly greater promise with significant reductions in the amount of circulating hormones and hormone-related symptoms but with minimal effects on overall tumor size or burden [10–13]. In addition, these tumors have also proven to be resistant to traditional external beam radiation.

Cytoreductive hepatic surgery

Cytoreductive surgery for NET refers to the planned operative resection and/or ablation of as much tumor as reasonably possible. Many investigators have suggested a minimum of 90% tumor reduction as optimal cytoreduction [14–17]. The intent is typically not to eliminate all gross tumor burden but rather to decrease it so that hormone production drops to clinically asymptomatic levels. Evidence suggests that patient survival may be extended with improved hormonal control [18].

Several features of NET make these malignancies particularly attractive for cytoreductive treatment. First, these tumors are characterized by slow tumor-doubling times. The reported 5-year survival rate for nontreated metastatic NET is 30% [19,20], a percentage roughly equivalent to that of resected metastatic colon cancer isolated to the liver [21–24]. Second, the dominant metastatic site for most NET disease is the liver. Directed anatomic and nonanatomic hepatic resections and ablative therapies can dramatically reduce the amount of active disease with relatively low morbidity and almost no mortality in contrast to other tumors that might require systemic resections and/or extensive peritoneal debulking to achieve adequate cytoreduction. In addition, the primary tumor can often be addressed during the same operation. Fortunately for the patient, the liver often remains the only site of significant metastatic disease for a long time. Third, the pattern of metastatic disease within the liver itself is often compatible with resection. The tumor rarely encases or invades large bile ducts, intrahepatic vessels, or other vital perihepatic structures. Most patients have enough residual healthy parenchyma to maintain adequate postresection hepatic function. Although bilobar disease is common, the bulk of disease is often confined to one lobe of the liver, with only segmental resection or ablation required for any additional lesions. Fourth, the immediate palliative effects of cytoreduction support its role even in the absence of long-term survival. Poorly controlled hormonal activity can severely impact quality of life and often antisecretory medications can only achieve partial symptomatic control. For instance, in classic carcinoid syndrome with severe, persistent flushing and refractory diarrhea, the somatostatin analog octreotide often initially controls symptoms but becomes dramatically less effective as the course of the disease progresses [25]. In addition, a significant percentage of these patients develop a carcinoid-induced heart disease, most often in the form of valvular dysfunction, further impacting overall quality of life [26].

Preoperative planning and approach

Patients referred for an opinion regarding hepatic cytoreduction of metastatic NET require a careful and comprehensive evaluation by the consulting surgeon. In addition to careful assessment of extent and location of disease, the surgeon must gauge the beneficial impact of a noncurative surgical intervention. What is the patient's overall health and current quality of life? How is the disease affecting the patient's well-being?

Initial workup should begin with a thorough patient history that meticulously documents current patient symptoms with an emphasis on those that impair quality of life. Both the patient and the surgeon should have a common understanding of what symptoms are secondary to excessive hormone production and would thereby be expected to improve with a reduction of circulating hormonal level and what other symptoms may not resolve after the cytoreduction. A physical exam should focus on findings that might place a patient at a higher than acceptable risk for a noncurative surgical intervention. For example, it is important to rule out valvular heart disease in a patient with carcinoid syndrome. Hepatic congestion secondary to right heart dysfunction can dramatically increase the risk of severe intraoperative bleeding and result in a prohibitive operative risk [27]. Several studies have documented the benefit and feasibility of a staged operative valvular replacement or repair before cytoreductive surgery [28,29].

Patients must also undergo a careful biochemical and radiographic workup. The functional nature of the patient's disease should be well understood from a biochemical and physiologic point of view. A patient with metastatic carcinoid and the carcinoid syndrome poses dramatically different perioperative challenges than a patient with metastatic insulinoma and refractory hypoglycemia. Before any consideration for cytroreductive therapy, all patients with metastatic NET should undergo total body imaging to fully document location and extent of disease. This should include CT scanning of the chest, abdomen, and pelvis with both oral and intravenous contrast as well as fine cuts through the perihepatic region. Complementary positron emission tomographic scanning as well as directed MRI may be helpful as well. Candidates for focused hepatic cytoreduction should have the bulk of their disease located in the liver and around the primary site. Because the goal of optimal cytoreduction is a 90% reduction in total tumor burden, the primary tumor and the bulk of metastatic disease should be in the abdomen to facilitate surgical resection.

Intraoperative findings should be used in a composite manner with preoperative imaging to remove as much tumor as possible with anatomic resection, wedge resection, ablative therapies, and any combination thereof, while preserving adequate hepatic function. Intraoperative ultrasound is a mandatory and indispensable tool that should be routinely used to help localize nonpalpable or undetected synchronous metastatic lesions. Our typical approach at the John Wayne Cancer Institute is to explore the patient through bilateral subcostal incisions, explore the peritoneal cavity, and fully mobilize the liver, followed by the use of intraoperative ultrasound. Formal resections are then performed to remove the most disease possible while preserving adequate functional liver. In a recent review of 63 patients who underwent hepatic cytoreduction for metastatic NET at our institution [30], the following anatomic resections were performed: right hepatectomy, left hepatectomy, extended right or left hepatectomy, and left lateral segmentectomy. Residual hepatic disease after formal anatomic resection was treated with nonanatomic wedge resection, radiofrequency ablation (RFA) or a combination of the two. In each case, all detectable hepatic disease was either removed or ablated. Although we prefer resection of disease whenever possible, we consider same-session ablations to be a legitimate form of cytoreduction that can be of great value in this patient population. Fig. 1 demonstrates intraoperative, ultrasound-guided RFA of a hepatic metastasis in a patient with NET that was not amenable to removal because of major contralateral hepatic resection.

Outcomes

The benefits of aggressive cytoreductive surgery in properly selected patients with highly symptomatic metastatic NET are well established. In recent years, many single-center studies have reported institutional experience with hepatic resection for cytoreduction in this setting [15,30–40]. Each has cited beneficial results both in terms of postoperative symptom control and prolonged survival times.

In 2003, Norton and colleagues [33] published results of hepatic resection for metastatic NET. Of 16 patients, 13 had metastatic carcinoid and 3 had metastatic gastrinoma. Most underwent synchronous resection of the primary tumor. Preoperative hormone-related symptoms resolved in all patients with the carcinoid syndrome and 5-year survival was 82%.

Osborne and his group [40], in their 2006 comparison paper of cytoreduction versus embolization for the treatment of hepatic metastatic NET, reported a 97% reduction in hormonal symptoms related to carcinoid and an 88% reduction in hormonal symptoms related to islet cell neoplasms after cytoreductive surgery.

A B

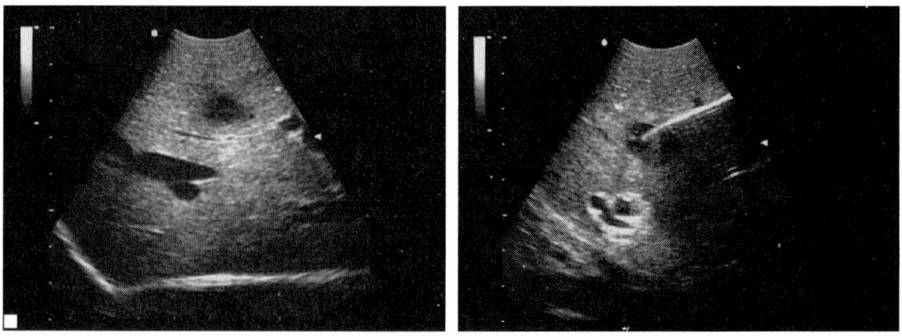

Fig. 1. (*A*) Intraoperative ultrasound demonstrating an isolated hepatic lesion in a patient undergoing major hepatic resection for cytoreduction of metastatic NET. The lesion was in a location that prevented inclusion in the planned resection. (*B*) Intraoperative, ultrasound-guided RFA of the same lesion. The RFA probe is seen entering the tumor just before ablation.

Sarmiento and colleagues [34] reviewed the Mayo Clinic experience with metastatic NET to the liver. Of 170 patients, 120 had metastatic carcinoid and 44% of the patients underwent resection of all gross disease. Seventy-six percent of the patients had bilobar hepatic metastases and 54% underwent a major hepatic resection. Either a partial or a full resolution of preoperative hormonal symptoms was noted in 96% of the patients and 5-year survival for the entire group was 61%.

We recently reported our experience with hepatic resection and RFA for hepatic-based metastatic NET [30]. The dominant indication for cytoreductive surgery included uncontrolled hormonal symptoms in 81% of the patients, tumor-related pain in 10% of the patients, and obstructive symptoms in the remaining 9%. Of the 63 patients, 60 had bilobar hepatic disease and 51 had metastatic carcinoid. Following cytoreduction, 90% of the patients reported full resolution of their dominant preoperative symptom. Among the 58 patients with elevated hormone levels before cytoreduction, the average hormone level decreased by 79% after surgery. Median overall survival was 48 months. Table 2 summarizes recently published results for cytoreduction in patients with hepatic-based metastatic NET.

Patient follow-up after cytoreduction

Most patients who undergo cytoreductive surgery for symptom palliation have residual areas or foci of metastatic disease. Even when all visible disease is resected, recurrence of disease and hormone-related symptoms is the expectation rather than the exception.

Table 2
Reported outcomes of hepatic cytoreductive surgery for metastatic neuroendocrine disease

Report	Study size (number of patients)	Symptomatic improvement/ resolution (percentage)	Operative mortality (number of patients)	Five-year survival (percentage)
Amersi (2007) [30]	63	90	0	NR
Hibi (2007) [31]	21	92	0	41
Musunuru (2006) [32]	13	100	0	NR
Knox (2004) [15]	13	100	NR	85
Norton (2003) [33]	16	100	0	82
Sarmiento (2003) [34]	170	96	2	61
Yao (2001) [35]	16	100	0	70
Jaeck (2001) [36]	13	100	0	68
Nave (2001) [37]	31	NR	0	47
Chamberlain (2000) [38]	34	90	2	76
Grazi (2000) [39]	19	95	0	92

Abbreviation: NR, not reported.

Using both serial postoperative imaging and assessment of hormone-related symptoms, Sarmiento and colleagues [34] demonstrated recurrence rates as high as 84% at 5 years, with no difference in patterns of recurrence for metastatic carcinoid versus metastatic islet cell neoplasms. There was a significant difference in rate of recurrence at 5 years after clinically complete versus incomplete cyoreduction.

In our own institutional review of 63 patients, 88% of the patients had a recurrence confirmed by imaging at a mean follow-up of 60 months. Most recurrences (73%) were intrahepatic and tended to occur in patients who had large (>4 cm) lesions, five or more lesions, or disease managed by ablation in combination with resection [30].

Because an optimal cytoreduction improves the duration and extent of symptom control, follow-up should evaluate the efficacy of cytoreduction. First, a comparison of preoperative and postoperative hormone levels should focus on those hormones most likely to correspond with clinical symptoms. For patients with metastatic carcinoid, levels of urinary and serum serotonin, 5-hydroxyindoleacetic acid (5-HIAA), and chromogranin should be tested within the first postoperative week. In those with metastatic pancreatic islet cell neoplasms, levels of serum glucagon, gastrin, and pancreatic polypeptide should be assessed as appropriate. Second, carefully established preoperative symptoms related to hormonal levels or disease bulk should be reevaluated for degree of resolution. This serves as an important reference point for deciding whether to repeat attempts at resection and/or ablation. Third, because patients eventually develop resistance to escalating doses of antisecretory or antihormonal drugs, attempts should be made to either reduce or eliminate them postoperatively.

The goals of long-term follow-up should include early detection of both local recurrence of resected disease and the development of resistance to antisecretory drugs. Laboratory and imaging studies should be updated at regular intervals with careful patient questioning about recurrent symptoms. In our practice, patients undergo laboratory testing 1 week postoperatively

Table 3
Standard follow-up at the John Wayne Cancer Institute after operative hepatic cytoreduction for metastatic neuroendocrine disease

First week	Monthly	Three-month intervals (For first 24 months)	Every 6 months (After first 24 months)
Initial postoperative abdominal CT scan	Second postoperative abdominal CT scan		
Liver function tests		Abdominal CT scan	Abdominal CT scan
Desired tumor markers	Desired tumor markers		
Symptom reassessment	Symptom reassessment		

and monthly thereafter. Imaging with abdominal CT is performed at the end of the first postoperative week and then at 1-month and 3-month intervals. After 2 years of stable disease, CT scans are performed every 6 months indefinitely. Detection of local recurrence and escalating hormonal levels in the setting of increasing symptoms should prompt evaluation for repeat attempts at surgical cytoreduction, percutaneous ablation and/or chemoembolization, and initiation of antisecretory therapies. Table 3 summarizes patient follow-up recommendations after cytoreductive surgery.

Summary

Patients with gut-based metastatic NET often present late in the course of their slowly progressive disease, when cancer has extended beyond the point of reasonable expectation for surgical cure. At this stage of disease, the tumor's overwhelming hormonal production often significantly impairs the patient's quality of life. Unlike many other malignancies that might involve a heavy burden of hepatic metastatic disease, many patients with metastatic NET continue to live for a long time despite escalating hormone-related symptoms. This establishes the justification and rationale for cytoreduction, a noncurative surgical intervention that reduces tumor burden and hormonal burden and thereby significantly increases symptom-free survival in the setting of an often slow but inevitable disease progression.

References

[1] Pearse AG. Common cytochemical and ultrastructural characteristics of cells producing polypeptide hormones (the APUD series) and their relevance to thyroid and ultimobranchial C cells and calcitonin. Proc R Soc Lond B Biol Sci 1968;170(18):71–80.
[2] Kvols LK, Perry RR, Vinik AI, et al. Neoplasms of the neuroendocrine system and neoplasms of the gastroenteropancreatic endocrine system. In: Kufe DW, Pollock RE, Weichselbaum RR, et al, editors. Cancer medicine. 6th edition. Houston (TX): B.C. Decker; 2003. p. 1121–72.
[3] Rindi G, Capella C, Solcia E. Cell biology, clinicopathological profile, and classification of gastro-enteropancreatic endocrine tumors. J Mol Med 1998;76(6):413–20.
[4] Vinik AI, Perry RR. Neoplasms of the gastroenteropancreatic endocrine system. In: Holland JF, Bast RC Jr, Morton DL, editors. Cancer Medicine 4th edition. vol. 1. Baltimore (MD): Williams and Wilkins; 1997. p. 1605–41.
[5] Modlin IM, Lye KD, Kidd M. A 5-decade analysis of 13,715 carcinoid tumors. Cancer 2003; 97(4):934–59.
[6] Williams ED, Sandler M. The classification of carcinoid tumors. Lancet 1963;1:238–9.
[7] Service FJ. Hypoglycemic disorders. N Engl J Med 1995;332(17):1144–52.
[8] Anthony LB. Long-acting formulations of somatostatin analogues. Ital J Gastroenterol Hepatol 1999;31:S216–8.
[9] Arnold R, Trautmann ME, Creutzfeldt W, et al. Somatostatin analogue octreotide and inhibition of tumor growth in metastatic endocrine gastroenteropancreatic tumours. Gut 1996;38(3):430–8.
[10] Biesma B, Willemse PH, Mulder NH, et al. Recombinant interferon alpha-2b in patients with metastatic apudomas: effect on tumours and tumour markers. Br J Cancer 1992; 66(5):850–5.

[11] Fjallskog ML, Sundin A, Westlin JE, et al. Treatment of malignant endocrine pancreatic tumors with a combination of alpha-interferon and somatostatin analogs. Med Oncol 2002; 19(1):35–42.
[12] Jacobsen MB, Hanssen LE, Kolmannskog F, et al. Interferon-alpha 2b, with or without prior hepatic artery embolization: clinical response and survival in mid-gut carcinoid patients. The Norwegian carcinoid study. Scand J Gastroenterol 1995;30(8):789–96.
[13] Moertel CG, Rubin J, Kvols LK. Therapy of metastatic carcinoid tumor and the malignant carcinoid syndrome with recombinant leukocyte A interferon. J Clin Oncol 1989;7(7):865–8.
[14] Wong RJ, DeCosse JJ. Cytoreductive surgery. Surg Gynecol Obstet 1990;170(3):276–81.
[15] Knox CD, Feurer ID, Wise PE, et al. Survival and functional quality of life after resection for hepatic carcinoid metastasis. J Gastrointest Surg 2004;8(6):653–9.
[16] Que FG, Nagorney DM, Batts KP, et al. Hepatic resection for metastatic neuroendocrine carcinomas. Am J Surg 1995;169(1):36–42.
[17] McEntee GP, Nagorney DM, Kvols LK, et al. Cytoreductive hepatic surgery for neuroendocrine tumors. Surgery 1990;108(6):1091–6.
[18] Norton JA, Doppman JL, Jensen RT. Curative resection in Zollinger-Ellison syndrome. Results of a 10-year prospective study. Ann Surg 1992;215(1):8–18.
[19] Proye C. Natural history of liver metastasis of gastroenteropancreatic neuroendocrine tumors: place for chemoembolization. World J Surg 2001;25(6):685–8.
[20] Moertel CG. Karnofsky memorial lecture. An odyssey in the land of small tumors. J Clin Oncol 1987;5(10):1502–22.
[21] Fong Y, Fortner J, Sun RL, et al. Clinical score for predicting recurrence after hepatic resection for metastatic colorectal cancer: analysis of 1001 consecutive cases. Ann Surg 1999; 230(3):309–18.
[22] Hughes KS, Simon R, Songhoradbodi S, et al. Resection of the liver for colorectal carcinoma metastases: a multi-institutional study of patterns of recurrence. Surgery 1986;100(2):278–84.
[23] Kato T, Yasui K, Hirai T, et al. Therapeutic results for hepatic metastasis of colorectal cancer with special reference to effectiveness of heatetomy: analysis of prognostic factors for 763 cases recorded at 18 institutions. Dis Colon Rectum 2003;46:S22–31.
[24] Scheele J, Stang R, Altendorf-Hofmann A, et al. Resection of colorectal liver metastases. World J Surg 1995;19(1):59–71.
[25] O'Toole D, Ruszniewski P. Chemoembolization and other ablative therapies for liver metastases of gastrointestinal endocrine tumours. Best Pract Res Clin Gastroenterol 2005;19(4): 585–94.
[26] Fox DJ, Khattar RS. Carcinoid heart disease: presentation, diagnosis, and management. Heart 2004;90(10):1224–8.
[27] Melendez JA, Arslan V, Fischer ME, et al. Perioperative outcomes of major hepatic resections under low central venous pressure anesthesia: blood loss, blood transfusion, and the risk of postoperative renal dysfunction. J Am Coll Surg 1998;187(6):620–5.
[28] McDonald ML, Nagorney DM, Connolly HM, et al. Carcinoid heart disease and carcinoid syndrome; successful surgical treatment. Ann Thorac Surg 1999;67(2):537–9.
[29] Stella M, Decian F, Mithieux F, et al. Ileal carcinoid with liver metastasis presenting after ten years with abdominal mass and right heart failure: report of a case. Tumori 2006;92(1):83–5.
[30] Amersi FF, Garza AM, Ahmed A, et al. Survival benefit of extensive hepatic cytoreduction for symptomatic metastases from neuroendocrine tumors. Ann Surg Oncol 2006;13(Suppl 2):14.
[31] Hibi T, Sano T, Sakamoto Y, et al. Surgery for hepatic neuroendocrine tumors: a single institutional experience in Japan. Jpn J Clin Oncol 2007;37(2):102–7.
[32] Musunuru S, Chen H, Rajpal S, et al. Metastatic neuroendocrine hepatic tumors: resection improves survival. Arch Surg 2006;141:1000–4.
[33] Norton JA, Warren RS, Kelly MG, et al. Aggressive surgery for metastatic liver neuroendocrine tumors. Surgery 2003;134(6):1057–63.
[34] Sarmiento JM, Heywood G, Rubin J, et al. Surgical treatment of neuroendocrine metastases to the liver: a plea for resection to increase survival. J Am Coll Surg 2003;197(1):29–37.

[35] Yao KA, Talamonti MS, Nemcek A, et al. Indications and results of liver resection and hepatic chemoembolization for metastatic for metastatic gastrointestinal neuroendocrine tumors. Surgery 2001;130(4):677–82.
[36] Jaeck D, Oussoultzoglou E, Bachellier P, et al. Hepatic metastases of gastroenteropancreatic neuroendocrine tumors: safe hepatic surgery. World J Surg 2001;25(6):689–92.
[37] Nave H, Mossinger E, Feist H, et al. Surgery as primary treatment in patients with liver metastases from carcinoid tumors: a retrospective, unicentric study over 13 years. Surgery 2001; 129:170–5.
[38] Chamberlain RS, Canes D, Brown KT, et al. Hepatic neuroendocrine metastases: does intervention alter outcomes? J Am Coll Surg 2000;190(4):432–45.
[39] Grazi GL, Cescon M, Pierangeli F, et al. Highly aggressive policy of hepatic resections for neuroendocrine liver metastases. Hepatogastroenterology 2000;47(32):481–6.
[40] Osborne DA, Zervos EE, Strosberg J, et al. Improved outcome with cytoreduction versus embolization for symptomatic hepatic metastases of carcinoid and neuroendocrine tumors. Ann Surg Oncol 2006;13(4):572–81.

ELSEVIER
SAUNDERS

Surg Oncol Clin N Am
16 (2007) 639–651

SURGICAL
ONCOLOGY CLINICS
OF NORTH AMERICA

Systemic and Regional Nonsurgical Therapy—What Is the Optimal Strategy for Metastatic Neuroendocrine Cancer?

Eric K. Nakakura, MD, PhD[a], Alan P. Venook, MD[b], Emily K. Bergsland, MD[b,*]

[a]*Department of Surgery, Division of Surgical Oncology, University of California, UCSF Comprehensive Cancer Center, 1600 Divisadero Street, A-724, San Francisco, CA 94143-1932, USA*

[b]*Department of Medicine, Division of Hematology/Oncology, University of California, UCSF Comprehensive Cancer Center, 1600 Divisadero Street, San Francisco, CA 94143-1705, USA*

At the time of diagnosis, most patients with neuroendocrine (NE) tumors have locally advanced or metastatic disease, so curative surgery is often not possible. For patients with isolated liver metastases, resection with or without ablation of all or most (>90%) of the disease is effective for controlling symptoms and appears to prolong survival. However, more than 90% of patients with hepatic NE tumor metastases have multifocal, bilobar disease, making it often impossible to achieve surgical resection of 90% or more of the tumor burden. The purpose of this chapter is to highlight the systemic and regional nonsurgical therapies available for patients suffering from metastatic NE tumors. We hope to provide clinicians with a useful framework for managing these patients. We also discuss the rationale for promising investigational therapies, which are desperately needed for improved palliation and survival of patients with advanced NE tumors.

E.K.N. is supported by an American College of Surgeons Faculty Research Fellowship and the James Ewing Foundation of the Society of Surgical Oncology.

* Corresponding author.
E-mail address: emilyb@medicine.ucsf.edu (E.K. Bergsland).

1055-3207/07/$ - see front matter © 2007 Elsevier Inc. All rights reserved.
doi:10.1016/j.soc.2007.04.019 **_surgonc.theclinics.com_**

Terminology

Much confusion exists in the literature regarding the terminology used to describe NE tumors. Subsequent to the first World Health Organization (WHO) classification of endocrine tumors, most pathologists used the term "carcinoid" for all tumors with NE features [1]. This created misunderstandings with clinicians who often understood the term "carcinoid" to refer to serotonin-producing neoplasms, the cause of the carcinoid syndrome. Because of the heterogeneity of NE tumors, the most recent WHO classification described three general categories: (1) well-differentiated NE tumors, which are benign or exhibit uncertain malignant potential; (2) well-differentiated NE carcinomas, which are low-grade malignant; and (3) poorly differentiated (typically small-cell) NE carcinomas, which are high-grade malignant [1]. Currently, the term "carcinoid" is commonly used to refer to a well-differentiated NE tumor or carcinoma of the gut. "Islet cell carcinoma" commonly refers to a well-differentiated NE carcinoma that arises from the pancreas or periampullary region (eg, duodenal gastrinoma).

Principles of treatment

For patients with locally advanced, well-differentiated NE tumors, long-term survival is common because of their indolent nature. Therefore, the potential benefit of any intervention must be carefully weighed against its potential toxicity. The rate of progression for metastatic well-differentiated NE tumors can vary greatly, so asymptomatic patients are initially observed to assess the tempo of disease. Indications for treatment include: (1) palliation of symptoms due to pain, tumor bulk, or hormonal excess; and (2) rapid disease progression. For these patients, regional, systemic, and investigational therapies should be strongly considered.

Poorly differentiated NE carcinomas behave like small-cell lung cancers, which are chemo-responsive but rapidly become resistant. Patients with poorly differentiated NE carcinomas are treated with the same combination chemotherapy used for small-cell lung cancer. Optimal treatment for patients with advanced NE tumors requires a multidisciplinary team with participation of medical oncology, surgical oncology, gastroenterology, interventional radiology, and pathology.

Biotherapy

Natural somatostatin-14 has diverse effects on the gastrointestinal (GI) tract, including inhibition of hormone secretion, pancreatic exocrine excretion, gallbladder contractility, and GI transit [2]. Somatostatin-14 also stimulates water and electrolyte absorption. These actions of somatostatin underlie the use of somatostatin analogs to ameliorate symptoms of hormonal excess in patients with functioning NE tumors. Moreover, these effects of somatostatin on the GI tract explain common adverse effects associated with their use. Because the half-life of somatostatin is only a few minutes, it must be administered as a continuous intravenous drip, precluding widespread use. Longer-acting somatostatin analogs permit convenient administration. For example, octreotide is administered subcutaneously three times a day. Slow-release octreotide and lanreotide are conveniently given intramuscularly every 4 weeks, and are as effective as short-acting octreotide in palliating hormone-mediated symptoms [3].

Somatostatin analogs exert their effects by binding to somatostatin receptor subtype 2, and, to a lesser extent, subtypes 3 and 5 [4]. Nearly 80% of NE tumors possess subtype 2 somatostatin receptors. Insulinomas, however, express somatostatin receptors in only 25% to 50%. Although somatostatin receptor scintigraphy (SRS) is sometimes used to predict who might benefit from somatostatin analog therapy, there is no clear correlation between SRS-avid tumors and clinical response to somatostatin analog use [5]. Most patients with functioning NE tumors who suffer from hormonally mediated symptoms benefit from somatostatin analog therapy. Unfortunately, with time, symptoms become refractory to somatostatin analog therapy in most patients.

Somatostatin analogs have little efficacy in causing tumor regression. In large clinical trials, an objective response with somatostatin analog treatment is observed in fewer than 5% of patients [6–8]. Approximately 25% to 50% of patients exhibit stable disease with somatostatin analog therapy. Whether disease stabilization is a direct result of somatostatin analog treatment or a reflection of the indolent nature of NE tumors is unclear. However, patients entered into these studies had evidence of progressive disease just before study entry, which suggests that somatostatin analog therapy may indeed promote disease stabilization.

Initially, common side effects from somatostatin analog therapy include nausea, abdominal cramps, flatulence, fat malabsorption, and diarrhea [2]. These symptoms usually resolve in 2 weeks. Patients are typically started on short-acting somatostatin analog therapy, and if it is well tolerated, long-acting agents are then given. Cholesterol gallstones occur in 20% to 50% of patients who receive long-term somatostatin analog therapy; however, only a minority of patients require urgent cholecystectomy for gallstone-related complications [9]. Therefore, prophylactic cholecystectomy should be considered for patients in whom long-term somatostatin analog therapy is planned and in whom surgery is undertaken for another reason.

In theory, because NE tumors may express all five somatostatin receptor subtypes at different levels and octreotide and lanreotide preferentially bind somatostatin receptor subtype 2, and, to a lesser degree, subtypes 3 and 5, improved efficacy may be achieved with novel agents that have expanded avidity to somatostatin receptor subtypes. A new somatostatin analog, SOM230, effectively binds somatostatin receptor subtypes 1, 2, 3, and 5 and is being evaluated in clinical trials [10]. Another treatment strategy under investigation involves radiolabeled somatostatin analogs. Preliminary results of peptide receptor radionuclide therapy are encouraging, but toxicity issues still need to be resolved [11,12].

Recombinant interferon-alpha activity in treating malignancies is thought to result from its immunomodulating and cytostatic effect [13]. Common adverse effects with interferon-alpha therapy include fatigue, flu-like symptoms, autoimmune reactions, and mental disturbances. Despite these adverse effects, interferon-alpha might be considered in patients who develop tachyphylaxis with somatostatin analogs [14]. Improved compliance and reduced adverse effects may be associated with longer-acting interferon-alpha preparations, such as pegylated interferon-alpha [15]. As with somatostatin analogs, interferon-alpha therapy rarely results in a radiologic response (<5%) and combination therapy with a somatostatin analog and interferon-alpha is no better than either agent alone in shrinking tumors [6]. In a phase II Eastern Cooperative Oncology Group (ECOG) study, interferon-gamma similarly failed to shrink tumors [16]. Symptomatic control and biochemical responses, such as decreases in hormone levels or chromogranin A, are variable with somatostatin analogs and/or interferon alpha [6]. However, usually modest control of hormonal symptoms can be achieved with acceptable adverse effects, making biotherapy a useful initial treatment to palliate hormone-mediated symptoms.

Chemotherapy

Despite decades of investigation, there is no commonly accepted chemotherapy regimen for patients with advanced NE tumors. Importantly, NE tumors are a heterogeneous group of neoplasms with unique biological properties. Numerous studies suggest that carcinoid tumors and islet cell carcinomas are biologically different. In general, islet cell carcinomas appear to be more responsive to chemotherapy than carcinoid tumors. Clearly, poorly differentiated NE tumors are biologically distinct and, as such, are treated differently from well-differentiated NE tumors.

In 1979, Moertel and Hanley [17] reported the results of an ECOG trial, which found that 14 (33%) of 42 of patients with advanced carcinoid tumors treated with streptozotocin and fluorouracil demonstrated an objective response. The median survival time was 11.2 months, and there was significant treatment-related toxicity. In response to the prohibitive toxicity found with streptozotocin/fluorouracil combination therapy, a subsequent ECOG trial increased the dosing interval between cycles [18]. Engstrom and colleagues reported response rates of 22% for streptozotocin/fluorouracil and 21% for doxorubicin, with median survival times of 64 and 48 weeks, respectively. A Southwest Oncology Group study of dacarbazine in patients with metastatic carcinoid tumors reported a response in 9 (16%) of 56 patients and a median survival of 20 months [19].

Based on these earlier results, a recent ECOG study randomized 248 patients with advanced carcinoid tumors to treatment with fluorouracil/streptozotocin or fluorouracil/doxorubicin [20]. After disease progression on either regimen, patients were "crossed over" to dacarbazine treatment. There was no difference in radiologic response rates between the two regimens (both were 16%). However, the median survival was 24.3 months for fluorouracil/streptozotocin, which was significantly longer than 15.7 months for fluorouracil/doxorubicin ($P = .03$). Approximately 8% of patients responded to crossover treatment with dacarbazine.

In summary, there is no clearly effective chemotherapy regimen for patients with advanced carcinoid tumors, and no standard regimen exists. In selected patients, existing data suggest that fluorouracil/streptozotocin is one potential chemotherapy option, but novel treatment strategies are clearly needed.

After an ECOG randomized trial in 1992 reported a 69% major objective response rate for patients with advanced islet cell carcinomas treated with streptozotocin/doxorubicin [21], this combination regimen gained initial acceptance as a standard therapy for this disease. The median survival with this regimen, however, was only 2.2 years. Recently, other groups have failed to confirm such a high objective response rate in this patient population when using this regimen along with modern radiologic response criteria, leading to controversy as to the relative merits of this regimen. Cheng and Saltz [22] reported only 1 (6%) of 16 patients with a major objective response. More recently, Kouvaraki and colleagues [23] found that 33 (39%) of 84 patients with advanced islet cell carcinomas had a major objective response to treatment with fluorouracil, doxorubicin, and streptozocin (FAS). Median survival was 3.4 years, and the median response duration was 9.3 months. Although these most recent reports were retrospective studies, they suggest that streptozocin-based therapy does have activity in this disease, but the efficacy data are inconsistent, ranging from 6% to 39% when modern radiologic response criteria are used. These reports also indicate that treatment-related toxicity is often limiting, and new therapies are needed.

Several recent studies have evaluated single- and multiagent chemotherapy for patients with advanced NE tumors. Regimens that have been found to be relatively inactive for this patient population include, gemcitabine [24], docetaxel [25], high-dose paclitaxel [26], and irinotecan/cisplatin [27]. Temozolamide, an oral and less-toxic alternative to dacarbazine, and thalidomide, which is believed to have antiangiogenic activity, have been used in combination for patients with metastatic NE tumors [28]. Overall, this regimen produced a 25% radiologic response rate and appeared to be more active for pancreatic endocrine tumors than carcinoid tumors. However, 55% of patients discontinued treatment because of treatment-related toxicity, including neuropathy, thrombocytopenia, infection, neutropenia, and rash. Median survival was not reached. Combination therapy with fluorouracil, epirubicin, and dacarbazine was associated with a 25% objective response in patients with metastatic NE tumors of diverse etiologies [29], which does not appear to be any better than treatment with dacarbazine alone.

Poorly differentiated NE carcinomas arise from a variety of primary sites, including the GI tract, prostate, kidney, skin (Merkell cell), and thyroid; however, often, the primary site is unknown. Most poorly differentiated NE carcinomas resemble small-cell lung cancer histologically. Others lack small-cell features but express general NE markers, such as chromogranin A, synaptophysin, and neuron-specific enolase, or exhibit neurosecretory granules using electron microscopy. Like small-cell lung cancers, poorly differentiated NE carcinomas are high-grade malignant.

Based on the known chemosensitivity of small-cell lung cancers to combination etoposide/cisplatin therapy, Moertel and colleagues [30] hypothesized that other NE carcinomas would also be susceptible to this regimen. In numerous retrospective series, treatment with etoposide/cisplatin produced an initial objective response in many patients with poorly differentiated NE carcinomas (Table 1) [30–32]. In contrast, patients with well differentiated NE carcinomas rarely responded to this treatment regimen. The duration of response to etoposide/cisplatin therapy in patients with poorly differentiated NE carcinomas was short, and, as was true for small-cell lung cancer, overall survival was limited.

These dismal results have led others to evaluate the efficacy of different drug combinations in patients with poorly differentiated NE carcinomas. Recently, Hainsworth and colleagues [33] reported the results of a phase II study of paclitaxel, carboplatin, and etoposide in patients with advanced

Table 1
Treatment of poorly differentiated neuroendocrine tumors

Treatment	Tumor type	N	OR, %	Median survival, mo	Reference
Etoposide/cisplatin	Carcinoid	13	0	11	Moertel et al [30]
	Islet cell	14	14	16	
	"Anaplastic"	18	67	19	
Etoposide/cisplatin	Well-differentiated	12	9	18	Mitry et al [31]
	Poorly differentiated	41	42	15	
Etoposide/cisplatin	Poorly differentiated or rapidly progressing	36	55	19	Fjallskog et al [32]
Etoposide/carboplatin/ paclitaxel (Phase II)	Poorly differentiated	78	53	15	Hainsworth et al [33]
Capecitabine/oxaliplatin (Phase II)	Well-differentiated	27	30	40	Bajetta et al [8,34]
	Poorly differentiated	13	23	5	

NE carcinomas (see Table 1). Similarly to prior anecdotal reports of etoposide/cisplatin, the three-drug regimen produced response rates in many patient (53%), but median survival was only 14.5 months. Response rates did not appear to differ between patients with known and unknown primary sites and between patients with or without small-cell features. This regimen was moderately toxic and was not clearly more efficacious than treatment with etoposide/cisplatin. The results from this study underlie the rationale for the investigational use of improved therapies for small-cell lung cancer for patients with advanced NE carcinomas. Finally, Bajetta and colleagues [34] recently studied the safety and efficacy of capecitabine and oxaliplatin (XELOX) in 40 patients with NE tumors. While the data revealed intriguing efficacy in patients with well-differentiated NE tumors progressing after somatostatin analog therapy (30% objective response rate), it also suggested that this regimen should not replace traditional platinum-based chemotherapy (ie, etoposide/cisplatin) in the first-line treatment of patients with poorly differentiated NE tumors.

Hepatic artery embolization/chemoembolization

Because NE liver metastases are hypervascular and derive most of their blood supply from the hepatic artery, hepatic arterial embolization (HAE) and hepatic arterial chemoembolization (HACE) have been used to palliate symptoms and control rapid growth of liver-dominant metastatic NE carcinoma. For both HAE and HACE, gelfoam powder or polyvinyl alcohol particles are administered via the hepatic artery until satisfactory embolization is achieved. For HACE, chemotherapy is given before embolization. To minimize adverse events such as postembolization syndrome, which is characterized by fever, nausea, abdominal pain, and liver failure, typically only one liver lobe (or part of one lobe) is embolized per session.

Recently, Gupta and colleagues [35] reported results of HAE/HACE for the treatment of a large series of patients with metastatic NE tumors. Patients with carcinoid tumors (n = 69) had better outcomes than patients with islet cell carcinomas (n = 54): radiologic response was 67% versus 35% ($P = .0001$); progression-free survival was 23 months versus 16 months ($P = .046$); and overall survival was 34 months versus 23 months ($P = .012$). In another report, 33 (63%) of 52 patients with liver-dominant metastatic carcinoid disease had a reduction in tumor-related symptoms including tumor bulk, pain, and hormonal excess [36]. Bile duct injury, which has the potential to be a source of infection and ultimately liver failure, was reported in 11% of patients after HACE in one recent study [37]. This complication is especially relevant in patients with indolent disease. To date, there are no conclusive data to suggest that HACE is more efficacious than HAE. Moreover, HAE/HACE does not clearly prolong survival of patients with advanced NE tumors.

Investigational therapies

Current options for treatment of patients with advanced NE tumors are inadequate. As a result, there is no standard treatment that is widely agreed upon. A better understanding of NE tumor biology may provide insight into their pathogenesis and suggest novel targets for treatment.

NE tumors and their metastases are highly vascular, and this observation has prompted interest in antiangiogenic agents as a novel therapeutic approach in this disease. Treatment with recombinant human endostatin, an endogenous peptide with antiangiogenic activity, was explored in a phase II study in patients with advanced pancreatic endocrine carcinomas or carcinoid tumors [38]. The drug was well tolerated, but no radiologic responses were seen. Expression of vascular endothelial growth factor (VEGF) and

Table 2
Selected clinical trials for neuroendocrine tumors

Trial	Phase	Tumor type	Sponsor/ Lead organization
FOLFOX with bevacizumab	II	Progressive carcinoid, islet cell carcinoma, poorly differentiated NE carcinoma	University of California San Francisco
Lanreotide autogel	II	Progressive well-differentiated NE tumor or carcinoma	Beaufour Ipsen International SNC
Panzem NCD with bevacizumab	II	Locally unresectable or metastatic carcinoid tumors	Entremed/Dana-Farber
Irinotecan/cisplatin	II	Poorly differentiated NE carcinoma of GI tract or unknown primary site	Pfizer/M. D. Anderson
Atiprimod	II	Progressive, symptomatic carcinoid, islet cell carcinoma	Callisto Pharmaceuticals
Yttrium Y90-DOTA-tyr3-octreotide	I	Children with advanced or refractory somatostatin receptor positive tumors	University of Iowa
Everolimus	II	Progressive islet cell carcinoma	Novartis
GW786034 (Pazopanib)	II	Advanced low-grade or intermediate-grade neuroendocrine carcinoma	NCI
Everolimus and Octreotide	III	Advanced carinoid tumor	Novartis

Adapted from National Cancer Institute. Clinical Trials. Available at: http://www.cancer.gov/clinicaltrials/search. Accessed May 16, 2007.

neuropilin-2, a coreceptor for a number of VEGF isoforms, has been detected in NE tumors of the pancreas and gut. In a mouse model of pancreatic NE carcinoma, knockout of the VEGF-A gene resulted in significantly impaired tumor angiogenesis and growth [39]. Treatment with a neutralizing antibody to VEGF also inhibited primary tumor growth and formation of liver metastases in a xenograft model of human NE carcinoma [40]. Preliminary results of a phase II study of bevacizumab, a humanized antibody against VEGF in patients with advanced carcinoid tumors, suggest that this antiangiogenic therapy may suppress blood flow, decrease urinary 5HIAA levels, and prolong progression-free survival [41].

Other potential molecular targets for NE tumors include the following members of the tyrosine kinase receptor family: c-KIT, platelet-derived growth factor receptors (PDGFRs) α and β, and epidermal growth factor receptor (EGFR). Most pancreatic NE carcinomas appear to express each of these receptors [42], and most malignant mid-gut carcinoid tumors express PDGFRβ and EGFR [43]. Preliminary results from a phase II trial with the oral multitargeted tyrosine kinase inhibitor SU11248 (sunitinib malate) for the treatment of advanced carcinoid and islet cell carcinomas revealed antiangiogenic and antitumor activity by specific inhibition of VEGFR, PDGFR, and c-KIT [44]. Treatment with SU11248 was well tolerated, but objective responses were rare, and most patients had stable disease.

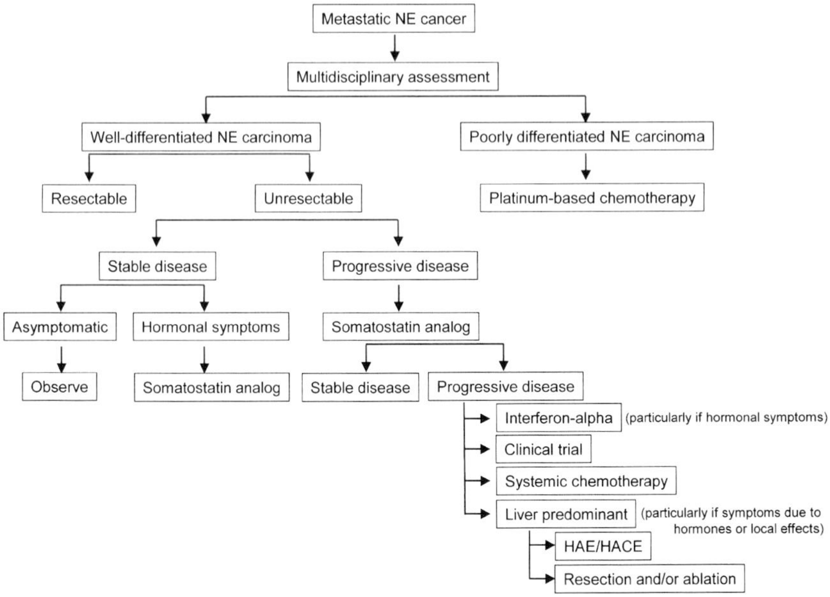

Fig. 1. Proposed algorithm for managing patients with metastatic neuroendocrine carcinomas. HAE, hepatic arterial embolization; HACE, hepatic arterial chemoembolization.

Finally, imatinib mesylate (Gleevec), a small molecule inhibitor of c-KIT, PDGFR, and c-ABL, was evaluated in patients (n = 15) with advanced NE tumors of diverse etiologies [45]. No objective responses were detected in this limited study with few patients and short duration of treatment due to adverse effects.

Currently, numerous other oral compounds are being investigated: gefitinib (EGFR inhibitor), FR901228 (histone deacetylase inhibitor), RAD001 (mTOR inhibitor), and sorafenib (RAF kinase inhibitor) (Table 2). Recently, in vitro studies showed that Raf pathway activation, rather than inhibition, suppresses hormone production and growth of carcinoid tumor cells [46], which suggests that sorafenib may not be an ideal agent for advanced NE tumors.

Summary

Optimal treatment of patients with metastatic NE tumors is challenging and requires a multidisciplinary team of physicians and surgeons. Early evaluation by a surgeon experienced in dealing with NE tumors is necessary to determine resectability and the potential role for surgical palliation. For patients who are not candidates for surgery, the main goals of therapy are to palliate symptoms and to improve survival. A proposed algorithm for managing patients with metastatic NE tumors is presented (Fig. 1). Clearly, a better understanding of NE tumor biology is required, which will lead to earlier detection of NE tumors and a greater chance for resection, as well as to more effective treatments for patients with advanced disease.

Acknowledgments

We thank Ms. Pamela Derish for expert editorial assistance.

References

[1] Kloppel G, Perren A, Heitz PU. The gastroenteropancreatic neuroendocrine cell system and its tumors: the WHO classification. Ann N Y Acad Sci 2004;1014:13–27.

[2] Lamberts SW, van der Lely AJ, de Herder WW, et al. Octreotide. N Engl J Med 1996;334(4): 246–54.

[3] Rubin J, Ajani J, Schirmer W, et al. Octreotide acetate long-acting formulation versus open-label subcutaneous octreotide acetate in malignant carcinoid syndrome. J Clin Oncol 1999; 17(2):600–6.

[4] Oberg K, Kvols L, Caplin M, et al. Consensus report on the use of somatostatin analogs for the management of neuroendocrine tumors of the gastroenteropancreatic system. Ann Oncol 2004;15(6):966–73.

[5] Vezzosi D, Bennet A, Rochaix P, et al. Octreotide in insulinoma patients: efficacy on hypoglycemia, relationships with Octreoscan scintigraphy and immunostaining with anti-sst2A and anti-sst5 antibodies. Eur J Endocrinol 2005;152(5):757–67.

[6] Faiss S, Pape UF, Bohmig M, et al. Prospective, randomized, multicenter trial on the antiproliferative effect of lanreotide, interferon alfa, and their combination for therapy of metastatic neuroendocrine gastroenteropancreatic tumors—the International Lanreotide and Interferon Alfa Study Group. J Clin Oncol 2003;21(14):2689–96.
[7] di Bartolomeo M, Bajetta E, Buzzoni R, et al. Clinical efficacy of octreotide in the treatment of metastatic neuroendocrine tumors. A study by the Italian Trials in Medical Oncology Group. Cancer 1996;77(2):402–8.
[8] Bajetta E, Procopio G, Catena L, et al. Lanreotide autogel every 6 weeks compared with Lanreotide microparticles every 3 weeks in patients with well differentiated neuroendocrine tumors: a Phase III Study. Cancer 2006;107(10):2474–81.
[9] Trendle MC, Moertel CG, Kvols LK. Incidence and morbidity of cholelithiasis in patients receiving chronic octreotide for metastatic carcinoid and malignant islet cell tumors. Cancer 1997;79(4):830–4.
[10] Schmid HA, Schoeffter P. Functional activity of the multiligand analog SOM230 at human recombinant somatostatin receptor subtypes supports its usefulness in neuroendocrine tumors. Neuroendocrinology 2004;80(Suppl 1):47–50.
[11] Kwekkeboom DJ, Mueller-Brand J, Paganelli G, et al. Overview of results of peptide receptor radionuclide therapy with 3 radiolabeled somatostatin analogs. J Nucl Med 2005; 46(Suppl 1):62S–6S.
[12] Valkema R, Pauwels S, Kvols LK, et al. Survival and response after peptide receptor radionuclide therapy with [90Y-DOTA0,Tyr3]octreotide in patients with advanced gastroenteropancreatic neuroendocrine tumors. Semin Nucl Med 2006;36(2):147–56.
[13] Niederhuber JE, Fojo T. Treatment of metastatic disease in patients with neuroendocrine tumors. Surg Oncol Clin N Am 2006;15(3):511–33, viii.
[14] Janson ET, Oberg K. Long-term management of the carcinoid syndrome. Treatment with octreotide alone and in combination with alpha-interferon. Acta Oncol 1993; 32(2):225–9.
[15] Pavel ME, Baum U, Hahn EG, et al. Efficacy and tolerability of pegylated IFN-alpha in patients with neuroendocrine gastroenteropancreatic carcinomas. J Interferon Cytokine Res 2006;26(1):8–13.
[16] Stuart K, Levy DE, Anderson T, et al. Phase II study of interferon gamma in malignant carcinoid tumors (E9292): a trial of the Eastern Cooperative Oncology Group. Invest New Drugs 2004;22(1):75–81.
[17] Moertel CG, Hanley JA. Combination chemotherapy trials in metastatic carcinoid tumor and the malignant carcinoid syndrome. Cancer Clin Trials 1979;2(4):327–34.
[18] Engstrom PF, Lavin PT, Moertel CG, et al. Streptozocin plus fluorouracil versus doxorubicin therapy for metastatic carcinoid tumor. J Clin Oncol 1984;2(11):1255–9.
[19] Bukowski RM, Tangen CM, Peterson RF, et al. Phase II trial of dimethyltriazenoimidazole carboxamide in patients with metastatic carcinoid. A Southwest Oncology Group study. Cancer 1994;73(5):1505–8.
[20] Sun W, Lipsitz S, Catalano P, et al. Phase II/III study of doxorubicin with fluorouracil compared with streptozocin with fluorouracil or dacarbazine in the treatment of advanced carcinoid tumors: Eastern Cooperative Oncology Group Study E1281. J Clin Oncol 2005; 23(22):4897–904.
[21] Moertel CG, Lefkopoulo M, Lipsitz S, et al. Streptozocin-doxorubicin, streptozocin-fluorouracil or chlorozotocin in the treatment of advanced islet-cell carcinoma. N Engl J Med 1992; 326(8):519–23.
[22] Cheng PN, Saltz LB. Failure to confirm major objective antitumor activity for streptozocin and doxorubicin in the treatment of patients with advanced islet cell carcinoma. Cancer 1999;86(6):944–8.
[23] Kouvaraki MA, Ajani JA, Hoff P, et al. Fluorouracil, doxorubicin, and streptozocin in the treatment of patients with locally advanced and metastatic pancreatic endocrine carcinomas. J Clin Oncol 2004;22(23):4762–71.

[24] Kulke MH, Kim H, Clark JW, et al. A Phase II trial of gemcitabine for metastatic neuroendocrine tumors. Cancer 2004;101(5):934–9.
[25] Kulke MH, Kim H, Stuart K, et al. A Phase II study of docetaxel in patients with metastatic carcinoid tumors. Cancer Invest 2004;22(3):353–9.
[26] Ansell SM, Pitot HC, Burch PA, et al. A Phase II study of high-dose paclitaxel in patients with advanced neuroendocrine tumors. Cancer 2001;91(8):1543–8.
[27] Kulke MH, Wu B, Ryan DP, et al. A Phase II trial of irinotecan and cisplatin in patients with metastatic neuroendocrine tumors. Dig Dis Sci 2006;51(6):1033–8.
[28] Kulke MH, Stuart K, Enzinger PC, et al. Phase II study of temozolomide and thalidomide in patients with metastatic neuroendocrine tumors. J Clin Oncol 2006;24(3):401–6.
[29] Bajetta E, Ferrari L, Procopio G, et al. Efficacy of a chemotherapy combination for the treatment of metastatic neuroendocrine tumours. Ann Oncol 2002;13(4):614–21.
[30] Moertel CG, Kvols LK, O'Connell MJ, et al. Treatment of neuroendocrine carcinomas with combined etoposide and cisplatin. Evidence of major therapeutic activity in the anaplastic variants of these neoplasms. Cancer 1991;68(2):227–32.
[31] Mitry E, Baudin E, Ducreux M, et al. Treatment of poorly differentiated neuroendocrine tumours with etoposide and cisplatin. Br J Cancer 1999;81(8):1351–5.
[32] Fjallskog ML, Granberg DP, Welin SL, et al. Treatment with cisplatin and etoposide in patients with neuroendocrine tumors. Cancer 2001;92(5):1101–7.
[33] Hainsworth JD, Spigel DR, Litchy S, et al. Phase II trial of paclitaxel, carboplatin, and etoposide in advanced poorly differentiated neuroendocrine carcinoma: a Minnie Pearl Cancer Research Network Study. J Clin Oncol 2006;24(22):3548–54.
[34] Bajetta E, Catena L, Procopio G, et al. Are capecitabine and oxaliplatin (XELOX) suitable treatments for progressing low-grade and high-grade neuroendocrine tumours? Cancer Chemother Pharmacol 2007;59(5):637–42.
[35] Gupta S, Johnson MM, Murthy R, et al. Hepatic arterial embolization and chemoembolization for the treatment of patients with metastatic neuroendocrine tumors: variables affecting response rates and survival. Cancer 2005;104(8):1590–602.
[36] Gupta S, Yao JC, Ahrar K, et al. Hepatic artery embolization and chemoembolization for treatment of patients with metastatic carcinoid tumors: the M.D. Anderson experience. Cancer 2003;9(4):261–7.
[37] Yu JS, Kim KW, Jeong MG, et al. Predisposing factors of bile duct injury after transcatheter arterial chemoembolization (TACE) for hepatic malignancy. Cardiovasc Intervent Radiol 2002;25(4):270–4.
[38] Kulke MH, Bergsland EK, Ryan DP, et al. Phase II study of recombinant human endostatin in patients with advanced neuroendocrine tumors. J Clin Oncol 2006;24(22):3555–61.
[39] Inoue M, Hager JH, Ferrara N, et al. VEGF-A has a critical, nonredundant role in angiogenic switching and pancreatic beta cell carcinogenesis. Cancer Cell 2002;1(2):193–202.
[40] Konno H, Arai T, Tanaka T, et al. Antitumor effect of a neutralizing antibody to vascular endothelial growth factor on liver metastasis of endocrine neoplasm. Jpn J Cancer Res 1998;89(9):933–9.
[41] Yao JC, Ng C, Hoff PM, et al. Improved progression free survival (PVS), and rapid, sustained decrease in tumor perfusion among patients with advanced carcinoid treated with bevacizumab [abstract 4007]. Presented at the Proceedings of the American Society of Clinical Oncology. Orlando, FL, May 13–15, 2007.
[42] Fjallskog ML, Lejonklou MH, Oberg KE, et al. Expression of molecular targets for tyrosine kinase receptor antagonists in malignant endocrine pancreatic tumors. Clin Cancer Res 2003;9(4):1469–73.
[43] Chaudhry A, Papanicolaou V, Oberg K, et al. Expression of platelet-derived growth factor and its receptors in neuroendocrine tumors of the digestive system. Cancer Res 1992;52(4):1006–12.

[44] Kulke M, Lenz HJ, Meropol NJ, et al. A phase 2 study to evaluate the efficacy and safety of SU11248 in patients (pts) with unresectable neuroendocrine tumors (NETs) [abstract 4008]. Presented at the Proc Am Soc Clin Oncol. 2005.
[45] Gross DJ, Munter G, Bitan M, et al. The role of imatinib mesylate (Glivec) for treatment of patients with malignant endocrine tumors positive for c-kit or PDGF-R. Endocr Relat Cancer 2006;13(2):535–40.
[46] Van Gompel JJ, Kunnimalaiyaan M, Holen K, et al. ZM336372, a Raf-1 activator, suppresses growth and neuroendocrine hormone levels in carcinoid tumor cells. Mol Cancer Ther 2005;4(6):910–7.

ELSEVIER
SAUNDERS

Surg Oncol Clin N Am
16 (2007) 653–666

SURGICAL
ONCOLOGY CLINICS
OF NORTH AMERICA

Cytoreductive Surgery for Peritoneal Malignancies—Development of Standards of Care for the Community

Jesus Esquivel, MD, FACS

Surgical Oncology, St. Agnes Hospital, 900 Caton Avenue, Baltimore, MD 21229, USA

Surgical resection remains the hallmark in the treatment of primary colon cancer. It allows the patients to become clinically disease free, provides proper staging, and determines who should receive adjuvant systemic chemotherapy. Treatment options for patients with unresectable metastatic disease have improved significantly in the past few years. The use of modern combination cytotoxic chemotherapy with biologic agents has resulted in an unprecedented improvement of the median survival for patients with stage IV colorectal cancer to nearly 2 years [1].

Peritoneal involvement in colorectal cancer occurs in approximately 30% of patients. In 8% of these patients peritoneal dissemination is diagnosed at the time of primary colorectal surgery and 25% present with recurrent disease confined to the peritoneal cavity [2]. Surgical therapy for stage IV colorectal cancer has evolved from the treatment of locally recurrent primary tumors to the routine resection of hepatic metastases, accounting for 5-year survival and cure seen in selected patients with stage IV colorectal cancer. As described in the previous chapters, the combination of systemic therapy with local ablative and/or surgical modalities has proven beneficial to an even larger group of patients with metastatic disease, including those with metastases in other sites than liver. Today, surgical therapy for stage IV colorectal cancer and other solid cancer metastases has evolved even further to embrace the concept of complete macroscopic surgical eradication and/or cytoreduction of metastatic disease. The aim of this chapter is to elucidate the concept of cytoreductive surgery in the treatment of peritoneal carcinomatosis. Our understanding of the biological and clinical behavior of peritoneal surface malignancies has helped to advance this therapeutic concept beyond clinical research into a viable treatment option with potential for broad application.

E-mail address: jesusesquivel@yahoo.com

1055-3207/07/$ - see front matter © 2007 Elsevier Inc. All rights reserved.
doi:10.1016/j.soc.2007.04.015 *surgonc.theclinics.com*

Pathophysiology of peritoneal carcinomatosis

Peritoneal surface malignancies represent a spectrum of diseases characterized by the rupture of the primary tumor with a predictable pattern of dissemination throughout the abdominal and pelvic regions [3]. However, the significance of free intraperitoneal cells is unknown since after seeding the peritoneal cavity, these cells must complete a series of steps to acquire the potential to form tumor deposits. First they need to survive in the peritoneal cavity by evading the immune system. In addition, they need to attach to secondary sites and develop a blood supply for their metabolic needs. Because of the complexity of this process, most tumor cells will fail to develop into a metastatic deposit.

The dissemination of tumor cells in the peritoneal cavity is governed by several factors. The physiologic flow of peritoneal fluid within the abdomen occurs in a clockwise fashion. This explains the predominance of tumor cell implants on the undersurface of the right hemidiaphragm as they are pulled into this region with every respiratory cycle. A second mechanism of dissemination is due to the phagocytic activity of both the greater and lesser omentum and the appendices epiploicae of the sigmoid colon. Infiltration of the greater omentum by tumor gives rise to the well-known "omental cake," a frequent hallmark of peritoneal malignancies. A third driving force of dissemination simply is gravity, resulting in tumor deposits in the pelvis causing pelvic outlet obstruction. In women, tumor cells will often attach to the ovaries, usually at the site of a ruptured follicle. Progressive invasion of the ovary leads to the clinical presentation of an ovarian mass. Once peritoneal tumor dissemination and growth has occurred, it will sustain itself through constant reimplantation. With sufficient accumulation of tumor cells in the greater omentum and the lymphatic lacunae of both diaphragms, physiologic flow and absorption of peritoneal fluid will cease and lead to malignant ascites. The protein-rich ascites further promote cancer growth.

Surgical intervention is an important contributor to the successful peritoneal implantation and growth of tumor cells. During resection of large primary lesions and in the presence of extensive lymph node involvement, large numbers of tumor cells are released into the peritoneal cavity. The inflammatory response induced by surgical trauma will entrap cancer cells and paradoxically protect them from destruction by the immune system. Trapped tumor cells benefit from the same micromilieu that is produced by the healing process following surgical intervention. Cancer growth is also promoted by fibroblast proliferation and local collagen production [4].

The concept of cytoreductive surgery and hyperthermic intraperitoneal chemotherapy

In the 1990s, Sugarbaker and colleagues proposed cytoreductive surgery and perioperative intraperitoneal chemotherapy as definitive treatment for peritoneal dissemination from appendiceal neoplasms and diffuse malignant peritoneal mesothelioma [5–7]. The successful treatment of peritoneal surface malignancies requires a combined approach that uses peritonectomy to remove all visible tumor nodules and intraperitoneal chemotherapy. The addition of perioperative intraperitoneal chemotherapy is thought to prevent the implantation of free intraperitoneal tumor cells and act against microscopic disease left behind after surgical resection of all macroscopic foci. Compared with systemic chemotherapy alone, novel regional intraperitoneal chemotherapy has shown favorable oncologic results and substantially changed the selection, treatment, and prognosis of patients with abdominal and pelvic malignancies such as peritoneal carcinomatosis, peritoneal sarcomatosis, and peritoneal mesothelioma [8,9]. Chemotherapy is given in the immediate perioperative setting and may be continued for the first 5 postoperative days. The size of the peritoneal implants is of critical importance for the success of this therapy. Only patients with small intraperitoneal tumor nodules that have a limited distribution within the abdomen and pelvis are likely to show prolonged benefit [10]. To properly balance the risks and benefits, judicious patient selection is essential. Both visceral and parietal peritonectomy are necessary for complete cytoreduction, a mandatory component of therapy [11]. Complete cytoreductive surgery is necessary before intraperitoneal chemotherapy instillation, and this is unlikely to be accomplished for advanced sarcomatosis or carcinomatosis. Normal peritoneum is preserved as much as possible and only areas grossly involved by tumor are removed.

Technique, standard protocols, and patient selection

A total of six subsets of peritonectomy procedures have been described. Their use depends on the distribution and extent of the disease within the peritoneal space. The following is a brief summary of the six peritonectomy procedures.

Parietal peritoneal stripping from the anterior abdominal wall

A single entry into the peritoneal cavity in the upper portion of the incision allows the surgeon to assess the need for a complete parietal peritonectomy. If tumor nodules are palpated on the parietal peritoneum, a complete parietal dissection is necessary. As the dissection proceeds to the peritoneum overlying the paracolic sulcus (line of Toldt) the dissection can proceed rapidly because of the loose connections of the peritoneum to the underlying fatty tissue.

Peritoneal stripping of the hemidiaphragms

The peritonectomy of the left and right upper quadrant is begun by progressive stripping of the posterior rectus sheath. Strong traction combined with ball-tip electrosurgical dissection allows separation of peritoneum and tumor deposits from all underlying normal tissue including the diaphragmatic muscle, the adrenal glands, and the superior half of the perirenal fat. The stripping of the diaphragmatic undersurface is continued until the bare area of the liver is encountered. At that point, tumor on the anterior and superior surface of the liver is electroevaporated until completely cleared. With ball-tipped electrosurgical dissection, a thick layer of tumor may be lifted off the dome of the liver by removing Glisson's capsule. The dissection proceeds laterally to the right until the perirenal fat is encountered and cleared. The right adrenal gland is exposed and injury to it carefully avoided as tumor is stripped from the right subhepatic space. Care is taken not to traumatize the vena cava or any of the short hepatic veins emanating from it, particularly those draining the caudate lobe.

Greater omentectomy and splenectomy

Greater omentectomy/splenectomy is performed to free the midabdomen from large tumor volumes. The greater omentum is elevated and separated from the transverse colon using electrocautery. The peritoneum covering the transverse mesocolon is carefully removed up to the inferior pancreatic edge. The gastroepiploic vessels on the greater curvature of the stomach and the short gastrics are divided. With traction on the spleen, tumor-bearing peritoneum anterior to the pancreas is stripped, exposing the splenic artery and vein at the tail of the pancreas. Injury to the main left gastric artery and vein must be avoided to preserve the sole remaining vascular supply to the stomach.

Cholecystectomy with stripping of the hepatoduodenal ligament

If the gallbladder is involved by tumor, a standard cholecystectomy is performed. Blunt dissection of Calot's triangle minimizes injury to the common bile duct and right hepatic artery and allows safe removal of any tumor deposits in this area. The triangular ligament of the left lobe of the liver is then resected, which allows retraction of the left lateral liver segments to expose the hepatogastric ligament in its entirety. A circumferential release of this ligament from the fissure between liver segments 1–3 and the lesser curvature of the stomach between right and left gastric arteries is required. After stripping the peritoneum of the lesser curvature, digital dissection with firm pressure from the surgeon's thumb and index finger separates lesser omental fat and tumor from the right and left gastric arteries. As much as possible of the anterior vagus nerve is spared.

Stripping the floor of the omental bursa

By anterior and superior retraction of the caudate lobe, the entire floor of the omental bursa is exposed. Electroevaporation of tumor from the posterior surface of the left caudate lobe portion may be necessary to achieve this exposure. Ball-tip electrosurgery is used to cautiously divide the peritoneal reflection of the liver onto the left side of the subhepatic vena cava. After the peritoneum is divided, Russian forceps assist in bluntly stripping the peritoneum from the superior recess of the omental bursa, the right diaphragmatic crus, and the portal vein. Electroevaporation of tumor from the liver surface that lies posterior to the hepatoduodenal ligament may be required. Care is taken while stripping the floor of the omental bursa to stay superficial to the right phrenic artery.

Resection of rectosigmoid colon, uterus, and cul-de-sac

First the sigmoid colon is divided with a linear stapler just above the superior extend of the carcinomatosis involving the pelvis, usually at the junction of sigmoid and descending colon. The inferior mesenteric artery and vein are divided, thus allowing retraction of the small bowel and the proximal descending colon into the upper abdomen. Ball-tipped electrosurgery is used to circumferentially dissect the peritoneum of the pelvic inlet. Extraperitoneal ligation of the uterine arteries is performed just above the ureter and close to the base of the bladder. In women, the bladder is moved gently off the cervix and the vagina is entered to complete the hysterectomy. Preservation of the lower half of the rectum will allow for a larger stool reservoir and diminish frequent bowel movements.

Criteria for complete cytoreduction

By definition, complete cytoreduction is equivalent to the eradication of all macroscopic residual tumor deposits greater than 2.5 mm. The ability to achieve a complete macroscopic removal of all tumors is assessed using the following clinical and radiographic criteria:

- Eastern Cooperative Oncology Group (ECOG) Performance status 2 or less
- No evidence of extra-abdominal disease
- No evidence of biliary obstruction
- No evidence of ureteral obstruction
- No evidence of intestinal obstruction at more than one site
- No evidence of gross disease in the small bowel mesentery and absence of several segmental sites of partial obstruction
- Small volume disease in the gastro-hepatic ligament

Hyperthermic intraperitoneal chemotherapy

To achieve a maximum cytotoxic effect after complete cytoreduction, the patient is subjected to hyperthermic intraperitoneal chemotherapy (HIPEC) with mitomycin C (15 to 35 mg/m^2) at a target intraperitoneal temperature of 39°C to 42°C for 60 to 120 minutes. Although mitomycin C is the most commonly used drug, other drugs such as oxaliplatin and combinations of mitomycin with cisplatin and doxorubicin are now being tested with promising early results [14].

The current technique for HIPEC begins with the preparation of the abdominal cavity for the chemotherapeutic perfusion. Either an open or closed method can be used. Each method has advantages and disadvantages. With the closed method the ability to control spillage of the perfusate and achieve and maintain higher temperatures in a shorter period of time is improved over the open method. With the open method, access to the intra-abdominal contents is easier, particularly in case of bleeding complications or functional problems with the perfusion catheters. The open approach also improves the ability to ensure adequate perfusion of all anatomic sites. With regard to its cytotoxic effect, both techniques are equivalent. With the open method, the patient's skin is lifted to the abdominal retractor creating a "coliseum," giving the surgeon access to the intra-abdominal contents during perfusion. With the closed technique, a watertight closure of the skin is accomplished before starting the perfusion.

After placing the perfusion catheters inside the abdomen along with two or three temperature probes, the catheters are connected to a roller pump and a heat exchanger and the warm chemotherapy solution (43°C) is perfused for 90 minutes. Creating a hyperthermia environment has several advantages. First, cancer cells are more heat sensitive than normal tissue. Temperatures between 40°C and 44°C are cytotoxic for cells in a low pO2 and pH environment. This condition is common in tumor tissues due to a hypoxic micromilieu. The preferential cytotoxic effect of hyperthermia on hypoxic tissue is augmented in hypovascular tumor tissue such as that found in peritoneal deposits. Second, hyperthermia increases the tissue penetration of chemotherapy agents. As tissues soften in response to heat, decreased interstitial pressure allows for improved drug penetration. Third and most importantly, heat increases the cytotoxicity of the chemotherapy agents. This synergism occurs only at the interface of the perfusate and the peritoneal/tumor surface.

Following completion of the perfusion, the perfusate is removed by suction and reconstructive surgery is begun. It is emphasized that no intra-abdominal sutures are placed until after the chemotherapy perfusion is complete with one exception: closure of the vaginal cuff to prevent leakage of the perfusate.

Under certain circumstances early postoperative intraperitoneal chemotherapy (EPIC) perfusion with 5-fluorouracil (5-FU) can be sustained for 5 days postoperatively. In patients with symptomatic ascites in whom adequate cytoreduction is impossible, HIPEC can be used for palliation of the intractable ascites. Finally, palliative incomplete cytoreduction has a role in individually selected patients.

Standardized surgical techniques, as described above, reproducible delivery methods for HIPEC, and observation of patient selection criteria are responsible for the recently published outcomes [12]. These results have spurred the establishment of numerous peritoneal surface malignancy treatment centers in the United States and Europe. Over the past 5 years, a number of international treatment centers have published their results using cytoreductive surgery and HIPEC for peritoneal carcinomatosis in patients with colorectal cancer [13–15]. In a randomized controlled trial reported in 2003, superior survival for cytoreductive surgery combined with HIPEC compared with systemic chemotherapy alone was demonstrated [16]. In 2004, a multi-institutional registry study from 28 international treatment centers demonstrated a median survival of 19 months and a 39% 3-year survival after cytoreductive surgery and HIPEC in 506 patients with colorectal peritoneal carcinomatosis [17]. In patients with low-volume peritoneal carcinomatosis of colonic origin, cytoreductive surgery and HIPEC can achieve long-term survival [17]. However, as pointed out by Yan and colleagues in a systematic review of 14 published series, only 2 were randomized controlled trials with one randomized comparative study. The remaining 11 reports consisted of observational studies without control groups [18]. Most importantly, the indications, the techniques, and the type of drugs used varied among the reported studies.

The Peritoneal Surface Malignancy Group (PSMG) has attempted to standardize the indications and techniques for the appropriate use of cytoreductive surgery and HIPEC in a recent consensus statement [19]. The statement lists the following principals of standardization with regard to operative technique and patient selection: (1) the goal of peritonectomy is to achieve complete macroscopic cytoreduction; (2) if complete surgical cytoreduction is achieved, HIPEC is a mandatory part of the treatment; (3) mitomycin C remains the drug of choice although recent data indicate the efficacy of intraperitoneal oxaliplatin combined with systemic biological therapy [14]; and (4) minor variations in dosage, temperature, and delivery method are allowed.

Proper patient selection remains a critically important aspect of the treatment for peritoneal dissemination from colorectal cancer. Long-term survival with cytoreductive surgery and HIPEC can only be achieved with complete cytoreduction. Current evidence clearly indicates that an incomplete cytoreduction of peritoneal disease confers no survival advantage over systemic chemotherapy alone. Therefore, patients do not benefit from this procedure if a complete cytoreduction cannot be accomplished [17].

Patients found to have peritoneal carcinomatosis and distant metastases should be considered for combinations of cytotoxic chemotherapy and biologic therapy. If they have a good response to systemic therapy and limited liver metastases as the only additional site of disease, cytoreductive surgery and intraperitoneal chemotherapy may be appropriate after a period of observation. There are currently no data indicating whether systemic chemotherapy should be given before or after cytoreductive surgery and HIPEC. However, it is important that patients with limited liver metastases who may be candidates for HIPEC are evaluated by specialized surgical oncologists before initiating systemic therapy alone.

Diagnostic evaluation

As outlined on the clinical pathway for the management of peritoneal surface malignancies of colonic origin (Fig. 1), once a patient is suspected or known to have colorectal cancer with peritoneal involvement, one of the most important steps in the diagnostic work-up is determining if the patient has peritoneal carcinomatosis with or without distant sites of dissemination. To evaluate the extent of peritoneal dissemination and to rule out any hematogenous metastases, a complete colonoscopy and a

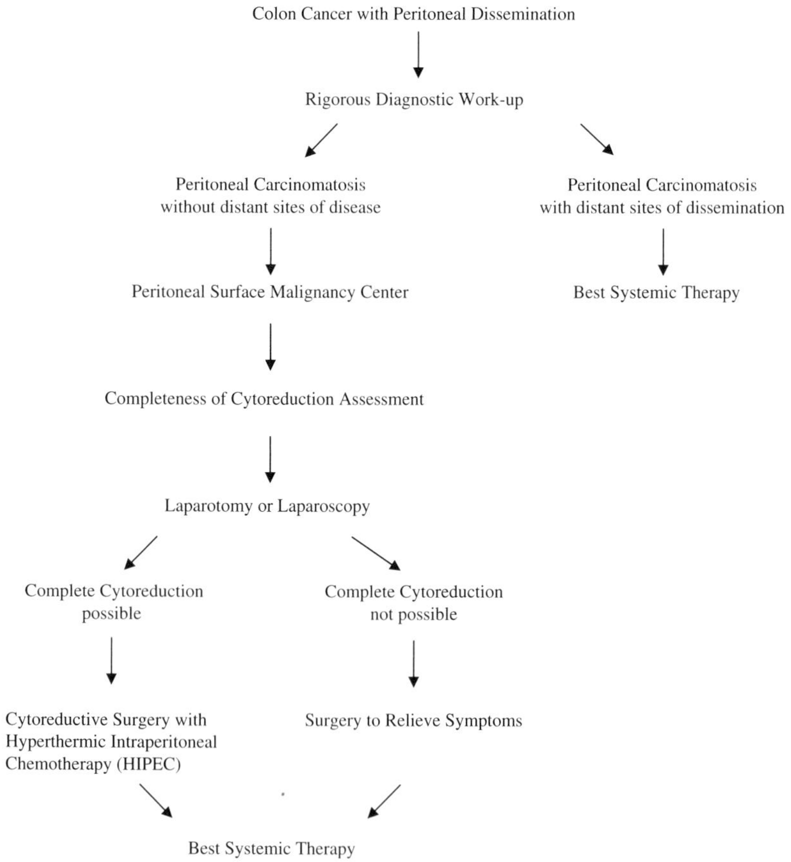

Fig. 1. Clinical pathway for the management of peritoneal surface malignancies of colonic origin.

contrast-enhanced CT scan of the chest, abdomen, and pelvis is performed. A positron emission tomography (PET) scan can be considered if there are any questions about hematogenous metastases or extensive retroperitoneal lymphadenopathy.

The role of CT scan in the evaluation of peritoneal carcinomatosis has been the subject of two published series [20,21]. The diagnostic accuracy of the CT for peritoneal carcinomatosis is limited, particularly for the detection of small bowel peritoneal implants. Routine CT scans are of limited value in excluding those patients with colorectal cancer peritoneal carcinomatosis that will not benefit from cytoreductive surgery with HIPEC. Therefore, alternative diagnostic methods to correctly stage patients with peritoneal malignancies are needed.

Role of laparoscopy in the evaluation of peritoneal carcinomatosis

Garofalo and Valle [22] reported on 97 cases of peritoneal carcinomatosis submitted to a staging laparoscopy. In 96 of 97 laparoscopic cases, they successfully assessed the Peritoneal Cancer Index. Only 2 of 96 cases were understaged. Correlation between laparoscopic and final open assessment of the Peritoneal Cancer Index was good. There was no mortality and no port sites metastases. Patients found to have massive small bowel and mesenteric involvement by staging laparoscopy were excluded from peritonectomy, establishing laparoscopy as a useful staging tool for peritoneal surface malignancies [22].

A group of French investigators evaluated the role of explorative laparoscopy in 11 patients with peritoneal carcinomatosis [23]. All patients successfully underwent laparoscopic evaluation. The median operating time for the laparoscopic portion of the procedure was 38 minutes (range 23 to 75 minutes). There were no complications. Three patients were judged unresectable by laparoscopy. Seven of the remaining 8 patients deemed resectable after laparoscopy were successfully resected. Only 1 out of 11 patients was understaged by laparoscopy.

These two studies demonstrate that laparoscopy staging is a valuable tool in the difficult selection of patients for complete cytoreduction and HIPEC.

Clinical results

Appendiceal malignancies are characterized by unique clinical features that make them particularly sensitive to peritonectomy and HIPEC. They therefore serve as the "role model" for this therapy and successful treatment has been documented [24]. Because of appendiceal obstruction and perforation, the manifestation of first tumor "spread" is the release of tumor cells into the free peritoneal cavity. In almost all patients with appendiceal malignancies, peritoneal seeding precedes the establishment of lymph node or liver metastases and therefore diagnosis is often established before lymphatic or hematogenous dissemination occurs. Appendiceal malignancies exhibit a large spectrum of invasion and biologic behavior. Some are minimally invasive (low-grade mucinous adenocarcinomas) and often can be completely resected using peritonectomy procedures even when every abdominopelvic region is involved by tumor. High-grade adenocarcinomas on the contrary are difficult to completely cytoreduce, particularly with involvement of the common bile duct or with ureteral encasement, even when smaller tumor volumes are encountered. The mucinous character of the majority of appendiceal malignancies facilitates a greater penetration of chemotherapy agents than in solid nonmucinous tumors. Finally, because dissemination is usually confined to the peritoneal space, HIPEC is often successful in eradicating all residual microscopic tumor and long-term survival is fairly common [24].

Traditionally, treatment of appendiceal adenocarcinoma and pseudomyxoma peritonei (PMP) consists of repeated debulking aimed at palliating symptoms with limited expectations for long-term survival or cure. Cytoreductive surgery and HIPEC appears to be a superior treatment method, but to this day it has not been tested in a randomized control trial. Most reports consist of observational studies from specialized tertiary referral centers and lack control groups. A review of these reports with more than 850 patients over the past 15 years shows that the study population in each series is quite heterogeneous. In the largest series by Sugarbaker and Chang [24], in which 205 patients with peritoneal malignancies originating from the appendix received cytoreductive surgery plus HIPEC, average 5-year survival was high (50%). Those who had a complete cytoreduction had a 5-year survival of 80% compared to 20% for those with incomplete cytoreduction. Similarly, survival in those with low-grade histology was 80% at 5 years versus 28% in those with high-grade tumors. Again, HIPEC therapy was not compared with traditional therapy. A phase III trial comparing cytoreductive surgery with HIPEC versus serial debulking would be ideal but is very difficult to conduct for a number of reasons. First, patients are unlikely to enroll in a trial comparing a treatment with intent to cure to a palliative procedure. Second, because of the low incidence of appendiceal malignancies, conducting a randomized trial is unlikely to be realized.

Recurrence of low-grade appendiceal mucinous adenocarcinomas after complete cytoreduction is not uncommon. This relapse in form of mucin reaccumulation has been correlated with a number of clinico-pathological parameters, including extent of initial disease, histology, and adequacy of cytoreduction. Pseudomyxoma peritonei is a disease of MUC 2 expressing goblet cells. MUC 2 expression accounts for the voluminous deposits of extracellular mucin (mucin-to-cell ratios exceeding 10:1). Increased steady-state mRNA is observed in pooled cases of pseudomyxoma peritonei but does not occur on the basis of gene rearrangement or gene amplification. Primary epithelial cell cultures obtained from pesudomyxoma peritonei express MUC 2, whose levels can be epigenetically regulated. Both immunocytochemical as well as in-situ hybridization studies with ancillary digital image analysis reveal that MUC 2 expression is independent of the degree of malignant transformation and, in fact, reflects the constitutive levels of expression observed in normal goblet cells of the appendix. These studies suggest that pseudomyxoma peritonei can be regarded as a disease of MUC 2–expressing goblet cells whose MUC 2 expression might be susceptible to targeted therapy. As pointed out by O'Connell and colleagues [25], *Pseudomyxoma peritonei,* with the abnormal MUC 2 gene regulation being responsible for the disease morbidity, offers the perfect setting for translational research.

Colon cancer with peritoneal carcinomatosis

Worldwide approximately 600 patients have been treated with cytoreductive surgery and HIPEC for colon cancer–induced peritoneal carcinomatosis. Current evidence suggests that best results require complete peritoneal cytoreduction and HIPEC [10]. This combined approach is based on the premise that all macroscopic disease is optimally removed and residual microscopic disease adequately addressed by HIPEC. In those patients in whom this is achieved, 2-year survival rates are close to 60% and 5-year survival rates approach 40% [12,14,26]. However, more so than for apendiceal malignancies, treatment success hinges on complete cytoreduction and those patients who are incompletely cytoreduced can only expect a average survival of 6 months [12,14].

At the present time, we lack universally accepted and easily reproducible prospective staging and scoring systems that address the quantity and location of the peritoneal dissemination and its impact on the ability to achieve a complete cytoreduction. We also do not have universal agreement on proper patient inclusion and exclusion criteria. Some centers consider patients with few liver metastases proper candidates for this procedure while others see them as an absolute contraindication. In the absence of a large prospective randomized trial that addresses all of the above-mentioned issues it is going to be difficult to demonstrate the true impact of cytoreductive surgery and HIPEC on the natural history of colorectal cancer with peritoneal dissemination.

Morbidity, mortality, and quality of life

The morbidity and mortality of 356 consecutive patients after cytoreductive surgery and HIPEC for peritoneal carcinomatosis has been reported [27]. Eighty-nine percent of the patients had a complete cytoreduction. Seven treatment-related deaths were seen (2%). Line sepsis (17%) and anemia (14%) were the two most common Grade III morbidities. Eleven percent of all patients required reoperation. The most common reasons for reexplorations were fistula (3.3%), anastomotic leak (2.2%), and bleeding (2%). The overall rate of grade III or IV complications was 40%. The median length of stay was 21 days (11 to 82 days). The median number of intraoperative blood transfusions was 2 (0 to 8). Two studies by McQuellon and colleagues [28,29] reported the short-term and long-term quality-of-life outcomes in patients with peritoneal carcinomatosis after cytoreductive surgery and HIPEC. In the short-term outcome study with 64 patients, the overall quality of life after surgery initially decreased but returned to baseline or better within 3 to 6 months after surgery [28]. A follow-up study of seventeen 3-year survivors demonstrated that more than 90% of patients had minimal to no limitations on their quality of life with functional assessments that compared favorably to national reference values for their respective age groups [29].

Future directions

Modern systemic therapy for patients with stage IV colorectal cancer generally consists of a combination of cytotoxic chemotherapy and biological agents. Many studies have shown the effectiveness of this approach in patients with solid organ colorectal metastases. Data on patients with colorectal cancer metastases limited to the peritoneum are scarce.

In the United States approximately 80 to 100 patients with peritoneal carcinomatosis from colorectal cancer are treated annually with cytoreductive surgery and HIPEC. This represents only a small portion of the true denominator, but presumably these patients are being treated with combinations of cytotoxic chemotherapy and biological agents. Clearly, better data are needed to determine the most appropriate therapy for these patients. At the present time, a Phase III trial with patients randomized to best systemic therapy versus cytoreductive surgery with HIPEC followed by best systemic therapy is being considered by the Peritoneal Surface Malignancy Group.

Summary

Cytoreductive surgery and HIPEC continue to play increasing roles in the management of peritoneal surface malignancies of gastrointestinal origin. The prognosis of patients and the responses to cytoreductive surgery and HIPEC depend on the histology, the degree of malignant transformation, the adequacy of the cytoreductive surgery, and the response to systemic therapy. Continuous interaction between medical and surgical oncologists is needed to identify the most appropriate patients for and the most efficient sequence of the available therapeutic modalities.

References

[1] Hurwitz HI, Fehrenbacher L, Hainsworth JD, et al. Bevacizumab in combination with fluorouracil and leucovorin: an active regimen for first-line metastatic colorectal cancer. J Clin Oncol 2005;23:3502–8.

[2] Sadeghi B, Arvieux C, Glehen O, et al. Peritoneal carcinomatosis from non-gynecologic malignancies: results of the EVOCAPE 1 multicentric prospective study. Cancer 2000;88: 58–63.

[3] Esquivel J, Sugarbaker PH. Clinical presentation of the *Pseudomyxoma peritonei* syndrome. Br J Surg 2000;87:1414–8.

[4] Zoetmulder F. Cancer cell seeding during abdominal surgery: experimental studies. In: Sugarbaker PH, editor. Peritoneal carcinomatosis: principles of management. Boston: Kluwer Academic Publishers; 1996. p. 155–61.

[5] Sugarbaker PH. New standard of care for appendiceal epithelial neoplasms and pseudomyxoma peritonei syndrome. Lancet Oncol 2006;7:69–76.

[6] Sugarbaker PH, Graves T, DeBruijn EA, et al. Rationale for early post-operative intraperitoneal chemotherapy (EPIC) in patients with advanced gastrointestinal cancer. Cancer Res 1990;50:5790–4.

[7] Look M, Chang D, Sugarbaker PH. Long-term results of cytoreductive surgery for advanced and recurrent epithelial ovarian cancers and papillary serous carcinoma of the peritoneum. Int J Gynecol Cancer 2004;14:35–41.

[8] Katz MH, Barone RM. The rationale of perioperative intraperitoneal chemotherapy in the treatment of peritoneal surface malignancies. Surg Oncol Clin N Am 2003;12:673–88.

[9] Sugarbaker PH, Yan TD, Stuart OA, et al. Comprehensive management of diffuse malignant peritoneal mesothelioma. Eur J Surg Oncol 2006;32:686–91.

[10] Verwaal VJ, van Tinteren H, van Ruth S, et al. Predicting the survival of patients with peritoneal carcinomatosis of colorectal origin treated by aggressive cytoreduction and hyperthermic intraperitoneal chemotherapy. Br J Surg 2004;91:739–46.

[11] Sugarbaker PH. Peritonectomy procedures. Ann Surg 1995;221:29–42.

[12] Glehen O, Cotte E, Schreiber V, et al. Intraperitoneal chemohyperthermia and attempted cytoreductive surgery in patients with peritoneal carcinomatosis of colorectal origin. Br J Surg 2004;91:747–54.

[13] Carmignani CP, Ortega-Perez G, Sugarbaker PH. The management of synchronous peritoneal carcinomatosis and hematogenous metastasis from colorectal cancer. Eur J Surg Oncol 2004;30:391–8.

[14] Elias D, Delperro JR, Sideris L, et al. Treatment of peritoneal carcinomatosis from colorectal cancer: impact of complete cytoreductive surgery and difficulties in conducting randomized trials. Ann Surg Oncol 2004;11:518–21.

[15] Elias D, Raynard B, Farkhondeh F, et al. Peritoneal carcinomatosis of colorectal origin: long-term results of intraperitoneal chemohyperthermia with oxaliplatin following complete cytoreductive surgery. Gastroenterol Clin Biol, in press.

[16] Verwaal VJ, van Ruth S, de Bree E, et al. Randomized trial of cytoreduction and hyperthermic intraperitoneal chemotherapy versus systemic chemotherapy and palliative surgery in patients with peritoneal carcinomatosis of colorectal origin. J Clin Oncol 2003;21:3737–43.

[17] Glehen O, Kwiatkowski F, Sugarbaker PH, et al. Cytoreductive surgery combined with perioperative intraperitoneal chemotherapy for the management of peritoneal carcinomatosis from colorectal cancer: a multi-institutional study. J Clin Oncol 2004;22:3284–92.

[18] Yan TD, Black D, Savady R, et al. A systemic review on the efficacy of cytoreductive surgery combined with perioperative intraperitoneal chemotherapy for peritoneal carcinomatosis from colorectal carcinoma. J Clin Oncol 2006;24:4011–9.

[19] Esquivel J, Sticca R, Sugarbaker PH, et al. Cytoreductive surgery and hyperthermic intraperitoneal chemotherapy in the management of peritoneal surface malignancies of colonic origin: a consensus statement. Ann Surg Oncol 2007;14(1):128–33.

[20] de Bree E, Koops W, Kroger R, et al. Preoperative computed tomography and selection of patients with colorectal peritoneal carcinomatosis for cytoreductive surgery and hyperthermic intraperitoneal chemotherapy. Eur J Surg Oncol 2005.

[21] Yan TD, Haveric N, Carmignani CP, et al. Computed tomographic characterization of malignant peritoneal mesothelioma. Tumori 2005;91:394–400.

[22] Garofalo A, Valle M. [Staging videolaparoscopy of peritoneal carcinomatosis]. Tumori 2003;89(4 Suppl):70–7 [Italian].
[23] Pomel C, Appleyard TL, Gouy S, et al. The role of laparoscopy to evaluate candidates for complete cytoreduction of peritoneal carcinomatosis and hyperthermic intraperitoneal chemotherapy. Eur J Surg Oncol 2005;31(5):540–3.
[24] Sugarbaker PH, Chang D. Results of treatment of 385 patients with peritoneal surface spread of appendiceal malignancy. Ann Surg Oncol 1999;6:727–31.
[25] O'Connell JT, Tomlinson JS, Roberts AA, et al. Pseudomyxoma peritonei is a disease of MUC2-expressing goblet cells. Am J Pathol 2002;161:551–64.
[26] Sugarbaker PH. Successful management of microscopic residual disease in large bowel cancer. Cancer Chemother Pharmacol 1999;43(Suppl):S15–25.
[27] Sugarbaker PH, Alderman R, Edwards G, et al. Prospective morbidity and mortality assessment of cytoreductive surgery plus perioperative intraperitoneal chemotherapy to treat peritoneal dissemination of appendiceal mucinous malignancy. Ann Surg Oncol 2006;13:1–11.
[28] McQuellon RP, Loggie BW, Fleming RA, et al. Quality of life after intraperitoneal hyperthermic chemotherapy (IPHC) for peritoneal carcinomatosis. Eur J Surg Oncol 2001;27: 65–73.
[29] McQuellon RP, Loggie BW, Lehman AB, et al. Long-term survivorship and quality of life after cytoreductive surgery plus intraperitoneal hyperthermic chemotherapy for peritoneal carcinomatosis. Ann Surg Oncol 2003;10:155–62.

ELSEVIER
SAUNDERS

Surg Oncol Clin N Am
16 (2007) 667–682

SURGICAL
ONCOLOGY CLINICS
OF NORTH AMERICA

Cytoreductive Surgery for Gynecologic Malignancies—New Standards of Care

Elizabeth Suh-Burgmann, MD[a,*],
C. Bethan Powell, MD[b]

[a]*Gynecologic Oncology, The Permanente Medical Group, 1425 S. Main Street, Walnut Creek, CA 94596, USA*
[b]*Division of Gynecologic Oncology, University of California, San Francisco, 1600 Divisidero, 4th floor, San Francisco, CA 94115, USA*

Cytoreductive surgery has long been recognized as an important component in the treatment of epithelial ovarian cancer. There is perhaps no other disease for which greater evidence of benefit from cytoreduction exists than advanced stage ovarian cancer. More recent evidence has been generated showing benefit of cytoreductive surgery in patients with stage IV endometrial cancer. Currently, the debate on the role of cytoreductive surgery for gynecologic cancers centers around the following questions: (1) what is the most appropriate definition of "optimal" cytoreduction, (2) how can the rates of optimal cytoreduction be maximized, (3) which patients benefit from cytoreduction, (4) who is a candidate for intraperitoneal chemotherapy, (5) what is the role of neoadjuvant chemotherapy, and (6) when is repeated, or "secondary" cytoreduction beneficial? This article will discuss these controversial issues and review the evolving standards for cytoreductive surgery in gynecologic cancer.

Overview of ovarian cancer

Based on recent Surveillance, Epidemiology, and End Results Program (SEER) data [1], epithelial ovarian cancer, which accounts for 70% of ovarian cancer cases, occurs in approximately 1 in 55 women. Approximately 60% of women diagnosed with epithelial ovarian cancer will die of the disease. Because there is no effective screening test and early

* Corresponding author.
E-mail address: betty.suh-burgmann@kp.org (E. Suh-Burgmann).

1055-3207/07/$ - see front matter © 2007 Elsevier Inc. All rights reserved.
doi:10.1016/j.soc.2007.04.017 ***surgonc.theclinics.com***

disease is difficult to identify, the majority of patients (70%) will have advanced stage disease at diagnosis. Prognosis is highly correlated to stage of disease, with 5-year survival in the 90% range for early-stage disease. The median survival times for women diagnosed with advanced disease has significantly lengthened over the past 2 decades. The most recent SEER data from 1993 to 1997 indicates that the 5-year survival for stage III or IV patients has increased from a historic 15% to almost 30% [2]. Recent trial data show median survival times for women with stage III disease of 50 to 66 months [3]. The combination of cytoreductive surgery, effective chemotherapy, and increased chemotherapeutic options for recurrent disease has contributed to the demonstrated improvement in survival.

Ovarian cancer is unique among cancers in that cytoreduction of advanced disease confers a proven survival benefit. The reason for this appears to be twofold. First, ovarian cancer is an unusually chemosensitive cancer with over 70% of patients with advanced disease responding to primary chemotherapy. Moreover, chemotherapy is more effective in smaller volume disease. Second, ovarian cancer metastasizes primarily via direct intra-abdominal dissemination from the ovarian tumor to peritoneal surfaces. Intraparenchymal liver, lung, bone, and brain metastases are relatively rare and usually occur late in the course of the disease. Consequently, for most patients, the sites of metastases are approachable via abdominal surgery and the potential often exists to remove either all visible disease or to reduce the disease to very small volume implants.

Tumor implants on the peritoneum, bowel surfaces, omentum, and diaphragm are hallmarks of the disease. Lymphatic spread is common, although bulky adenopathy is unusual, but hematogenous spread to distant organs is relatively rare. Splenic involvement is found in approximately 6% of cases [4]. The most common manifestation of stage IV disease is malignant pleural effusion.

These disease characteristics apply also to extraovarian papillary serous adenocarcinoma, commonly referred to as primary peritoneal cancer. Most trials of patients with advanced ovarian cancer have included women with primary peritoneal cancer, since the distinction between these two entities can be difficult to make. Primary peritoneal cancer was first recognized as a clinical entity in 1959 and should not be confused with mesothelioma or pseudomyxoma peritoneii, which each have a distinct histopathology and clinical course [5]. The diagnosis usually rests on the observation of tumor involvement of the ovaries that is confined to the surface epithelium with no evidence to suggest a primary tumor in either ovary itself. The histology, biology, chemosensitivity, and natural course of disease of primary peritoneal cancer mirrors that of advanced papillary serous ovarian carcinoma [6–9]. In addition, this disease has been observed after prophylactic oophorectomy in women at increased genetic risk of breast or ovarian cancer [10].

Definition of "optimal" cytoreduction

The importance of cytoreduction in the treatment of advanced ovarian cancer was first recognized by Munnel [11] in 1969. He demonstrated that "maximum surgical effort" was associated with improved survival. In 1975 Griffiths [12] was the first to show that the volume of residual disease after surgery was inversely related to survival, and since then, many other studies have found a similar correlation between the volume of residual disease and length of survival. Historically, the definition of "optimal" has evolved as more data have become available. In 1986, the Gynecologic Oncology Group (GOG) conducted a chemotherapy dose intensity trial in patients with sub-optimal cytoreduction, defined as residual disease greater than 1 cm. Hoskins and colleagues [13], reporting for the GOG, observed a significant improvement in survival for patients with less than 2 cm residual disease compared with those with greater than 2 cm residual tumor volume, but no difference was seen between patients with greater than 2 cm residual disease compared with exploration without any debulking. This has been widely accepted as evidence that a surgical survival benefit can only be realized with "optimal" debulking, defined as residual disease of less than 2 cm. Based on this study, residual disease of less than 2-cm volume became the working definition of optimal cytoreduction. Leaving residual disease greater than 2 cm behind may confer a palliative benefit to patients with relief of bowel obstruction and other symptoms, but cannot be expected to carry a survival benefit.

Multiple additional studies have not only confirmed the correlation between optimal cytoreduction and survival, but have shown that there is a continuous relationship between both, with patients with only microscopic disease having improved survival over those with residual macroscopic disease less than 5 mm, who in turn do better than patients with residual disease less than 1 cm [14–23]. The GOG found that patients with microscopic residual disease only have a 60% 5-year survival compared with 35% for patients with macroscopic small volume disease [13]. Another study found that among patients with stage IIIC ovarian cancer, those without visible residual disease had a median survival of 106 months compared with 66 months for those with residual disease volumes up to 0.5 cm, 48 months for disease residuals of 0.6 to 1.0 cm, and only 34 months for residual disease greater than 2 cm [24]. Several meta-analyses have examined the benefit of optimal cytoreduction on survival [25–27]. The most recent analysis by Bristow and colleagues [27] found that for every 10% increase in cytoreduction, median survival increased 5.5%.

Today, the generally accepted definition of optimal cytoreduction is a residual tumor diameter no greater than 1 cm. This definition is used by GOG in reporting and analyzing outcomes of trials. However, it is important to recognize that the 1-cm cut-off is somewhat arbitrary along a continuum and that, therefore, one should always attempt to achieve complete cytoreduction to a level of no visible disease or microscopic disease.

How can the rate of optimal cytoreduction be maximized?

Epithelial ovarian cancer most commonly spreads by direct extension to other pelvic tissues and by intraperitoneal dissemination to other surfaces in the abdominal cavity. The surgical procedures required to achieve complete cytoreduction depend on the disease distribution. The most common areas of tumor involvement are the paracolic gutters, small bowel serosal and mesentery surfaces, diaphragmatic and pelvic peritoneum, the greater and lesser omentum with extension to the transverse colon, and the sigmoid colon affected by direct extension from the ovary. At a minimum, total abdominal hysterectomy, bilateral salpingo-oophorectomy and gastrocolic omentectomy are performed. In approximately 25% to 35% of cases, additional colon resection is required. In cases of extensive tumor involvement, complete cytoreduction may involve a radical pelvic en bloc resection of all involved peritoneal surfaces, the uterus, ovaries, tubes, cervix, sigmoid colon, and upper rectum. Disease rarely extends below the levator muscle, allowing anastomosis to the rectum in most cases.

Retroperitoneal node dissection is performed in cases of bulky adenopathy. Splenectomy should be included when involvement is present, as associated morbidity is acceptably low [28–31]. In a recent series from the Mayo clinic, splenectomy was required in approximately 6% of cases, with half of these due to intraparenchymal splenic disease and half due to capsular involvement [4]. Diaphragmatic disease is usually confined to the right side and can be managed by mobilization of the liver and stripping of the entire diaphragmatic peritoneum. On occasion, tumor invades the diaphragmatic muscle and a partial full-thickness resection is necessary [32].

One of the more controversial issues regarding cytoreduction is the handling of diffuse small-volume disease or miliary dissemination, typically located on the bowel, mesentery, peritoneal, and diaphragmatic surfaces. The significance of the number of nodules on the overall benefit of aggressive surgery is unclear. Presumably, small nodules are well penetrated by chemotherapy; on the other hand, they reflect a greater burden of disease and their cumulative volume can be significant. Addressing this type of diffuse small-volume disease surgically is challenging. Different ablative techniques such as argon beam coagulation (ABC) and cavitational ultrasonic surgical aspiration (CUSA) are commonly used in this setting. Eisenkop and colleagues [33] found that attempts at complete ablation of diffuse small-volume disease improved survival. In his study, he used argon beam coagulation to vaporize small implants and thin sheets of tumor deposits. Because the electrical energy is conducted through an ionized beam of gas rather than through direct tissue contact, damage to adjacent or underlying structures is minimized. To rapidly fulgurate nodules on surfaces such as the diaphragm, liver, and mesentery, the ABC is set at high power (100 to 150 W and gas flow rates of 10 L/min), whereas lower wattage (40 W for brief periods) is relatively safe on bowel surfaces. The CUSA uses ultrasonic energy to selectively fragment tissue of high water and low collagen content (tumor) while sparing tissues with higher collagen content (connective tissue). Collateral damage is very small, making it an excellent choice for ablation of lesions on the bowel surface [34].

The ability to achieve optimal cytoreduction depends on many factors, including patient fitness, surgeon experience, and aggressiveness. That, combined with the inherently subjective measurement of residual disease, makes reported "rates" of optimal cytoreduction difficult to interpret. Heintz and colleagues [35] reported optimal tumor reduction rates of 87%. In 20% of cases bowel resection was required. In a study by Piver and Baker [36], 75% of patients were optimally cytoreduced, with 36% of them requiring bowel resection. Eisenkop and colleagues [37] reported an 85% complete resection of all visible disease in 163 consecutive patients. Optimal debulking to less than 1 cm was achieved in an additional 14% of patients, with only 1% left with unresectable bulky disease. Clearly, optimal cytoreduction is possible in the vast majority of cases, but the reported rates vary, depending on both surgeon experience and patient selection.

Similarly, a wide variation of complication rates for aggressive cytoreductive surgery has been published. Liu and colleagues [38], in their series of 47 patients, found a major complication rate of 8%. In contrast, Guidozzi and Ball [39] reported a 43% serious postoperative complication rate in 30 patients with advanced ovarian cancer undergoing aggressive cytoreductive surgery. In one of the largest and most detailed clinical studies of cytoreduction by Michel and colleagues [40], comprising 152 patients, rectosigmoid resection was required in 35%, small bowel resection in 19%, splenectomy in 13%, and resection of liver parenchymal metastases in 2 patients. Lower urinary tract resection was necessary in 10% of cases. Pelvic and para-aortic lymph node metastases were found in at least 50% of patients. Ninety-one percent of patients achieved optimal debulking defined as less than 2 cm. The authors noted that the main reasons for suboptimal debulking were the presence of unresectable upper abdominal disease and poor functional status of the patient. The authors report a 33% complication rate. In 38 patients, repeat laparotomy was necessary. In 14 patients repeat laparotomy was necessary because of an anastomotic leak, for an overall anastomotic failure rate of 9%. Other studies reported much lower anastomotic failure rates in patients after colon resection for advanced ovarian cancer, ranging from 1.4% to 3.2% [41–46]. As with any surgery, advanced age, poor functional status, and poor nutritional state increase the risk of complications and, therefore, decisions about the appropriateness of aggressive surgery must be individualized.

Delivery of care for ovarian cancer by a gynecologic oncologist has been associated with superior outcomes including appropriate staging, extent of debulking, achievement of optimal residual disease, delivery of postoperative chemotherapy, and, most importantly, survival. In a review of the SEER data from 1992 to 1999, Earle and colleagues [47] found that the proportion of patients with ovarian cancer undergoing surgery by a gynecologic oncologist was 33%, by a gynecologist 45%, and by a general surgeon 27% of cases. Patients with advanced stage disease were more likely to undergo cytoreductive surgery if the initial surgery was performed by a gynecologic oncologist (58%), compared with gynecologists (50%) or general surgeons (40%). Despite treating patients with more advanced disease, gynecologic oncologists had better outcomes and patient survival than general surgeons or gynecologists. In a study of 263 women undergoing surgery for advanced ovarian cancer, the most significant predictor of survival by multivariate analysis was the presence of a gynecologic oncologist at the operation ($P < .0001$) [48]. A Dutch study also found superior cytoreduction rates, improved survival, and closer adherence to standard surgical guidelines when the initial surgery was performed by a gynecologic oncologist versus a gynecologist [49]. Not surprisingly, treatment results also correlate with case volume. Cytoreductive surgery rates at low-volume centers were found to be at a low 20% compared with 90% at high-volume centers [50]. Therefore, the involvement of specialty trained gynecologic oncologists performing at high-volume centers maximizes the likelihood of a patient to receive optimal cytoreduction and survival benefit.

Cytoreduction for gynecologic cancer: who benefits?

Because most patients diagnosed with ovarian cancer present with stage III disease, studies on surgical cytoreduction are mostly composed of these patients and those with advanced primary peritoneal cancer. The association of aggressive cytoreduction in patients with stage III ovarian or peritoneal cancer with improved survival has been demonstrated in many studies. Best survival was observed in patients after optimal cytoreduction followed by adjuvant cisplatin-based chemotherapy.

One of the criticisms of the data supporting the benefit of cytoreductive surgery is that optimal cytoreduction may not be an independent prognostic marker but rather dependent on inherent tumor biology. Because of ethical concerns, a randomized trial to answer this question is unrealistic and one has to rely on retrospective data. Several studies have found that the volume of residual disease is highly correlated with survival, whereas the volume of initial disease is not [51,52]. The need to perform extensive upper abdominal surgery to achieve optimal cytoreduction was not associated with a worse prognosis in a recent study [53]. Another study showed that patients whose disease was successfully cytoreduced to microscopic disease had the same survival as patients who initially presented with microscopic disease [54]. The presence of clinically detectable ascites or poor histologic grade did not negate the survival benefit of optimal cytoreductive surgery [55]. Although tumor biology may be a confounding factor in the relationship between survival and optimal cytoreduction, the available data overwhelmingly supports the view that optimal cytoreduction is an independent factor for survival in women with ovarian cancer. It should be considered the standard of care to attempt optimal cytoreduction unless the patient is medically unfit for surgery.

In the past, women with stage IV disease—malignant pleural effusion and liver metastases being the most common determinants—were felt to have such poor prognosis that aggressive cytoreduction was considered ineffective and not indicated. Recent studies, however, have challenged this assumption. Curtin and colleagues [56] found a 22-month survival advantage for stage IV patients who were cytoreduced to a residual disease of less than 2 cm compared with those not cytoreduced. Optimal abdominal tumor debulking was particularly beneficial in patients with pleural effusion as their only manifestation of stage IV disease, as shown by Liu and colleagues [38]. In his study of 47 women, of whom 55% had stage IV disease solely on the basis of pleural effusion cytology, optimal cytoreduction conferred a median survival of 37 months compared with only 17 months after nonoptimal cytoreduction. The remaining 45% of patients in this study had parenchymal liver or other extra-abdominal metastases. Munkara and colleagues [57] reported on 108 women with stage IV cancer. The median survival among optimally debulked patients was 25 months compared with 15 months in those not receiving optimal surgery. In this series, approximately half of the patients had stage IV disease based on pleural involvement only. For patients with intraparenchymal liver involvement, options for treatment have expanded over the past 10 years. As with other cancers, liver metastases from ovarian cancer are amenable to a variety of treatment modalities, including radiofrequency ablation and surgical resection [58–60]. Treatment in these particular cases must be highly individualized as the survival benefit is less certain and will depend on the overall disease distribution, chemosensitivity, and the patient's functional status. In carefully selected women with stage IV disease, an attempt at optimal cytoreduction is indicated and, if successful, can improve survival.

Cytoreduction for endometrial cancer

Although most of the data on the benefit of cytoreductive surgery are derived from patients with ovarian and peritoneal cancer, recent studies have shown benefit in advanced stage endometrial cancer [61,62]. In particular, uterine papillary serous adenocarcinoma (UPSC), which comprises 10% to 15% of endometrial cancers, has a clinical course similar to that of ovarian carcinoma with an aggressive biologic behavior and a higher propensity for intra-abdominal spread and recurrence. These similarities have naturally led to an extension of the principles of ovarian cancer treatment to these patients as well. Bristow and colleagues [63] reported on 31 patients with stage IV UPSC who underwent primary cytoreductive surgery and found a significant survival improvement associated with optimal cytoreduction (26.2 versus 9.6 months). Similar to ovarian cancer, there is an inverse correlation between survival and residual disease volume. Patients with only microscopic residual disease achieve significantly longer median survival (30.4 months) compared to those with macroscopic residual disease (20.5 months). Whether these patients benefit from intraperitoneal chemotherapy in addition to systemic chemotherapy, as shown for ovarian cancer, remains unclear.

For patients with advanced endometrioid-type endometrial cancer, the benefit of cytoreductive surgery is more controversial, in part because these cancers are typically less chemosensitive. However, some studies indicate that aggressive cytoreductive surgery significantly improves survival for these patients as well. Lambrou and colleagues [64] reported their experience with cytoreduction in 88 patients with stage III and IV endometrioid-type endometrial cancer. Of these, 72% (33 stage IIIC and 9 stage IV) underwent optimal cytoreduction and had a median survival of 17.8 months, compared to 6.7 months for patients with suboptimal cytoreduction. Chi and colleagues [65] found that patients with stage IV disease who underwent optimal debulking had a median survival of 31 months, compared to 12 months for those who had suboptimal debulking, and 3 months for those who had no debulking. No survival differences were seen for histologic grade of tumor, presence of extra-abdominal disease, or age.

Intraperitoneal chemotherapy—the new standard of care?

The concept of intraperitoneal (IP) chemotherapy has developed into one of the most promising therapeutic options for ovarian cancer since its inception in the 1960s and first application in the clinical realm in the 1980s [66–68]. Building on earlier randomized trials using intraperitoneal chemotherapy, the GOG-172 trial published in early 2006 demonstrated the longest survival times ever reported for patients with stage III ovarian or peritoneal cancer at 65.6 months [3]. In this study, 429 patients with stage III ovarian or peritoneal cancer were randomized after optimal cytoreductive surgery to either standard intravenous chemotherapy with cisplatin and paclitaxel or combined intravenous and intraperitoneal chemotherapy with the same drugs. Optimal cytoreduction was defined as residual disease less than 1 cm. Progression-free survival was significantly prolonged (23.8 versus 18.3 months), overall survival was improved from 49.7 to 65.6 months in the IP arm, and risk of death was significantly reduced by 25% after IP therapy. Previous GOG randomized trials comparing IP to systemic chemotherapy after cytoreduction have shown a sequential improvement in overall survival for each arm (IV versus IP): GOG-104: 41versus 49 months; GOG-114: 52.2 versus 63.2 months; GOG-172: 49.7 versus 65.6 months [66–68]. However, these trials are somewhat difficult to compare because of changes in definition of progression-free survival, rates of negative second-look operations, and, most importantly, differences in regimens for both IV and IP chemotherapy. The outstanding results of IP therapy seen in this latest trial were achieved with an IP regimen that used a more intense and frequent dosing schedule than those previously used and increased toxicity was observed. Of the women randomized to receive the IP regimen, only 42% successfully completed all six IP cycles. The early termination of IP chemotherapy was due to toxicity in two thirds of cases, and to IP catheter-related issues in one third of cases [69]. However, despite that less than one half of the women in the IP group received the assigned therapy, the group as a whole still showed the impressive improvement in median survival, suggesting that the benefit of IP chemotherapy may come early in the course of chemotherapy. The impressive results of GOG-172 led to a National Cancer Institute Clinical Announcement recommending that "consideration should be given to a regimen containing IP cisplatin and taxane" in these patients [70]. Although the announcement of the study resulted in a surge of IP therapy for women with advanced ovarian cancer, there are reasons to proceed cautiously. First, the administration of IP chemotherapy requires special training of both physicians and nurses to minimize complications. Second, patient selection is of great importance because of the increased toxicity of this regimen. In addition to successful optimal cytoreduction to less than 1 cm tumor volume, normal renal function, absence of significant peritoneal adhesions and abdominal infection, and a strong commitment by the patient to this treatment modality are required. Third, while the results of GOG-172 are impressive, the intravenous arm of the trial consisted of cisplatin and 24-hour paclitaxel, rather than carboplatin and 3-hour paclitaxel, which is the current standard of care. As shown by the GOG-158 trial, which compared intravenous carboplatin/paclitaxel to cisplatin/paclitaxel, the carboplatin-containing regimen is associated with superior progression-free (20.7 versus 19.4 months) and overall survival (57.4 versus 48.7 months) [71]. Therefore, a randomized trial comparing an IP regimen to the current standard of care of intravenous carboplatin and paclitaxel regimen must be done before IP chemotherapy can be declared the new standard of care for these patients. In the meantime, the use of IP chemotherapy should be reserved to eligible patients after being fully informed and accepting of the potential risks and benefits.

What is the role of neo-adjuvant chemotherapy?

In the past, surgery was the essential tool to establish the diagnosis of advanced ovarian cancer. With the availability of modern CT scanning and interventional radiology techniques, many patients with advanced ovarian cancer are diagnosed before a planned surgical intervention. This development has opened the door to the concept of neo-adjuvant chemotherapy, raising the question of whether "up front" surgery is always the best first treatment modality. The debate as to whether neo-adjuvant chemotherapy followed by surgery is an equivalent or even superior strategy has continued over the past decade. Clearly, upfront surgical cytoreduction has several advantages: (1) accurate identification of all tumor sites, (2) improvement in the delivery of chemotherapy after cytoreduction, (3) stimulation of residual tumor to enter a growth phase and therefore increase their sensitivity to chemotherapy, (4) relief of potential obstructive symptoms and avoidance of bowel obstruction, (5) lowering the chance of developing chemoresistance due to reduced tumor volume, (6) improvement in patient's sense of well-being, and (7) ability to administer adjuvant intraperitoneal chemotherapy. The potential advantages of neoadjuvant systemic chemotherapy are: (1) reduced impact of surgery due to preoperative "downstaging," (2) improved functional and/or nutritional status as disease regresses, and (3) resolution of ascites, potentially improving postoperative recovery.

The European Organization for Research and Treatment of Cancer (EORTC) conducted a Phase III randomized trial of patients with advanced ovarian or peritoneal cancer who had undergone suboptimal debulking (residual tumor greater than 1 cm). After receiving 3 cycles of cisplatin-based chemotherapy, patients were randomized to either repeat debulking surgery followed by chemotherapy versus chemotherapy alone [72]. There was a significant survival advantage seen in the patients who underwent repeat cytoreductive surgery.

Although patients with suboptimal primary debulking surgery do not show a survival benefit compared with those who have only chemotherapy, it has been difficult to establish criteria to predict which patients will not be successfully debulked at initial surgery. Currently, CA125 levels, volume of ascites, and various radiologic criteria do not reliably identify patients in whom disease cannot be optimally debulked. In one study, it was estimated that one of every three patients deemed to have unresectable disease could actually undergo optimal cytoreduction [73]. The EORTC is currently conducting a randomized trial of upfront surgery versus upfront chemotherapy to further assess the value of neoadjuvant chemotherapy in these patients.

When is repeated or "secondary" cytoreduction beneficial?

Reoperation for ovarian cancer most often falls into one of two categories: (1) early reoperation in women who initially undergo a suboptimal surgery and (2) reoperation for recurrent disease. The question of early reoperation typically occurs when initial surgery is performed by surgeons who are not expecting and are not prepared for the degree of disease present. Patients faced with this situation often elect to start chemotherapy postoperatively rather than undergo a repeat laparotomy. The EORTC found a significant survival benefit for a second attempt at cytoreduction in patients who had undergone initial suboptimal debulking followed by three cycles of chemotherapy [72]. In contrast, Rose and colleagues [74] reporting for the GOG found that patients who had a previous "maximal effort" surgery but significant residual disease did not benefit from "secondary" cytoreduction after three cycles of chemotherapy. In this study, "maximal effort" constituted a laparotomy with removal of as much gross disease as possible. Most patients had residual disease of less than 5 cm. In contrast, in the EORTC study, the extent of surgery was not specified and less than one third of patients had residual disease of less than 5 cm at enrollment. These studies suggest that patients, in whom the intent at initial surgery is not optimal cytoreduction, may benefit from reoperation, whereas those patients in whom optimal cytoreduction was intended but not achieved, do not benefit from a second attempt.

The role of "secondary" cytoreduction in the setting of recurrent disease has been evaluated with an attempt to define selection criteria for patients most likely to benefit from reoperation. Onda and colleagues [75] identified four favorable predictors of survival in a retrospective review of 44 patients who underwent secondary cytoreduction for recurrent disease: (1) disease-free interval (DFI) longer than 12 months, (2) solitary tumor, (3) no liver metastases, and (4) tumor size less than 6 cm. While other studies have mostly confirmed these findings, the significance of a long disease-free interval remains controversial [76–80]. In a series of 117 patients with a disease-free interval before recurrence of at least 3 months, Zang and colleagues [81] found no difference in survival between a DFI of 3 to 12 months compared with 13 to 23 months. Optimal cytoreduction was the only significant predictor of survival. Similarly, Chi and colleagues [82] in their series of 153 patients found DFI, number of recurrent sites, and residual disease to be significant prognostic factors. Patients who had a DFI of 6 to 12 months had a median survival of 30 months compared to 39 months for patients with a DFI of 13 to 30 months. Moreover, patients with an isolated recurrence had a survival of 60 months compared with 42 months for patients with multiple sites and 29 months for patients presenting with diffuse disease. Cytoreduction to less than 0.5 cm residual disease was associated with a 56-month median survival compared to 27 months for larger residual disease. Therefore, for appropriately selected patients, an optimal "secondary" cytoreduction for recurrent tumor can provide significant extension of survival.

Summary

The definition for "optimal" cytoreduction in the treatment of gynecologic cancer is generally accepted to be residual disease less than 1 cm in diameter. However, resection of all macroscopic disease is the goal for cytoreductive surgery and is associated with the best survival, even in cases of initial bulky disease. Upfront cytoreductive surgery now has the additional benefit of adding intraperitoneal chemotherapy, which can further extend survival and has become the current standard of care at many centers.

A surgical effort to achieve optimal cytoreduction should also be offered to selected women with advanced endometrial cancer and recurrent ovarian and endometrial disease, as it has been shown to confer a significant survival benefit. A wide range of surgical procedures can be used to achieve optimal cytoreduction, including radical en bloc resection of all involved pelvic viscera and associated peritoneum, bowel resection, splenectomy, and diaphragmatic, and liver resection. The benefit of such aggressive surgery outweighs the risk of morbidity in the vast majority of patients. Because of the compelling body of evidence demonstrating a survival benefit of aggressive cytoreductive surgery for women with advanced gynecologic cancer, better access to appropriate care is needed. Current data indicate that only 20% to 40% of ovarian cancer patients in the United States have access to gynecologic oncologists, who are the most likely to perform optimal primary cytoreduction [83,84]. Realizing the best possible outcomes will depend on improving awareness of and access to aggressive cytoreductive surgery for all women with advanced gynecologic cancer.

References

[1] National Cancer Institute, Division of Cancer Control and Population Sciences, Surveillance Research Program, Cancer Statistics Branch. Surveillance, Epidemiology, and End Results (SEER) Program, Public-Use Data (1973–2004). Available at: http://www.cancer.gov. Accessed May 24, 2007.

[2] Chan JK, Cheung MK, Husain A, et al. Patterns and progress in ovarian cancer over 14 years. Obstet Gynecol 2006;108:521–8.

[3] Armstrong DK, Bundy B, Wenzel L, et al. Gynecologic Oncology Group. Intraperitoneal cisplatin and paclitaxel in ovarian cancer. N Engl J Med 2006;354:34–43.

[4] Magtibay PM, Adams PB, Silverman MB, et al. Splenectomy as part of cytoreductive surgery in ovarian cancer. Gynecol Oncol 2006;102:369–74.

[5] Bloss JD, Liao SY, Buller RE, et al. Extraovarian peritoneal serous papillary carcinoma: a case-control retrospective comparison to papillary adenocarcinoma of the ovary. Gynecol Oncol 1993;50(3):347–51.

[6] Bloss JD, Brady MF, Liao SY, et al. Gynecologic Oncology Group Study. Extraovarian peritoneal serous papillary carcinoma: a phase II trial ofcisplatin and cyclophosphamide with comparison to a cohort with papillary serous ovarian carcinoma—a Gynecologic Oncology Group Study. Gynecol Oncol 2003;89(1):148–54.

[7] Ayhan A, Taskiran C, Yigit-Celik N, et al. Long-term survival after paclitaxel plus platinum-based combination chemotherapy for extraovarian peritoneal serous papillary carcinoma: is it different from that for ovarian serous papillary cancer? Int J Gynecol Cancer 2006;16(2): 484–9.

[8] Dubernard G, Morice P, Rey A, et al. Prognosis of stage III or IV primary peritoneal serous papillary carcinoma. Eur J Surg Oncol 2004;30(9):976–81.

[9] Killackey MA, Davis AR. Papillary serous carcinoma of the peritoneal surface: matched-case comparison with papillary serous ovarian carcinoma. Gynecol Oncol 1993;51(2):171–4.

[10] Koutselini HA, Lazaris AC, Thomopoulou G, et al. Papillary serous carcinoma of peritoneum: case study and review of the literature on the differential diagnosis of malignant peritoneal tumors. Adv Clin Path 2001;5:99–104.

[11] Munnell EW. The changing prognosis and treatment in cancer of the ovary. Am J Obstet Gynecol 1969;100:790–805.

[12] Griffiths CT. Surgical resection of tumor bulk in the primary treatment of ovarian carcinoma. Natl Cancer Inst Monogr 1975;42:101–4.
[13] Hoskins WJ, McGuire WP, Brady MF, et al. The effect of diameter of largest residual disease on survival after primary cytoreductive surgery in patients with suboptimal residual epithelial ovarian carcinoma. Am J Obstet Gynecol 1994;170:974–9.
[14] Vogl SE, Pagano M, Kaplan BH, et al. Cisplatin based combination chemotherapy for advanced ovarian cancer: high overall response rate with curative potnetial only in women with small tumor burden. Cancer 1983;51:2024–30.
[15] Delgado G, Oram DH, Petrilli ES. Stage III epithelial ovarian cancer: the role of maximal surgical reduction. Gynecol Oncol 1984;18:293–8.
[16] Conte PF, Sertoli MR, Bruzzone M, et al. Cisplatin, methotrexate and 5-fluorouracil combination chemotherapy for advanced ovarian cancer. Gynecol Oncol 1985;5: 290–7.
[17] Posada JG Jr, Marantz AB, Yeung KY, et al. The cyclophosphamide, hexamethylmelamine, 5-fluorouracil (CHF) regimen in the treatment of advanced and recurrent ovarian cancer. Gynecol Oncol 1985;20:23–31.
[18] Neijt JP, ten Bokkel Huinink WW, van der Burg ME, et al. Long-term survival in ovarian cancer: mature data from The Netherlands Joint Study Group for Ovarian Cancer. Eur J Cancer 1991;27:1367–72.
[19] Hainsworth JD, Grosh WW, Burnett LS, et al. Advanced ovarian cancer: long-term results of treatment with intensive cisplatin-based chemotherpay of brief duration. Ann Intern Med 1988;108:165–70.
[20] Piver MS, Lele SB, Marchetti DL, et al. Surgical documented response to intraperitoneal cisplatin, cytarabine, and bleomycin after intravenous cisplatin-based chemotherapy in advanced ovarian adenocarcinoma. J Clin Oncol 1988;6:1679–84.
[21] Sutton GP, Stehman FB, Einhorn LH, et al. Ten-year follow-up of patients receiving cisplatin, doxorubicin, and cyclophosphamide chemotherapy for advanced epithelial ovarian carcinoma. J Clin Oncol 1989;7:223–9.
[22] Bertelsen K. Tumor reduction surgery and long-term survival in advanced ovarian cancer: a DACOVA study. Gynecol Oncol 1990;38:203–9.
[23] Gershenson DM, Wharton JT, Copeland LJ. Treatment of advanced epithelial ovarian cancer with cisplatin and cyclophosphamide. Gynecol Oncol 1989;32:336–51.
[24] Chi DS, Eisenhauer EL, Lang J, et al. What is the optimal goal of primary cytoreductive surgery for bulky stage IIIC epithelial ovarian carcinoma (EOC)? Gynecol Oncol 2006;103(2): 559–64 [Epub 2006 May 22].
[25] Allen DG, Heintz Ap, Touw FW. A meta-analysis of residual disease and survival in stage III and IV carcinoma of the ovary. Eur J Gynaecol Oncol 1995;16:349–56.
[26] Hunter RW, Alexander ND, Soutter WR. Meta-analysis of surgery in advance ovarian carcinoma: Is maximum cytoreductive surgery an independent determinant of prognosis? Am J Obstet Gynecol 1992;166:504–11.
[27] Bristow RE, Tomacruz RS, Armstrong DK, et al. Survival effect of maximal cytoreductive surgery for advanced ovarian carcinoma during the platinum era: a meta-analysis. J Clin Oncol 2002;20:1248–59.
[28] Eisenkop SM, Spirtos NM, Lin WC. Splenectomy in the context of primary cytoreductive operations for advanced epithelial ovarian cancer. Gynecol Oncol 2006;100: 344–8.
[29] Chi DS, Franklin CC, Levine DA, et al. Improved optimal cytoreduction rates for stages IIIC and IV epithelial ovarian, fallopian tube, and primary peritoneal cancer: a change in surgical approach. Gynecol Oncol 2004;94:650–4.
[30] Chen LM, Leuchter RS, Lagasse LD, et al. Splenectomy and surgical cytoreduction for ovarian cancer. Gynecol Oncol 2000;77:362–8.
[31] Scarabelli C, Campagnutta E, Zarelli A, et al. Splenectomy in cytoreductive surgery in ovarian cancer. Minerva Ginecol 1993;45:19–25.

[32] Aletti GD, Dowdy SC, Podratz KC, et al. Surgical treatment of diaphragm disease correlates with improved survival in optimally debulked advanced stage ovarian cancer. Gynecol Oncol 2006;100:283–7.
[33] Eisenkop SM, Nalick Rh, Wang HJ, et al. Peritoneal implant elimination during cytoreductive surgery of ovarian cancer: impact on survival. Gynecol Oncol 1993;51:224–9.
[34] Rose PG. The cavitational ultrasonic surgical aspirator for cytoreduction in advanced ovarian cancer. Am J Obstet Gynecol 1992;166:843–6.
[35] Heintz APM, Hacker NF, Berek JS, et al. Cytoreductive surgery in ovarian carcinoma: feasibility and morbidity. Obstet Gynecol 1986;67:783–8.
[36] Piver MS, Baker T. The potential for optimal (<2 cm) cytoreductive surgery in advanced ovarian carcinoma at a tertiary medical center: a prospective study. Gynecol Oncol 1986; 24:1–8.
[37] Eisenkop SM, Friedman RL, Wang HJ. Complete cytoreductive surgery is feasible and maximizes survival in patients with advanced epithelial ovarian cancer: a prospective study. Gynecol Oncol 1998;69:103–8.
[38] Liu PC, Benjamin I, Morgan MA, et al. Effect of surgical debulking on survival in stage IV ovarian cancer. Gynecol Oncol 1997;64:4–8.
[39] Guidozzi F, Ball JHS. Extensive primary cytoreductive surgery for advanced epithelial ovarian cancer. Gynecol Oncol 1994;53:326–30.
[40] Michel G, De Iaco P, Castaigne D, et al. Extensive cytoreductive surgery in advanced ovarian carcinoma. Eur J Gynaecol Oncol 1997;18:9–15.
[41] Mourton SM, Temple LK, Abu-Rustum NR, et al. Morbidity of rectosigmoid resection and primary anastomosis in patients undergoing primary cytoreductive surgery for advanced epithelial ovarian cancer. Gynecol Oncol 2005;99:608–14.
[42] Obermair A, Hagenauer S, Tamandl D, et al. Safety and efficacy of low anterior en bloc resection as part of cytoreductive surgery for patients with ovarian cancer. Gynecol Oncol 2001;83:115–20.
[43] Bristow RE, del Carmen MG, Kaufman HS, et al. Radical oophorectomy with primary stapled colorectal anastomosis for resection of locally advanced anastomosis for resection of locally advanced epithelial ovarian cancer. J Am Coll Surg 2003;197:565–74.
[44] Eisenkop SM, Nalick RH, Teng NN. Modified posterior exenteration for ovarian cancer. Obstet Gynecol 1991;78:879–85.
[45] Park JY, Seo SS, Kang S, et al. The benefits of low anterior en bloc resection as part of cytoreductive surgery for advanced primary and recurrent epithelial ovarian cancer patients outweigh morbidity concerns. Gynecol Oncol 2006;103:977–84.
[46] Tebes SJ, Cardosi R, Hoffman MS. Colorectal resection in patients with ovarian and primary peritoneal carcinoma. Am J Obstet Gynecol 2006;195:585–9.
[47] Earle CC, Schrag D, Neville BA, et al. Effect of surgeon specialty on processes of care and outcomes for ovarian cancer patients. J Natl Cancer Instit 2006;98:172–80.
[48] Eisenkop SM, Spirtos NM, Montag TW, et al. The impact of subspecialty training on the management of advanced ovarian cancer. Gynecol Oncol 1992;47:203–9.
[49] Engelen MJ, Kos HE, Pax HB, et al. Surgery by consultant gynecologic oncologists improves survival in patients with ovarian carcinoma. Cancer 2006;106:589–98.
[50] Aletti GD, Dowdy SC, Gostout BS, et al. Aggressive surgical effort and improved survival in advanced stage ovarian cancer. Obstet Gynecol 2006;107:77–85.
[51] Berek JS, Hacker NF, LaGasse LD, et al. Second-look laparotomy in stage III epithelial ovarian cancer: clinical variables associated with disease status. Obstet Gynecol 1984;64: 207–12.
[52] Redman JF, Petroni GR, Saigo PE, et al. Prognostic factors in advanced ovarian carcinoma. J Clin Oncol 1986;4:515–23.
[53] Eisenhauer EL, Abu-Rustum NR, Sonoda Y, et al. The addition of extensive upper abdominal surgery to achieve optimal cytoreduction improves survival in patients with stages IIIC–IV epithelial ovarian cancer. Gynecol Oncol 2006;103:1083–90.

[54] Le T, Krepart GV, Lotocki RJ, et al. Does debulking surgery improve survival in biologically aggressive ovarian carcinoma? Gynecol Oncol 1997;67:208–14.
[55] Hacker NF, Berek JS, Lagasse LD, et al. Primary cytoreductive surgery for epithelial ovarian cancer. Obstet Gynecol 1983;61:413–20.
[56] Curtin JP, Malik R, Venkatraman ES, et al. Stage IV ovarian cancer: impact of surgical debulking. Gynecol Oncol 1997;64:9–12.
[57] Munkarah AR, Hallum AV 3rd, Morris M, et al. Prognostic significance of residual disease in patients with stage IV epithelial ovarian cancer. Gynecol Oncol 1997;64:13–7.
[58] Gervais DA, Arellano RS, Mueller PR. Percutaneous radiofrequency ablation of ovarian cancer metastasis to the liver: indications, outcomes, and role in patient management. AJR Am J Roentgenol 2006;180:746–50.
[59] Mateo R, Singh G, Jabbour N, et al. Optimal cytoreduction after combined resection and radiofrequency ablation of hepatic metastases from recurrent malignant ovarian tumors. Gynecol Oncol 2005;97:266–70.
[60] Yoon SS, Jarnagin WR, Fong Y, et al. Resection of recurrent ovarian or fallopian tube carcinoma involving the liver. Gynecol Oncol 2003;91:383–8.
[61] Memarzadeh S, Holschneider CH, Bristow RE, et al. FIGO stage III and IV uterine papillary serous carcinoma: impact of residual disease on survival. Int J Gynecol Cancer 2002;12: 454–8.
[62] Geisler JP, Geisler HE, Melton ME, et al. What staging surgery should be performed on patients with uterine papillary serous carcinoma? Gynecol Oncol 1999;74:465–7.
[63] Bristow RE, Duska LR, Montz FJ. The role of cytoreductive surgery in the management of stage IV uterine papillary serous carcinoma. Gynecol Oncol 2001;81:92–9.
[64] Lambrou NC, Gomez-Marin O, Mirhashemi R, et al. Optimal surgical cytoreduction in patients with Stage III and Stage IV endometrial carcinoma: a study of morbidity and survival. Gynecol Oncol 2004;93:653–8.
[65] Chi DS, Welshinger M, Venkatraman ES, et al. The role of surgical cytoreduction in Stage IV endometrial carcinoma. Gynecol Oncol 1997;67:56–60.
[66] Alberts DS, Liu PY, Hannigan EV, et al. Intraperitoneal cisplatin plus intravenous cyclophosphamide versus intravenous cisplatin plus intravenous cyclophosphamide for stage III ovarian cancer. N Engl J Med 1996;335:1950–5.
[67] Markman M, Bundy BN, Alberts DS, et al. Phase III trial of standard-dose intravenous cisplatin plus paclitaxel versus moderately high-dose carboplatin followed by intravenous paclitaxel and intraperitoneal cisplatin in small-volume stage III ovarian carcinoma: an intergroup study of the Gynecologic Oncology Group, Southwestern Oncology Group, and Eastern Cooperative Oncology Group. J Clin Oncol 2001;19: 1001–7.
[68] Shapiro F, Schneider J, Markman M, et al. High-intensity intravenous cyclophosphamide and cisplatin, interim surgical cytoreductive, and intraperitoneal cisplatin in advanced ovarian carcinoma: a pilot trial with ten-year follow-up. Gynecol Oncol 1997;67:39–45.
[69] Walker JL, Armstrong DK, Huang HQ, et al. Intraperitoneal catheter outcomes in a phase III trial of intravenous versus intraperitoneal chemotherapy in optimal stage III ovarian and primary peritoneal cancer: a Gynecologic Oncology Group Study. Gynecol Oncol 2006;100: 27–32.
[70] Trimble E. NCI clinical announcement on intraperitoneal chemotherapy in ovarian cancer. Available at: http://ctep.cancer.gove/highlights/ovarian.html. Accessed January 6, 2006.
[71] Ozols RF, Bundy BN, Greer BE, et al. Phase III trial of carboplatin and paclitaxel compared with cisplatin and paclitaxel in patients with optimally resected stage III ovarian cancer: a Gynecologic Oncology Group study. J Clin Oncol 2003;21:3194–200.
[72] van der Burg ME, van Lent M, Buyse M, et al. The effect of debulking surgery after induction chemotherapy on the prognosis in advanced epithelial ovarian cancer. N Engl J Med 1995; 332:629–34.

[73] Bristow RE, Eisenhauer EL, Santillan A, et al. Delaying the primary surgical effort for advanced ovarian cancer. A systematic review of neoadjuvant chemotherapy and interval cytoreduction. Gynecol Oncol 2007;104:480–90.
[74] Rose PG, Nerenstone S, Brady MF, et al. Secondary surgical cytoreduction for advanced ovarian carcinoma. N Engl J Med 2004;351:2489–97.
[75] Onda T, Yoshikawa H, Yasugi T, et al. Secondary cytoreductive surgery for recurrent epithelial ovarian carcinoma: proposal for patients selection. Br J Cancer 2005;92:1026–32.
[76] Berek JS, Hacker NF, LaGasse LD, et al. Survival of patients following secondary cytoreductive surgery in ovarian cancer. Obstet Gynecol 1983;61:189–93.
[77] Morris M, Gershenson DM, Wharton JT, et al. Secondary cytoreductive surgery for recurrent epithelial ovarian cancer. Gynecol Oncol 1989;34:334–8.
[78] Janicke F, Holscher M, Kuhn W, et al. Radical surgical procedure improves survival time in patients with recurrent ovarian cancer. Cancer 1992;70:2129–36.
[79] Gadducci A, Iacconi P, Cosio S, et al. Complete salvage surgical cytoreduction improves further survival of patients with late recurrent ovarian cancer. Gynecol Oncol 2000;79:344–9.
[80] Eisenkop SM, Friedman RL, Wang HJ. Secondary cytoreduction for recurrent ovarian cancer. A prospective study. Cancer 1995;76:1606–14.
[81] Zang RY, Zhang ZY, Li ZT, et al. Effect of cytoreductive surgery on survival of patients with recurrent epithelial ovarian cancer. J Surg Oncol 2000;75:24–30.
[82] Chi DS, McCaughty K, Diaz JP, et al. Guidelines and selection criteria for secondary cytoreductive surgery in patients with recurrent, platinum-sensitive epithelial ovarian carcinoma. Cancer 2006;106:1933–9.
[83] Nguyen HN, Averette HE, Hoskins W, et al. National Survey of Ovarian Carcinoma: V. The impact of physician's specialty on patients' survival. Cancer 1993;72:3663–70.
[84] Elit L, Bondy SJ, Paszat, et al. Oucomes in surgery for ovarian cancer. Gynecol Oncol 2002; 887:260–7.

ELSEVIER
SAUNDERS

Surg Oncol Clin N Am
16 (2007) 683–693

SURGICAL
ONCOLOGY CLINICS
OF NORTH AMERICA

Cytoreductive Surgery for Melanoma

James M. McLoughlin, MD[a],
Jonathan S. Zager, MD[b],
Vernon K. Sondak, MD[b,c,*]

[a]*Division of Surgical Oncology, Department of Surgey, Medical College of Georgia, Augusta, GA 30912, USA*
[b]*Division of Cutaneous Oncology, Department of Interdisciplinary Oncology, University of South Florida College of Medicine, Tampa, FL 33612, USA*
[c]*Department of Surgery, University of South Florida College of Medicine, Tampa, FL 33612, USA*

Cytoreductive surgery, sometimes called "debulking," represents a therapeutic attempt to improve patient outcomes by the removal of either as much tumor as possible or all tumor masses greater than a certain minimum size, even when complete tumor removal is impossible. Explicit in this approach is the recognition that there must be a therapeutic goal that cannot be met by treating the patient nonsurgically or with neoadjuvant (preoperative) therapy. For instance, a larger tumor burden might exert an immunosuppressive effect that precludes response to immunotherapy presumed to be effective against a smaller amount of the same tumor. Alternatively, certain symptoms of advanced tumor, such as active bleeding or intestinal obstruction, may be worsened by available therapies (eg, bleeding exacerbated by chemotherapy-induced thrombocytopenia) and/or so difficult to control with nonoperative means as to preclude effective treatment without surgical correction of the problem. In any case, cytoreductive surgery should always be differentiated from complete resection of oligometastatic tumor. The latter is done with curative intent and often involves no other modalities of (adjuvant) therapy. Cytoreductive surgery should also be differentiated from "prophylactic" surgical attempts to prevent symptoms from developing in asymptomatic patients. By definition, it is impossible to palliate an asymptomatic patient and, unless the risk or the consequences of the potential symptoms are dramatic, it is difficult to justify the

* Corresponding author. H. Lee Moffitt Cancer Center & Research Institute, 12902 Magnolia Drive, Tampa, FL 33612.
E-mail address: vernon.sondak@moffitt.org (V.K. Sondak).

1055-3207/07/$ - see front matter © 2007 Elsevier Inc. All rights reserved.
doi:10.1016/j.soc.2007.04.007 **surgonc.theclinics.com**

morbidity, expense, and time away from home and family that such surgical prophylaxis entails.

Complete resection for metastatic melanoma

Metastatic melanoma is a highly lethal malignancy with few good treatment options. Sometimes heroic surgical undertakings are justified solely on the basis of a presumed dismal outcome in the absence of surgery. But the lack of good alternatives does not justify the use of other bad alternatives, so any surgical intervention in metastatic melanoma should be carefully considered and its therapeutic intent clearly understood. In fact, carefully selected patients with isolated, resectable metastatic disease may derive long-term benefit from complete resection of all identifiable tumor sites, even in the absence of any additional nonsurgical therapy. In these selected patients, the percentage of individuals achieving a long-term disease-free state appears to be better after surgery than after any other available treatment option for metastatic melanoma. This subject has been extensively reviewed in several recent publications [1–5], and general principles governing resection of metastatic melanoma have emerged:

- Advances in imaging provide the opportunity to exclude patients who are unlikely to be rendered disease-free by surgery. Most patients being considered for complete resection of metastatic melanoma should have a preoperative evaluation including a whole-body positron emission tomographic scan or CT scan and an MRI of the brain, as well as appropriate studies aimed at delineating the local extent of lesions to be resected [6,7].
- A long disease-free interval from primary diagnosis to the diagnosis of metastases, fewer metastatic lesions, and limited numbers of organ systems involved by disease all identify patients that are more likely to have prolonged survival after surgical intervention. Patients with isolated resectable metastatic melanoma in the absence of a known primary site are also appropriate candidates for an aggressive surgical approach. Patients with hepatic metastases rarely if ever achieve long-term disease-free status after liver resection and are considered poor candidates for a resection approach [3,8].
- Complete resection of all identifiable disease should always be considered the goal in asymptomatic patients with metastatic melanoma, as it is only after complete resection that patients have a significant chance for prolonged disease-free survival (Fig. 1). Surgery for palliation is rarely effective in melanoma, but some exceptions are recognized as described in detail below. Surgery has a palliative role in patients with bleeding or obstructing intestinal metastases, provided there are only a few lesions within the gastrointestinal tract [1,9]. Patients with symptomatic brain metastases, particularly when the symptoms are due to

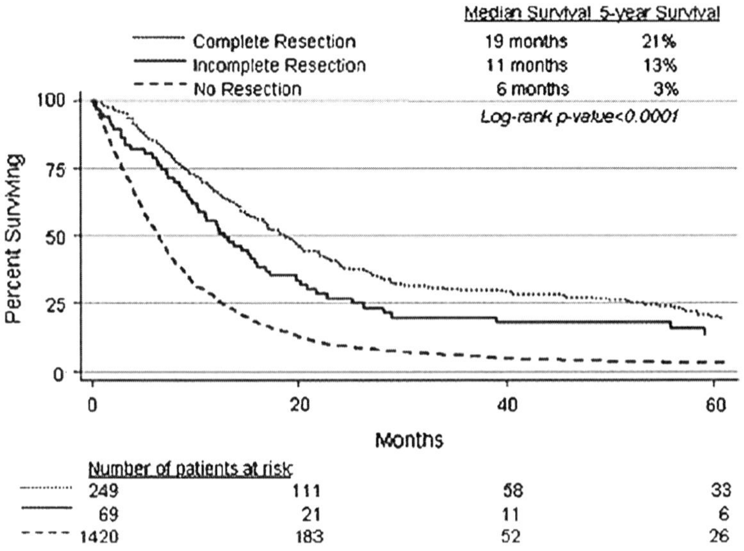

Fig. 1. Overall survival by complete resection, incomplete resection, and nonsurgical treatment (n = 1720). (*From* Petersen RP, Hanish SI, Haney JC, et al. Improved survival with pulmonary metastasectomy: an analysis of 1720 patients with pulmonary metastatic melanoma. J Thorac Cardiovasc Surg 2007;133(1):107; with permission. Copyright © 2007, The American Association for Thoracic Surgery.)

intracranial bleeding, also can be successfully palliated with surgery [10,11]. Despite these exceptions, in most symptomatic patients with metastatic melanoma, surgery has little to offer and should be used judiciously.

- No adjuvant therapy has been proven useful after resection of metastatic melanoma beyond the regional nodes. While nonrandomized studies using historical controls have often suggested a possible benefit [12–14], to date no prospective randomized trial data exist to document such benefit. Indeed, the intervention with the strongest nonrandomized data to support its use after resection of stage IV melanoma, the Canvaxin allogeneic melanoma vaccine, showed no benefit compared with placebo in a recent randomized trial [15]. High-dose interferon alfa is the only adjuvant therapy approved by the US Food and Drug Administration (FDA) for "high risk" melanoma patients, but has never been prospectively tested in patients after resection of stage IV melanoma. Moreover, many patients who develop resectable stage IV melanoma have already received adjuvant interferon for stage IIB/C or stage III melanoma. Nonetheless, resected stage IV melanoma patients who have never had adjuvant interferon previously should be considered for high-dose interferon therapy, and all eligible patients should be offered the opportunity to participate in prospective clinical trials.

Palliation of symptomatic melanoma by cytoreductive surgery

Even patients with symptomatic melanoma metastases are best served by complete resection of all evident disease. Only a few undisputed indications exist for surgical palliation of metastatic melanoma when complete resection is judged impossible. Surgical palliation is a realistic goal for appropriately selected patients with symptomatic brain and gastrointestinal metastases, particularly when bleeding or intestinal obstruction is present. Pulmonary metastases are rarely symptomatic, and when they cause dyspnea at rest, any palliative surgical effort comes too late. Symptomatic pleural effusions and ascites from melanoma metastases are also associated with a grave prognosis and are almost always best managed nonsurgically. When hemoptysis is caused by an endoluminal pulmonary metastasis, surgical palliation can be effectively achieved when other measures, such as endoscopic treatment, have failed.

Wornom and colleagues [14] reported on 65 patients treated surgically for melanoma metastases and evaluated the nature of preoperative symptoms, if any, and the degree to which they were relieved by surgery. Of 17 patients undergoing resection of lung metastases, 2 were symptomatic (persistent cough), and both had resolution of their cough after surgery. Symptoms of intraabdominal metastases were relieved by surgery in 100% of the patients. The abdominal surgeries were most commonly performed for small bowel obstruction or anemia. All patients developed progression of disease in other organs during follow-up. For 17 patients with symptomatic brain metastases, 14 had complete relief of symptoms and 2 had partial relief, but 2 patients died from surgical complications. Among the survivors, more than two-thirds developed recurrent disease in the brain, and more than half developed non–central-nervous-system metastases. Patients with soft tissue disease presented with symptoms of pain, itching, burning, or bleeding. Most palliative soft tissue resections resulted in relief of symptoms (44 out of 50, 88%), but 92% of patients subsequently developed disease in other organs.

Ollila and colleagues [1] reported on 124 patients with metastases to the gastrointestinal tract, of whom 69 were operated on with either curative or palliative intent. Of the 69 surgical patients, 23 patients were treated for palliation. Symptoms requiring operation included crampy abdominal pain, anemia and/or acute gastrointestinal bleeding, and high-grade obstruction. Overall, 67 of the 69 patients had their presenting symptoms relieved by operative intervention, indicating the palliative value of surgical resection in selected patients. Median survival was the same for patients treated nonoperatively compared with patients treated by palliative resection (5.7 months versus 5.4 months respectively), but it was noticeably better for those treated by complete resection (48.9 months). No patients survived beyond 25 months in the palliative or nonoperative group, whereas the 5-year survival in the complete resection group was 41%.

Haigh and colleagues [2] evaluated 27 patients operated for melanoma metastases to the adrenal gland. Of these, 9 underwent successful surgery solely for palliation of symptoms, such as adrenal hemorrhage and intractable pain. Again, no survival advantage was seen compared with nonoperative treatment. The median survival was 9.2 months with 8 of the 9 patients developing additional metastases during follow-up.

Patients with cerebral metastases often present with headaches, motor and sensory deficits, visual deficits, seizures, or decreased mentation. Stereotactic radiotherapy can offer palliation in up to 50% of patients as well as reduce the dependence on corticosteroids. Palliative surgery can also offer symptomatic relief and diminish the need for steroids. It may be the preferred approach for patients with a single metastasis in a "silent" area of the brain and when symptoms are due to intracranial hemorrhage [16–18].

Unresectable regional metastases can also cause significant symptoms, particularly from bleeding and ulceration. Isolated limb perfusion is a useful tool for loco-regional control in patients symptomatic from extremity disease. Reported response rates are as high as 90% [19]. The duration of responses, however, may be shorter than previously appreciated [20]. Takkenberg and colleagues [21] followed 8 patients treated with isolated limb perfusion for palliation of symptomatic limb disease. One patient had no response, 1 had a complete response, and 6 had partial tumor response. Six of the 8 patients experienced successful palliation of symptoms. A study performed by Fraker and colleagues [22] followed 15 patients treated with isolated limb perfusion for palliation of symptoms. Nine of 11 patients with painful lesions had symptom resolution, whereas 6 of 6 patients with edema had symptom resolution. Bleeding was eliminated in 5 of 6 patients. Careful patient selection is required because the morbidity of the intervention is significant. Palliative surgery offers an alternative therapeutic approach for isolated or limited symptomatic cutaneous lesions, with relatively low morbidity and the promise of rapid resolution of symptoms. Although the duration of symptomatic relief is generally short, repeated resections are often practical.

The available data support the judicious use of palliative surgery for carefully selected patients with symptomatic melanoma metastases, but the actual magnitude of benefit patients derive is difficult to ascertain. Objective reports of outcome results for palliative surgery are notoriously difficult to find in the literature, especially for melanoma patients. The Palliative Surgery Outcome Score was devised to assess the impact and success rate of treatment in this setting [23]. The determination of success is based on the ratio of the number of symptom-free, nonhospitalized days compared with the number of days in the hospital. If 70% of the days are symptom-free, the palliative intervention is considered successful. Other useful measures include the Functional Assessment of Cancer Therapy and the European Organization for Research and Treatment of Cancer questionnaires. Future studies of palliative surgery in melanoma patients should make use of these objective tools, which facilitate comparisons with other studies and with nonsurgical modalities. Patient selection criteria should be defined as clearly as possible. Given the major limitations and inconsistent success rates of palliative surgery in melanoma, the decision to surgically intervene requires clear and realistic communication with the patient on therapy goals and potential outcomes.

Cytoreductive surgery in melanoma

Notwithstanding the value of surgery in the management of carefully selected patients with isolated or symptomatic metastatic lesions, most patients with metastatic melanoma have widespread or unresectable metastases and hence are not candidates for definitive surgery. These patients would be potential candidates for cytoreductive surgery if it could be shown that (1) effective therapy for metastatic melanoma were available to patients with limited residual tumor burden but not to patients with intact widespread metastases and (2) surgical intervention could reliably reduce the tumor burden to a treatable level with acceptable morbidity and low mortality. To date, no clinical evidence exists in humans with melanoma that would support either of these required principles. Some have suggested that data from immunotherapy trials showing better outcomes for patients with less advanced tumors imply a role for cytoreduction [24]. Others cite preclinical evidence from animal models to support the theoretical principle of cytoreductive surgery facilitating immunotherapy—under the premise that a large tumor burden correlates to a significant degree with systemic immunosuppression.

Rationale for cytoreductive surgery before immunotherapy

Tumors, including melanoma, produce inhibitory cytokines and other substances that suppress the host immune system [25–28]. Cancer cells are known to shed tumor antigens into the bloodstream, which in turn may interact with antibodies to form complexes that can directly inhibit antitumor antibodies and/or cytotoxic lymphocytes. Tumor cells also produce cytokines that can down-regulate the activity of cytotoxic T cells [29–31]. Therefore, a surgical reduction of the tumor burden should theoretically allow the host's immune system to recover from the inhibitory effects produced by tumor cells and improve the ability of the innate immune system to control residual macroscopic and microscopic disease [32,33].

Emms [33] have shown that, compared with debulking alone, the combination of melphalan chemotherapy with debulking of anal sac tumors and clinically positive nodal disease in dogs leads to improved survival. These results were compared with historical reported controls of surgical treatment alone. Janssen and colleagues [34] have shown similar results in a cytoreduction model of ovarian cancer in mice treated with radio-immunotherapy using ^{90}yttrium, ^{186}rhenium, or ^{131}iodine labeled murine monoclonal antibody directed against the MUC1 glycoprotein found on more than 90% of ovarian carcinomas.

Another reason for cytoreduction before immunotherapy comes from the recognition that antigenic heterogeneity increases with increasing tumor burden [35,36]. With increasing tumor burden, the likelihood increases that some tumor cells will not express the tumor rejection antigens necessary for immune-mediated destruction. Many questions remain about this rationale for cytoreduction. No data exist to indicate how much tumor must be removed to cross a threshold below which antigenic heterogeneity is likely to be significant. In fact, evidence suggests that clinically relevant antigenic heterogeneity and immunosuppressive mechanisms are present even in the earliest detectable melanoma micrometastases within sentinel nodes [37–39]. These findings make it unlikely for cytoreductive surgery—which intentionally leaves macroscopic residual metastatic melanoma in place—to improve the prospects of immunotherapy based on either elimination of suppressive factors or reduction in antigenic heterogeneity.

Adjuvant immunotherapy—failure to date of the "ultimate" in cytoreduction

To date, no clinical trial in melanoma patients has prospectively evaluated the impact of cytoreductive surgery on any immunologic or clinical parameter. The published immunotherapy trials require gross total tumor resection before adjuvant immunotherapy. Patients who cannot be completely resected are excluded from participation in adjuvant immunotherapy clinical trials. These clinical trials are nonetheless instructive, as they provide data on adjuvant immunotherapy after "ultimate" cytoreduction. We know that even after complete removal of all grossly evident metastatic melanoma, disease recurrence rates are very high. If cytoreduction is a valid theoretical concept, we should see evidence that immunologic therapies improve outcome in this "minimal residual disease" setting. In the absence of positive data after complete resection, it is difficult to expect a positive impact on outcome after cytoreduction, which by definition would leave macroscopic disease behind.

Unfortunately, the large phase-III adjuvant vaccine trials that have been reported in melanoma patients have uniformly produced disappointing results. Perhaps most disappointing of all were the results of the Canvaxin allogeneic melanoma vaccine. In two randomized controlled trials, this polyvalent whole-cell melanoma vaccine plus bacillus Calmette-Guèrin (BCG) was compared with placebo vaccine plus BCG after complete surgical resection of either stage III or stage IV melanoma. The trials showed that patients on the placebo arm fared as well as those receiving the vaccine [40]. Since the vaccine could not control the microscopic residual disease that was present in the majority of these patients, the same approach is expected to be equally ineffective if gross residual disease had been left behind. While it is possible that autologous melanoma vaccines might fare better than the allogeneic vaccines that have been most extensively tested to date, no evidence yet supports that conjecture. Given our current state of knowledge, no patient with unresectable metastatic melanoma should be subjected to surgery with the sole intent of procuring tumor for allogeneic vaccination outside of the setting of carefully conducted clinical trials.

Adjuvant therapy with high-dose interferon alfa has been shown to improve outcomes for stage III melanoma patients rendered surgically free of disease [41–43]. This therapy has never been prospectively tested in patients with resected stage IV melanoma, in part because many such patients in the United States have already received high-dose interferon before the development of stage IV disease. Still, completely resected stage IV melanoma patients who have never received high-dose interferon should at least be informed about and offered this therapy, which remains the only FDA-approved adjuvant therapy available for melanoma. Evidence does not support recommending cytoreductive surgery short of complete resection before administration of interferon or any other cytokine, nor does evidence support recommending high-dose interferon in patients with known unresected or gross residual melanoma.

One small but interesting study has evaluated neoadjuvant interferon alfa given intravenously for 1 month to patients with grossly evident nodal metastases before definitive lymphadenectomy. Even after this relatively brief exposure, a surprising 11 of 20 patients (55%) responded with shrinkage or disappearance of their nodal tumor [44]. Other phase II studies have promising survival rates with neoadjuvant immunotherapy of various types [45,46]. Hence, neoadjuvant interferon therapy certainly merits further investigation. Other neoadjuvant approaches may warrant consideration for patients who have already received or who are not candidates for high-dose interferon.

Summary

Patients with limited, resectable metastatic melanoma should be considered candidates for surgery not for cytoreduction, but rather in an attempt to control their disease and occasionally cure it. Patients who have been resected to a disease-free state should be considered for adjuvant therapy with high-dose interferon or participation in a prospective clinical trial. Palliative operations may also have value in carefully selected patients with symptomatic metastatic melanoma, but relatively few patients are appropriate candidates for palliative surgery. To date, no adjuvant immunologic or chemotherapeutic intervention has been shown to improve relapse-free or overall survival for patients with stage IV melanoma after complete resection. Because of this, cytoreductive surgery or "debulking," which is the planned resection of only a portion of the grossly evident disease in hopes of improving the outcome of subsequent therapies, cannot be recommended for melanoma patients in any current clinical context. Interest in this approach remains strong because, if cytoreduction combined with vaccination or other adjuvant immunotherapies is going to work in any human malignancy, melanoma remains one of the best potential candidates. Better immunologic therapies and a better understanding of the consequences of tumor burden on host immune response are clearly needed if cytoreductive surgery is going to achieve clinical success.

References

[1] Ollila DW, Essner R, Wanek LA, et al. Surgical resection for melanoma metastatic to the gastrointestinal tract. Arch Surg 1996;131(9):975–80.

[2] Haigh PI, Essner R, Wardlaw JC, et al. Long-term survival after complete resection of melanoma metastatic to the adrenal gland. Ann Surg Oncol 1999;6(7):633–9.

[3] McLoughlin JM, Zager JS, Sloan AS, et al. Melanoma: surgical approach to metastatic disease. In: Silberman H, Silberman AW, editors. Principles and practice of surgical oncology: a multidisciplinary approach to difficult problems. 2nd edition. Baltimore (MD): Lippincott Williams & Williams; 2007.

[4] Essner R, Lee JH, Wanek LA, et al. Contemporary surgical treatment of advanced-stage melanoma. Arch Surg 2004;139(9):961–6 [discussion: 966–7].

[5] Sondak VK, Liu PY, Warnecke J, et al. Surgical resection for stage IV melanoma: a Southwest Oncology Group Trial (S9430). Proc Amer Soc Clin Oncol 2006;24:457S.

[6] Fogarty GB, Tartaguia C. The utility of magnetic resonance imaging in the detection of brain metastases in the staging of cutaneous melanoma. Clin Oncol (R Coll Radiol) 2006;18(4): 360–2.

[7] Brady MS, Akhurst T, Spanknebel K, et al. Utility of preoperative ^{18}F-fluorodeoxyglucose-positron emission tomography scanning in high-risk melanoma patients. Ann Surg Oncol 2006;13(4):525–32.

[8] Pawlik TM, Zorzi D, Abdalla EK, et al. Hepatic resection for metastatic melanoma: distinct patterns of recurrence and prognosis for ocular versus cutaneous disease. Ann Surg Oncol 2006;13(5):712–20.

[9] Agrawal S, Yao TJ, Coit DG. Surgery for melanoma metastatic to the gastrointestinal tract. Ann Surg Oncol 1999;6(4):336–44.

[10] Mandybur TI. Intracranial hemorrhage caused by metastatic tumors. Neurology 1977;27(7): 650–5.

[11] Tran P, Fogarty G, Phillips C, et al. Worthwhile palliation with surgery for symptomatic haemorrhage from brain metastasis. ANZ J Surg 2005;75(5):366.

[12] Spitler LE, Grossbard ML, Ernstoff MS, et al. Adjuvant therapy of stage III and IV malignant melanoma using granulocyte-macrophage colony-stimulating factor. J Clin Oncol 2000;18(8):1614–21.

[13] Hsueh EC, Essner R, Foshag LJ, et al. Prolonged survival after complete resection of disseminated melanoma and active immunotherapy with a therapeutic cancer vaccine. J Clin Oncol 2002;20(23):4549–54.

[14] Wornom IL 3rd, Smith JW, Soong SJ, et al. Surgery as palliative treatment for distant metastases of melanoma. Ann Surg 1986;204(2):181–5.

[15] Morton DL, Mozzillo N, Thompson JF, et al. An international randomized, double-blind, phase 3 study of the specific active immunotherapy agent, onamelatucel-L (Canvaxin™),

compared to placebo as a post-surgical adjuvant in AJCC stage IV melanoma. Ann Surg Oncol 2006;13(Suppl 2):5.
[16] Bezjak A, Adam J, Barton R, et al. Symptom response after palliative radiotherapy for patients with brain metastases. Eur J Cancer 2002;38(4):487–96.
[17] Bezjak A, Adam J, Panzarella T, et al. Radiotherapy for brain metastases: defining palliative response. Radiother Oncol 2001;61(1):71–6.
[18] Fife KM, Colman MH, Stevens GN, et al. Determinants of outcome in melanoma patients with cerebral metastases. J Clin Oncol 2004;22(7):1293–300.
[19] Fraker DL. Management of in-transit melanoma of the extremity with isolated limb perfusion. Curr Treat Options Oncol 2004;5(3):173–84.
[20] Noorda EM, Vrouenraets BC, Nieweg OE, et al. Safety and efficacy of isolated limb perfusion in elderly melanoma patients. Ann Surg Oncol 2002;9(10):968–74.
[21] Takkenberg RB, Vrouenraets BC, van Geel AN, et al. Palliative isolated limb perfusion for advanced limb disease in stage IV melanoma patients. J Surg Oncol 2005;91(2):107–11.
[22] Fraker DL, Alexander HR, Andrich M, et al. Palliation of regional symptoms of advanced extremity melanoma by isolated limb perfusion with melphalan and high-dose tumor necrosis factor. Cancer J Sci Am 1995;1(2):122–30.
[23] McCahill LE, Smith DD, Borneman T, et al. A prospective evaluation of palliative outcomes for surgery of advanced malignancies. Ann Surg Oncol 2003;10(6):654–63.
[24] Petersen RP, Hanish SI, Haney JC, et al. Improved survival with pulmonary metastasectomy: an analysis of 1720 patients with pulmonary metastatic melanoma. J Thorac Cardiovasc Surg 2007;133(1):104–10.
[25] Mukherji B, Nashed AL, Guha A, et al. Regulation of cellular immune response against autologous human melanoma. II. Mechanism of induction and specificity of suppression. J Immunol 1986;136(5):1893–8.
[26] Mukherji B, Wilhelm SA, Guha A, et al. Regulation of cellular immune response against autologous human melanoma. I. Evidence for cell-mediated suppression of in vitro cytotoxic immune response. J Immunol 1986;136(5):1888–92.
[27] Chakraborty NG, Twardzik DR, Sivanandham M, et al. Autologous melanoma-induced activation of regulatory T cells that suppress cytotoxic response. J Immunol 1990;145(7):2359–64.
[28] Hsueh EC, Nathanson L, Foshag LJ, et al. Active specific immunotherapy with polyvalent melanoma cell vaccine for patients with in-transit melanoma metastases. Cancer 1999;85(10):2160–9.
[29] Rabinovich GA, Gabrilovich D, Sotomayor EM. Immunosuppressive strategies that are mediated by tumor cells. Annu Rev Immunol 2007;25:267–96.
[30] Gajewski TF. Identifying and overcoming immune resistance mechanisms in the melanoma tumor microenvironment. Clin Cancer Res 2006;12(7):2326S–30S.
[31] Sakatsume M, Harada Y, Ling X, et al. Autoreactive T-cell clones which suppress cytotoxic T cell responses. Int Immunol 1991;3(4):377–84.
[32] Moiseyenko VM, Danilov AO, Baldueva IA, et al. Phase I/II trial of gene therapy with autologous tumor cells modified with tag7/PGRP-S gene in patients with disseminated solid tumors: miscellaneous tumors. Ann Oncol 2005;16(1):162–8.
[33] Emms SG. Anal sac tumours of the dog and their response to cytoreductive surgery and chemotherapy. Aust Vet J 2005;83(6):340–3.
[34] Janssen ML, Pels W, Massuger LF, et al. Intraperitoneal radioimmunotherapy in an ovarian carcinoma mouse model: effect of the radionuclide. Int J Gynecol Cancer 2003;13(5):607–13.
[35] Jarnicki AG, Lysaght J, Todryk S, et al. Suppression of antitumor immunity by IL-10 and TGF-beta-producing T cells infiltrating the growing tumor: influence of tumor environment on the induction of CD4+ and CD8+ regulatory T cells. J Immunol 2006;177(2):896–904.

[36] Uno K, Mitsuishi Y, Tanigawa M, et al. A series of immune responses leading to the induction of T cell IL-12/IL-18 responsiveness in patients with relatively large tumor burdens. Cancer Immunol Immunother 2003;52(1):33–40.
[37] Yamshchikov GV, Barnd DL, Eastham S, et al. Evaluation of peptide vaccine immunogenicity in draining lymph nodes and peripheral blood of melanoma patients. Int J Cancer 2001;92(5):703–11.
[38] Shu S, Cochran AJ, Huang RR, et al. Immune responses in the draining lymph nodes against cancer: implications for immunotherapy. Cancer Metastasis Rev 2006;25(2):233–42.
[39] Vuylsteke RJ, Molenkamp BG, van Leeuwen PA, et al. Tumor-specific CD8+ T cell reactivity in the sentinel lymph node of GM-CSF-treated stage I melanoma patients is associated with high myeloid dendritic cell content. Clin Cancer Res 2006;12(9):2826–33.
[40] Faries MB, Morton DL. Therapeutic vaccines for melanoma: current status. BioDrugs 2005; 19(4):247–60.
[41] Kirkwood JM, Strawderman MH, Ernstoff MS, et al. Interferon alfa-2b adjuvant therapy of high-risk resected cutaneous melanoma: the Eastern Cooperative Oncology Group Trial EST 1684. J Clin Oncol 1996;14(1):7–17.
[42] Kirkwood JM, Ibrahim JG, Sondak VK, et al. High- and low-dose interferon alfa-2b in high-risk melanoma: first analysis of intergroup trial E1690/S9111/C9190. J Clin Oncol 2000; 18(12):2444–58.
[43] Kirkwood JM, Ibrahim JG, Sosman JA, et al. High-dose interferon alfa-2b significantly prolongs relapse-free and overall survival compared with the GM2-KLH/QS-21 vaccine in patients with resected stage IIB-III melanoma: results of intergroup trial E1694/S9512/ C509801. J Clin Oncol 2001;19(9):2370–80.
[44] Moschos SJ, Edington HD, Land SR, et al. Neoadjuvant treatment of regional stage IIIB melanoma with high-dose interferon alfa-2b induces objective tumor regression in association with modulation of tumor infiltrating host cellular immune responses. J Clin Oncol 2006;24(19):3164–71.
[45] Buzaid AC, Colome M, Bedikian A, et al. Phase II study of neoadjuvant concurrent biochemotherapy in melanoma patients with local-regional metastases. Melanoma Res 1998;8(6):549–56.
[46] Lewis KD, Robinson WA, McCarter M, et al. Phase II multicenter study of neoadjuvant biochemotherapy for patients with stage III malignant melanoma. J Clin Oncol 2006; 24(19):3157–63.

ELSEVIER
SAUNDERS

Surg Oncol Clin N Am
16 (2007) 695–701

SURGICAL
ONCOLOGY CLINICS
OF NORTH AMERICA

A Critical Appraisal: Providing Care for Patients with Solid Tumors Metastases—Challenges Across Academic and Community Practice

Pascal Fuchshuber, MD, PhD, FACS[a,*],
Nicholas Petrelli, MD, FACS[b]

[a]*The Permanente Medical Group, Kaiser Medical Center, 1425 South Main, Walnut Creek, CA 94596, USA*
[b]*Department of Surgery, Christiana Care Health System, Helen F. Graham Cancer Center, 4701 Ogletown Stanton Road, Newark, DE 19713, USA*

As a growing number of new therapeutic options have become available for the treatment of advanced-stage solid tumors, the number of patients eligible for cancer-directed surgical intervention is rapidly increasing. For example, the outlook for patients with metastatic colorectal cancer (CRC), once thought of as nearly uniformly fatal, has now changed drastically. Major advances in systemic biologic and cytotoxic therapies as well as surgical oncology approaches have increased the proportion of CRC patients with liver metastases eligible for potentially curative surgical therapy from about 3% to more than 10%. Assuming 150,000 new CRC patients annually, an increase from roughly 4000 patients to more than 15,000 patients that are candidates for metastasectomy in the United States. Similarly, emerging new therapies have increased the number of patients with other treatable advanced-stage solid tumors. Standardized protocols for regional and systemic cytotoxic treatments are available and accepted by national consensus. The challenge to the treating oncologist, particularly the surgical oncologist, has become rather daunting as the traditional boundary between palliative and curative resections has become less distinct. The surgical oncologist at the crossroad of palliation, cytoreduction, debulking, and curative metastasectomy is faced with the task to select patients appropriately,

* Corresponding author.
E-mail address: pascal.fuchshuber@kp.org (P. Fuchshuber).

1055-3207/07/$ - see front matter © 2007 Elsevier Inc. All rights reserved.
doi:10.1016/j.soc.2007.04.006 surgonc.theclinics.com

coordinate multimodality treatment to minimize complications and maximize surgical benefit, and provide state-of-the art surgical therapy with acceptable mortality and morbidity. Further responsibilities such as teaching the next generation of surgeons in this field, participating in randomized clinical trials, and leadership within the multimodality treatment team need to be addressed as well.

With surgeons now less fearful of side effects from systemic chemotherapy and radiation therapy, the optimal integration of surgical, medical, and radiation oncology for patients with advanced solid tumor metastases has become paramount. This chapter attempts to identify and discuss how to address the complex needs for the care of these patients. What are the outcomes of community versus academic practices, what role does volume and surgeon expertise play, and is there a need for regionalization and standardization of care?

Metastasectomy for colorectal cancer

The most critical determinants of clinical outcome for CRC metastasectomy are patient selection, appropriate timing and integration of systemic therapy, and technical ability to achieve complete metastasectomy with satisfactory morbidity and mortality. Proper patient selection hinges on appropriate pretreatment imaging and evaluation of surgical risk. Even though there are no data comparing academic and community practice, there is good reason to believe that these parameters can be equally well established in both. High-quality imaging modalities are now routinely available in community practice, and surgical risk assessment does not require specialized services restricted to academic centers. Adequate timing and coordination of systemic chemotherapy with surgical resection is a critical issue in the treatment of most of these patients because 1) of the hepatotoxic effects of cytotoxic agents potentially threatening good surgical outcome and 2) the lack of data supporting one approach over another such as preoperative versus postoperative therapy and cytotoxic versus combined cytotoxic and biologic therapy [1,2]. For patients with CRC metastases, particularly in the curative setting, treatment results are likely to depend on the quality of the multimodality team (ie, on the timely coordination between surgeon and medical oncologist) and the adherence to a particular protocol. Even though evidence suggests that surgical outcomes for liver and lung resections are not different between community and academic practices [3–6], well-integrated academic multimodality teams are more likely to provide the necessary coordination of multimodality care for cases with high complexity, such as patients with large tumor burden, initially unresectable metastatic disease, and limited hepatic or pulmonary reserve. Clearly, community-based practices that want to provide care for CRC patients with complex metastatic disease need to emulate the multimodality approach of tertiary academic centers.

The technical ability to achieve a complete metastasectomy is not anymore the sole domain of the surgeon. For advanced metastatic colorectal cancer to the liver "downstaging" by neoadjuvant systemic therapy, interventional radiology techniques such as portal vein embolization and percutaneous ablations, staged hepatectomies, and lung resections are instrumental in making a complete resection possible and require a team approach of multiple providers. The surgeon needs to be facile with advanced hepatobiliary techniques and oncologic principles. The advent of minimally invasive surgical techniques has further complicated the playing field and increased the level of required surgical competency. If community-based health care systems want to meet the increased demand for surgical treatment in patients with advanced CRC metastatic disease, they need to invest appropriately in such surgical expertise to assure satisfactory outcome.

Even though the surgical approach is but one of many steps in a highly complex treatment algorithm that may include patients with extrahepatic or extrapulmonary disease for potential curative intent surgery, the surgeon needs to be involved from the beginning of the therapeutic planning. A priori, surgical resection gives the patient the best chance for complete metastasectomy and should always be preferred over nonresectional modalities. Therefore, the surgeon should select what modality to use for metastasectomy to avoid inappropriate use of nonsurgical techniques with high recurrence rates for potentially curable patients [7,8]. Poorly executed multimodality treatment plans can lead to higher recurrence rates, inability to surgically resect disease because of overtreatment by chemotherapy, and underutilization of cancer-directed surgery [2]. Conversely, even patients with relatively limited tumor burden in whom complete resection can be achieved with simple subsegmentectomies or wedge resections are likely to benefit from a multimodality approach [9].

Adequate integration of multimodality care for patients with metastatic CRC is essential for optimal oncologic outcome and to overcome disparities in use of cancer-directed care. Although tertiary and academic referral centers are, for the most part, well equipped to meet this demand, community-based practices should emulate at least a well-coordinated multimodality approach with appropriate surgical, oncologic, radiologic, and radiation therapy expertise and equipment.

Metastasectomy and cytoreduction for noncolorectal cancer

Contrary to CRC, evidence for metastasectomy in noncolorectal cancer is scant and utility less well defined. In most cases, surgery is the only potentially curative or palliative modality and effective systemic therapy nonexistent. Therefore, clinical decision making is less complex and essentially relies on selecting those patients most likely to benefit from resection. These are in essence patients with limited metachronous disease that are amenable to margin-negative resection or significant hepatic debulking. In most instances, the goal of surgery is palliative or for prolongation of a disease-free state rather than cure. Experienced community-based and academic oncologic surgeons should be equally qualified to provide care for these patients. Because of the low number of eligible patients and the wide spectrum of clinical scenarios, only large multi-institutional trials are likely to change the current approach to treating these patients. Patients with neuroendocrine metastases may require referral to a specialized surgeon experienced in extensive cytoreductive surgery for palliation. Cytoreductive surgery for both melanoma and neuroendocrine tumors will remain palliative in nature until effective systemic therapy is available.

Cytoreductive surgery for peritoneal and gynecologic malignancies

Cytoreductive surgery for peritoneal surface and gynecologic malignancies successfully evolved from an experimental procedure restricted to a few centers to become a part of the standard armamentarium of surgical and gynecologic oncology. In both arenas, broadly accepted standards of care protocols have been developed while the procedure has been successfully adapted for community practice [10,11]. The requirement for highly motivated, well-organized and super-specialized surgical and intensive care teams will assure that these procedures remain restricted to tertiary referral centers in the academic and community settings. Evidence-based national consensus statements on the appropriateness of this approach will no doubt spur the establishment of community-based subspecialty centers for these treatments. Evidence also suggests that outcomes are similar between academic and community-based referral centers, a proof of the concept that community-based systems, by investing in appropriate equipment and treatment teams, can achieve results and support advanced clinical research similar to that of academic centers.

Minimally invasive surgery for metastasectomy and cytoreduction

The impact of minimally invasive surgery on the development of surgical oncology for advanced solid tumors is very difficult to assess and predict. These techniques have obvious advantages in the palliative setting of cancer patients because of their ability to reduce postoperative pain and hospital stay. Metastasectomy of liver, lung, and other solid organ sites are now performed routinely by advanced laparoscopic surgeons, although the benefits and equivalence in oncologic outcome have not been established by clinical trial. The interesting and challenging aspect of minimally invasive surgery is that it is not preferentially done at large tertiary referral centers or within the setting of a multimodality cancer treatment team. Few leaders in this field are trained as surgical oncologists or hepatobiliary surgeons with special expertise in the treatment of cancer patients. Clearly, these modalities are going to be developed further and may play an increasing role in the surgical management of advanced-stage solid cancer patients. Surgical oncologists have the responsibility to assure training in these techniques and participate actively in setting the standards for minimally invasive procedures.

Regionalization and training

The treatment of patients with advanced metastatic disease to the liver and peritoneal surfaces require very complex surgical and multimodality approaches. Because of the need for specialized teams with much focused knowledge of how to orchestrate all involved treatment modalities, care for these patients is best provided in regionalized centers of excellence. By design, academic referral centers can easily provide such an environment. For community-based practices to do the same requires investment into regionalized centers of excellence. Regionalization into high-volume centers of care has been shown to improve outcome, decrease length of stay, and increase the use of community-based services, particularly for cancer-directed surgeries [3,12–15]. Establishing large regional centers of excellence for complex cancer-directed surgery in the current health care environment is difficult to imagine. Likely only very large nonacademic hospital systems will be able to cover all needed aspects of care for patients with advanced solid tumor metastases. It will require the leadership of professional organizations such as the Society of Surgical Oncology, American Society of Clinical Oncology, American Hepato-Pancreato-Biliary Association, and Society of American Gastrointestinal Endoscopic Surgeons to establish appropriate training and regionalized care models to provide access to and meet the growing demand for subspecialty surgical care of these patients. Standardization of subspecialty fellowship programs for hepatobiliary surgery by the AHPBH are a step in the right direction. Similar efforts are needed to integrate minimal invasive surgery and cytoreductive surgery into the training of surgical oncologist. As an example the University of California at San Francisco-East-Bay residency training program has piloted a program of subspecialty rotations for senior surgical residents for hepatobiliary and thoracic surgery. If one takes into consideration that treatment of patients with liver metastases is provided by surgical oncologists, transplant surgeons, general surgeons, colorectal surgeons, minimally invasive surgeons, and interventional radiologists in tertiary referral centers as well as in community practices, one of the ultimate goals of regionalization and training should be to overcome the disparity in cancer-directed care caused by the diversity of providers and competing health care systems [16,17].

Summary

Metastasectomy and cytoreductive surgery are evolving rapidly for those advanced-stage solid tumors for which there are effective systemic treatments. The best example—colorectal cancer—stays in contrast to melanoma, for which there currently is no effective systemic therapy, and cytoreductive surgery plays only a minor role. Emerging therapies and the growing number of therapeutic options available for some of the solid cancers have led to a large number of patients eligible for these surgical approaches. It is likely that within the current health care structure, academic tertiary referral centers alone are not going to be able to accommodate the growing number of patients that are potential beneficiaries. Community-based practices will have to develop strategies to meet the demand for appropriate multimodality treatment teams to address the needs of these patients. Regionalization of care into high-volume centers of excellence and hiring of appropriately trained physicians present a challenge for both the health care system and professional organizations.

References

[1] Zorzi D, Laurent A, Pawlik TM, et al. Chemotherapy-associated hepatotoxicity and surgery for colorectal liver metastases. Br J Surg 2007;94(3):274–86.

[2] Aloia T, Sebagh M, Plasse M, et al. Liver histology and surgical outcomes after preoperative chemotherapy with fluorouracil plus oxaliplatin in colorectal cancer liver metastases. J Clin Oncol 2006;24(31):4983–90.

[3] Simunovic M, Rempel E, Theriault ME, et al. Influence of hospital characteristics on operative death and survival of patients after major cancer surgery in Ontario. Can J Surg 2006; 49(4):251–8.

[4] Yanaga K, Wakasugi K, Matsusaka T, et al. Hepatic resection without mortality at a community hospital. Int Surg 2003;88(2):87–91.

[5] Metreveli RE, Sahm K, Denstman F, et al. Hepatic resection at a major community-based teaching hospital can result in good outcome. Ann Surg Oncol 2005;12(2):133–7.

[6] Ston ME Jr, Rehman SU, Conaway G, et al. Hepatic resection at a community hospital. J Gastrointest Surg 2000;4(4):349–53.

[7] Abdalla EK, Adam R, Bilchik AJ, et al. Improving resectability of hepatic colorectal metastases: expert consensus statement. Ann Surg Oncol 2006;13(10):1271–80.

[8] Aloia TA, Vauthey JN, Loyer EM, et al. Solitary colorectal liver metastasis: resection determines outcome. Arch Surg 2006;141(5):460–6.

[9] Petrelli NJ. Systemic chemotherapy should be the primary treatment of synchronous colorectal metastases in the asymptomatic patient. Ann Surg Oncol 2006;13(2):137–9.

[10] Esquivel J, Sticca R, Sugarbaker P, et al. Cytoreductive surgery and hyperthermic intraperitoneal chemotherapy in the management of peritoneal surface malignancies of colonic origin: a consensus statement. Ann Surg Oncol 2007;14(1):128–33.

[11] Trimble E. NCI clinical announcement on intraperitoneal chemotherapy in ovarian cancer. 2006. Available at: http://ctep.cancer.gove/highlights/ovarian.html. Accessed January 5, 2006.

[12] Hollenbeck BK, Dunn RL, Miller DC, et al. Volume-based referral for cancer surgery: informing the debate. J Clin Oncol 2007;25(1):91–6.

[13] Dimick JB, Wainess RM, Cowan JA, et al. National trends in the use and outcomes of hepatic resection. J Am Coll Surg 2004;199(1):31–8.

[14] Hamilton SM, Johnston WC, Voaklander DC. Outcomes after the regionalization of major surgical procedures in the Alberta Capital Health Region (Edmonton). Can J Surg 2001; 44(1):51–8.

[15] Birkmeyer JD, Lucas FL, Wennberg DE. Potential benefits of regionalizing major surgery in Medicare patients. Eff Clin Pract 1999;2(6):277–83.
[16] Tan J, Coburn N, Kiss a, et al. Surgical resection of intrahepatic cholangiocarcinoma: a population based study [abstract 130]. Gastrointestinal Cancers Symposium, American Society of Clinical Oncology. Orlando, FL, January 19–21, 2007.
[17] Govindarajan A, Coburn NG, Kiss A, et al. Population-based assessment of the surgical management of locally advanced colorectal cancer. J Natl Cancer Inst 2006;98(20): 1474–81.

ELSEVIER
SAUNDERS

Surg Oncol Clin N Am
16 (2007) 703–710

SURGICAL
ONCOLOGY CLINICS
OF NORTH AMERICA

Index

Note: Page numbers of article titles are in **boldface** type.

1055-3207/07/$ - see front matter © 2007 Elsevier Inc. All rights reserved.
doi:10.1016/S1055-3207(07)00072-5

E

M

Moving?

Make sure your subscription moves with you!

To notify us of your new address, find your **Clinics Account Number** (located on your mailing label above your name), and contact customer service at:

E-mail: elspcs@elsevier.com

800-654-2452 (subscribers in the U.S. & Canada)
407-345-4000 (subscribers outside of the U.S. & Canada)

Fax number: 407-363-9661

Elsevier Periodicals Customer Service
6277 Sea Harbor Drive
Orlando, FL 32887-4800

*To ensure uninterrupted delivery of your subscription, please notify us at least 4 weeks in advance of move.

ELSEVIER